KU-740-107

OXFORD MEDICAL PUBLICATIONS

Oxford Handbook of
Gastroenterology
and Hepatology

Published and forthcoming Oxford Handbooks

Oxford Handbook of Clinical Medicine 6/e
(also available for PDAs and in a Mini Edition)
Oxford Handbook of Clinical Specialties 7/e
Oxford Handbook of Accident and Emergency Medicine 2/e
Oxford Handbook of Acute Medicine 2/e
Oxford Handbook of Anaesthesia 2/e
Oxford Handbook of Applied Dental Sciences
Oxford Handbook of Cardiology
Oxford Handbook of Clinical and Laboratory Investigation 2/e
Oxford Handbook of Clinical Diagnosis
Oxford Handbook of Clinical Haematology 2/e
Oxford Handbook of Clinical Immunology and Allergy 2/e
Oxford Handbook of Clinical Surgery 2/e
Oxford Handbook of Critical Care 2/e
Oxford Handbook of Dental Patient Care 2/e
Oxford Handbook of Dialysis 2/e
Oxford Handbook of Endocrinology and Diabetes
Oxford Handbook of ENT and Head and Neck Surgery
Oxford Handbook for the Foundation Programme
Oxford Handbook of Gastroenterology and Hepatology
Oxford Handbook of General Practice 2/e
Oxford Handbook of Genitourinary Medicine, HIV and AIDS
Oxford Handbook of Geriatric Medicine
Oxford Handbook of Medical Sciences
Oxford Handbook of Obstetrics and Gynaecology
Oxford Handbook of Oncology
Oxford Handbook of Ophthalmology
Oxford Handbook of Palliative Care
Oxford Handbook of Practical Drug Therapy
Oxford Handbook of Psychiatry
Oxford Handbook of Public Health Practice 2/e
Oxford Handbook of Rehabilitation Medicine
Oxford Handbook of Respiratory Medicine
Oxford Handbook of Rheumatology
Oxford Handbook of Tropical Medicine 2/e
Oxford Handbook of Urology

Oxford Handbook of
Gastroenterology
and Hepatology

Stuart Bloom

Consultant Gastroenterologist
University College London Hospitals
NHS Foundation Trust London, UK

and

George Webster

Consultant Gastroenterologist/Hepatologist
University College London Hospitals
NHS Foundation Trust London, UK

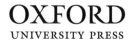

OXFORD
UNIVERSITY PRESS

OXFORD
UNIVERSITY PRESS

Great Clarendon Street, Oxford OX2 6DP

Oxford University Press is a department of the University of Oxford.
It furthers the University's objective of excellence in research, scholarship,
and education by publishing worldwide in

Oxford New York

Auckland Cape Town Dar es Salaam Hong Kong Karachi
Kuala Lumpur Madrid Melbourne Mexico City Nairobi
New Delhi Shanghai Taipei Toronto

With offices in
Argentina Austria Brazil Chile Czech Republic France Greece
Guatemala Hungary Italy Japan Poland Portugal Singapore
South Korea Switzerland Thailand Turkey Ukraine Vietnam

Oxford is a registered trade mark of Oxford University Press
in the UK and in certain other countries

Published in the United States
by Oxford University Press Inc., New York

British Library Cataloguing in Publication Data
Data available

Library of Congress Cataloging in Publication Data
Data available

Typeset by Newgen Imaging Systems (P) Ltd., Chennai, India
Printed in Italy
on acid-free paper by LegoPrint S.p.A

ISBN 0–19–856652–2 (flexicover: alk. paper)
       978–0–19–856652–6 (flexicover: alk. paper)

10 9 8 7 6 5 4 3 2 1

Preface

Why write another textbook?

There are many excellent textbooks of gastroenterology and hepatology, and many calls on our time. Apart from the fact that the commissioning editor, Alison Langton, asked us very nicely and persistently, a few considerations raised us from our naturally indolent state and gave us the energy to contemplate the task:

- The format and portability of the Oxford Handbooks is attractive and the series has not, to date, included a text on gastroenterology and hepatology. Even with white coats out of fashion, the Handbooks are easily transportable in rucksacks or handbags and do not induce herniae on opening.
- Gastroenterology and hepatology involve many organ systems. Most textbooks are organized anatomically (i.e. start at the mouth and move south), which often relates poorly to how patients present to doctors (e.g. the jaundiced patient—due to hepatitis A, gallstones, or pancreatic cancer?). This may lead to both repetition through the text, and a need for large complicated indices to help search for relevant information.
- It seemed to us that there is a need for up-to-date information on how to approach both clinical scenarios (e.g. abnormal liver tests; lower GI bleeding), and specific conditions in GI and liver practice, both common and uncommon. This information needs to be organized in such a way that it can be easily obtained in the clinic, on the way to a ward to see a patient referred with an exotic or unfamiliar condition, or when telephoned for advice by a colleague—or a patient.

Who is it written for?

- This book is aimed at all those interested in the presentation and management of patients with gastrointestinal and liver disease. This includes some but not all medical students, most junior doctors training in hospital medicine and in general practice, and all those training in gastroenterology/hepatology, one of the most challenging and fast developing of the medical specialties.
- We hope it will also appeal to many senior doctors immersed in busy practice who may find it useful to be reminded of the salient points of commonly (and less commonly) encountered conditions and problems in the field.
- Finally we hope that in the age of multidisciplinary teams the book will be of value to those working in nursing and professions allied to medicine, particularly clinical nurse specialists and nurse consultants and those involved in pharmaceutical practice and dietetics.

How is it different from other textbooks?

We have organized the book into a series of colour-coded sections. Underlinings represent an entry in the relevant section and will enable hyperlinking in electronic version of the book (if it's successful).

- <u>Red for emergencies</u>

A section on GI emergencies offering help on acute management based on clinical priorities.

- <u>Green for approaches to common clinical problems</u>

A section on the approach to various clinical problems and scenarios encountered in the clinic and on the wards

- <u>Black for A to Z of topics</u>

Most of the book is dedicated to an A to Z of conditions and problems in gastroenterology and hepatology. This is (to our knowledge) a new way of organizing a text on the subject, but we hope it will enable readers in accessing information. Throughout this section, there are text links to other related topics, and to the emergencies and approaches section, highlighted by red and green links respectively.

- <u>SMALL CAPITALS FOR PARTICULAR DRUGS</u>

An index of drugs commonly used in gastroenterology and hepatology. This is not intended to duplicate or replace information in crucial and authoritative texts such as the *British National Formulary*, but rather to give key facts of dosage, methods of administration and common cautions, side effects and interactions. Practice points are also included, drawing on our combined experience in the specialty.

Acknowledgements

We learnt a lot from reading other volumes in the Oxford Handbook series with overlapping content (*the Oxford Handbook of Clinical Medicine* and the *Oxford Handbook of Tropical Medicine* in particular). We are grateful to our colleagues at University College London Hospitals and UCL, who kindly reviewed the book, and particular thanks to Daniel Marks, Ailsa Hart, and Raza Malik, who carefully read, edited and improved the text. Thanks as ever, also goes to our families, who remained incredibly supportive throughout, even with the realization that writing a little book never takes a little time!

Finally

So here's the result, and we hope you find this book of practical use, fun, and informative. We would welcome feedback, which can be directed to us via the OUP website www.oup.co.uk/academic/medicine/handbooks/comments

Stuart Bloom and George Webster
University College London Hospitals
2006

Contents

Detailed contents

2 An A to Z of gastroenterology and hepatology   123

Abbreviations

AAD	antibiotic-associated diarrhoea
Ab	antibody
ACE	angiotensin-converting enzyme *or* antegrade colonic enema
ACTH	adrenocorticotrophic hormone
ADH	antidiuretic hormone
AF	atrial fibrillation
AFLP	acute fatty liver of pregnancy
AFP	alpha fetoprotein
AGA	American Gastroenterology Association
AIDS	acquired immune deficiency syndrome
AIH	autoimmune hepatitis
AIP	acute intermittent porphyria *or* autoimmune pancreatitis
ALA	amino-laevulinic acid
ALF	acute liver failure
ALP	alkaline phosphatase
ALT	alanine aminotransferase
AMA	anti-mitochondrial antibodies
AMP	adenosine monophosphate
ANA	anti-nuclear antibody
AP	acute pancreatitis
APC	adenomatous polyposis coli (gene) *or* argon plasma coagulation
apo-B	apolipoprotein B
APTT	activated partial thromboplastin time
APUD	amine precursor uptake and decarboxylation (cells)
ASA	American Society of Anesthesiology
5-ASA	5-aminosalicylates
ASD	atrial septal defect
ASM	anti-smooth muscle (antibodies)
AST	aspartate aminotransaminase
AV	arteriovenous
AXR	abdominal X-ray
BCS	Budd–Chiari syndrome
bd	twice a day
BDS	bile duct stones

BM	Boehringer Mannheim (in glucose BM, i.e. blood monitoring for glucose)
BMD	bone mineral density
BMI	body mass index
BMR	basal metabolic rate
Bn	bilirubin
BNF	*British National Formulary*
BP	blood pressure
BSG	British Society of Gastroenterology
Bx	biopsy
cAMP	cyclic adenosine monophosphate
CBD	common bile duct
CDAI	Crohn's disease activity index
CDC	Center for Disease Control (US)
CDEIS	Crohn's disease endoscopic inflammation score
CEA	carcinoembryonic antigen
CF	cystic fibrosis
CFTR	cystic fibrosis transmembrane conductance regulator
CGD	chronic granulomatous disease
CLO	*Clostridium*-like organisms (test for)
CMV	cytomegalovirus
CNS	central nervous system
CO	carbon monoxide *or* cardiac output
COX-2	cyclo-oxygenase 2
CREST	calcinosis–Raynaud's–oesophageal dysmotility–sclerodactyly–telangiectasia (syndrome)
CRP	C-reactive protein
CSF	cerebrospinal fluid
CSU	catheter specimen of urine
CT	computerized tomography
CTD	connective tissue disease
CVA	cerebrovascular accident
CVP	central venous pressure
CXR	chest X-ray
DAEC	diffusely adhering *E. coli*
DBE	double-balloon enteroscopy
DCC	deleted in colorectal cancer (gene)
DEXA	dual energy X-ray absorptiometry
DF	discriminant function
DIC	disseminated intravascular coagulation
DT	delirium tremens

DU	duodenal ulcer
DVT	deep vein thrombosis
EAggEC	entero-aggregatory *E. coli*
EBV	Epstein–Barr virus
ECG	electrocardiogram
EGC	early gastric cancer
EGF	epidermal growth factor
EGG	electrogastrography
EHEC	enterohaemorrhagic *E. coli*
EIA	enzyme immunoassay
EIEC	enteroinvasive *E. coli*
ELISA	enzyme-linked immunosorbent assay
EMR	endoscopic mucosal resection
ENT	ear, nose, and throat
EPEC	enteropathogenic *E. coli*
ERCP	endoscopic retrograde cholangiopancreatography
ESR	erythrocyte sedimentation rate
EST	endoscopic sclerotherapy
ESWL	extracorporeal shock wave lithotripsy
ETEC	enterotoxigenic *E. coli*
EUS	endoscopic ultrasound
FAP	familial adenomatous polyposis
FBC	full blood count
FDG	2-fluoro-2-deoxy-D-glucose
FE1	faecal elastase type 1
FFP	fresh frozen plasma
FNA	fine needle aspiration
FNH	focal nodular hyperplasia
FOBT	faecal occult blood test
FSH	follicle-stimulating hormone
5FU	fluorouracil
GABA	γ-aminobutyric acid
GAVE	gastric antral vascular ectasia
GBS	Guillain–Barré syndrome
GDA	gastroduodenal artery
GGT	gammaglutamyl transpeptidase
GH	genetic haemochromatosis
GI	gastrointestinal
GIST	gastrointestinal stromal tumours
GMP	guanosine monophosphate
GORD	gastro-oesophageal reflux disease

G6PD	glucose 6-phosphate dehydrogenase
GTN	glyceryl trinitrate
GU	gastric ulcer
GvHD	graft versus host disease
HAART	highly active antiretroviral therapy
H & E	haematoxylin and eosin
HAS	human albumin solution
HAV	hepatitis A virus
Hb	haemoglobin
HBcAg	hepatitis B core antigen
HBeAg	hepatitis B envelope antigen
HBsAg	hepatitis B surface antigen
HBV	hepatitis B virus
HCC	hepatocellular carcinoma
β-HCG	beta human chorionic gonadotrophin
HCV	hepatitis C virus
HDL	high-density lipid
HDU	high dependency unit
HDV	hepatitis D virus
HE	hepatic encephalopathy
HELLP	haemolysis–elevated liver enzymes–low platelets (syndrome)
HEV	hepatitis E virus
HGD	high grade dysplasia
HGV	hepatitis G virus
5-HIAA	5 hydroxy indole acetic acid
HIDA	hepatobiliary iminodiacetic acid (hepatobiliary scintigraphy)
HII	hepatic iron index
HIV	human immunodeficiency virus
HNIG	human normal immunoglobulin
HNPCC	hereditary non-polyposis cancer
HOCM	hypertropic obstructive cardiomyopathy
HP	*Helicobacter pylori*
HPV	human papillomavirus
HR	heart rate
H2RA	H2-receptor antagonist
HRQL	health-related quality of life
HRS	hepatorenal syndrome
HRT	hormone replacement therapy
HSV	herpes simplex virus
5-HT	5-hydroxytryptamine (serotonin)

HV	hepatic vein
HVPG	hepatic venous pressure gradient
IBS	irritable bowel syndrome
ICP	intracranial pressure
IF	intrinsic factor
IFN-α	interferon alpha
IL	interleukin (IL-2, etc.)
IM	intramuscular
INR	international normalized ratio
IPAA	ileal pouch–anal anastomosis
IPMT	intraductal papillary mucinous tumour
IPSID	immunoproliferative small intestinal disease (alpha chain disease)
ITU	intensive therapy unit
IU	international units
IV	intravenous
JVP	jugular venous pressure
KS	Kaposi's sarcoma
LBx	liver biopsy
LC	laparoscopic cholecystectomy
LCHAD	3-hydroxyacyl coenzyme A dehydrogenase
LCT	long-chain triglyceride
LDH	lactate dehydrogenase
LDL	low-density lipid
LFT	liver function test
LGD	low grade dysplasia
LH	luteinizing hormone
LKM1	liver–kidney microsomes, type 1
LOS	lower oesophageal sphincter
MAC	*Mycobacterium avium complex*
MAI	*Mycobacterium avium intracellulare*
MALT	mucosa-associated lymphoid tissue
MAP	mean arterial pressure
MARS	molecular absorbance recirculation system
MCH	mean corpuscular haemoglobin
MCHC	mean corpuscular haemoglobin concentration
MCN	mucinous cystic neoplasm
MCT	medium-chain triglyceride
MCTD	mixed connective tissue disease
MCV	mean corpuscular volume
MDP	muramyl dipeptide

MELD	model for end-stage liver disease (score)
MEN	multiple endocrine neoplasia (e.g. MEN-1)
MI	myocardial infarction
MIBG	metaiodobenzylguanidine
6-MP	6-mercaptopurine
MRCP	magnetic resonance cholangiopancreatography
MRI	magnetic resonance imaging
MS	multiple sclerosis
MSU	mid-stream urine
MTB	mycobacterium tuberculosis
NADPH	nicotinamide adenine dinucleotide phosphate (reduced form).
NAFLD	non-alcoholic fatty liver disease
NASH	non-alcoholic steatohepatitis
NBM	nil by mouth
NET	neuroendocrine tumours
NF	neurofibramotosis
NG	nasogastric (tube)
NHL	non-Hodgkin's lymphoma
NHS	National Health System (UK)
NICE	National Institute for Clinical Excellence (UK)
NRH	nodular regenerative hyperplasia
NSAID	nonsteroidal anti-inflammatory drug
OATP	organic anion transporting polypeptide
OC	open cholecystectomy
OCP	oral contraceptive pill
od	once a day
OGD	oesophago-gastro-duodenoscopy
OHCM	*Oxford Handbook of Clinical Medicine*
OLT	orthotopic liver transplantation
ORS	oral rehydration solution
PA	postero-anterior *or* pernicious anaemia
PABA	para-aminobenzoic acid
PAN	polyarteritis nodosa
PaO_2	arterial oxygen tension
PAS	para-aminosalicyclic acid
PBC	primary biliary cirrhosis
PBG	porphobilinogen
PCR	polymerase chain reaction
PCT	porphyria cutanea tarda
PDAI	pouchitis disease activity index

PDT	photodynamic therapy
PE	pulmonary embolism
PEG	percutaneous endoscopic gastrostomy *or* polyethylene glycol
PET	positron emission tomography *or* pancreatic endocrine tumour
PHG	portal hypertensive gastropathy
PICC	peripherally inserted central catheters
PMC	pseudomembranous colitis
PNS	peripheral nervous system
PO	by mouth (*per os*)
PPI	proton pump inhibitor
PPPD	pylorus-preserving pancreaticoduodenectomy
PR	by (per) rectum
prn	as required
PSA	prostate-specific antigen
PSC	primary sclerosing cholangitis
PT	prothrombin time
PTD	percutaneous transhepatic drainage
PTH	parathyroid hormone
PTLD	post-transplant lymphoproliferative disorder
PUD	peptic ulcer disease
PUO	pyrexia of unknown origin
PV	by (per) vagina
PVT	portal vein thrombosis
qds	four times a day
RA	rheumatoid arthritis
RCT	randomized control trial
RIBA	recombinant immunoblot assay
SAAG	serum to ascites albumin gradient
SACE	serum angiotensin-converting enzyme
SAMe	S-adenosylmethionine
SBE	subacute bacterial endocarditis
SBP	spontaneous bacterial peritonitis
SBT	Sengstaken–Blakemore tube
SCA	sickle cell anaemia
SCC	squamous cell carcinoma
SCFA	short chain fatty acids
SD	standard deviation
SeHCaT	selenium-75 labelled homotaurocholic acid test
SLA	soluble liver antigen

SLE	systemic lupus erythematosus
SMA	superior mesenteric artery
SOD	sphincter of Oddi dysfunction
SOM	sphincter of Oddi manometry
SSRI	selective serotonin reuptake inhibitor
SVC	superior vena cava
SVR	sustained virological response *or* systemic vascular resistance
TACE	transcatheter chemoembolization
TB	tuberculosis
tds	three times a day
TG	triglyceride
TGF	transforming growth factor
Th1	T helper cell type 1
TIBC	total iron binding capacity
TIPSS	transjugular intrahepatic portosystemic shunt
TMP-SMX	trimethoprim–sulphamethoxazole
TNF	tumour necrosis factor
TNM	tumour–node–metastasis (staging system for cancer)
TOF	tracheo-oesophageal fistula
TPMT	thiopurine methyltransferase
TPN	total parenteral nutrition
TSH	thyroid-stimulating hormone
UC	ulcerative colitis
UDCA	ursodeoxycholic acid
U & E	urine and electrolytes
UGT	uridine diphosphate glucuronyl transferase
ULN	upper limits of normal
U/S	ultrasound
UTI	urinary tract infection
VBL	variceal band ligation
VIP	vasoactive intestinal polypeptide
VOD	veno-occlusive disease
VTEC	verocytotoxin-producing *E. coli*
WCC	white cell count
WDP	Wilson's disease protein
WE	Wernicke's encephalopathy
WHO	World Health Organization
ZES	Zollinger–Ellison syndrome

Section 1

Approaches to common clinical problems

Acute diarrhoea (less than 14 days)

Most cases of acute diarrhoea are due to infections; in immunocompetent patients these are usually self-limiting and intervention may be limited to oral rehydration if there are no signs of significant fluid loss. Diarrhoea lasting more than 14 days is usually described as persistent or chronic and is usually due to some other cause (exceptions in immunocompetent patients include _Giardia_ and _Yersinia_). Diagnosis and management are addressed in Approach to chronic diarrhoea.

Key questions in the history
- How long is the history?
- Are there systemic symptoms (fever, tachycardia) or vomiting?
- Is there recognizable blood in the stool?
- How frequent are the stools?
- Presence and location of any associated abdominal pain?
- Any contact with possible infected food or water?
- Recent travel history?
- Any contact with similarly ill people? Anyone in the family unwell?
- On examination, always look for signs of dehydration and malnutrition.

Risk factors
- Age. During and after weaning the protective effects of breast milk are lost. The elderly may have declining immune competence, but also reduced acid secretion (e.g. due to pernicious anaemia, _Helicobacter_ infection, drugs such as PPIs).
- Immune deficiency: includes patients with HIV (see HIV and the gut), and those on anti-cancer chemotherapy.
- Medication, including antibiotics: (see antibiotic-associated diarrhoea).
- Travel (see below).
- Infected food and water: either a true infection with ingestion of enteropathogens that multiply in the gut, or ingestion of pre-formed toxin in food contaminated with an enterotoxin-producing microorganism.
- Known sensitivity to certain foods: see food allergy/intolerance.

Classifying acute diarrhoea

Subdivide acute diarrhoeal diseases into the presence or absence of blood in the stool, since the causes are largely different (but remember _Shigella_ and _Campylobacter_ can present as acute watery diarrhoea).

Causes of acute diarrhoea with blood

- Bacillary dysentery (shigellosis)
- Enterohaemorrhagic *E. coli*
- *Campylobacter*
- *Salmonella*
- *Yersinia*
- Amoebic dysentery
- Antibiotic-associated colitis
- Rarely, *Schistosoma* (*mansoni* or *japonicum*) and *Tricuris*

Causes of acute diarrhoea without blood

- Viruses (rotavirus, Norwalk, astrovirus, adenovirus)
- Bacteria
  - Mild infection with *Shigella*, *Salmonella*, or *Campylobacter*
  - *E. coli* (enterotoxigenic, enteropathogenic, enteroaggregative)
  - Cholera, Clostridia spp.
- Protozoa: *Giardia*, cryptosporidiosis, *Cyclospora*
- *Strongyloides*
- Food toxins
- Malaria

Also consider whether the process involves mostly the small intestine.

Pathogens targeting the small bowel include toxigenic bacteria, viruses, and the parasite *Giardia lamblia* (see giardiasis). They all produce large volume watery diarrhoea and mid-abdominal pain. Blood and faecal leucocytes are rare (see upper table on p3).

Pathogens targeting the large bowel are usually invasive organisms like *Shigella*, *Campylobacter*, and enteroinvasive and enterohaemorrhagic *E. coli* (EIEC and EHEC). They produce lower abdominal or rectal pain (tenesmus), mucoid or bloody diarrhoea with many faecal leucocytes, and inflamed rectal mucosa (see food poisoning).

A few pathogens (e.g. *Salmonella* and *Yersinia*) infect the lower small bowel but can invade the colon as well. They can present with a spectrum from watery diarrhoea to colitis (see lower table on p3).

Infectious agents targeting small bowel

	Agent	Source and incubation period
Viruses	Rotavirus, Norwalk agent, calcivirus, torovirus, enteric adenovirus	Short incubation (1–3 d) for rotavirus and Norwalk agent, longer (8–10 d) for adenovirus. Norwalk occurs in shellfish
Bacteria that colonize the gut	Vibrio cholerae	2–144 hours. See cholera.
	Vibrio parahaemolyticus	Raw fish or seafood, 2–48 hrs. Usually short illness
	Yersinia enterocolitica Salmonella	Principally invade the lower small bowel but may invade the colon. The clinical spectrum varies from watery diarrhoea to colitis
	E. coli (ETEC, EPEC)	See Escherichia coli
	Giardia	See giardiasis

Infectious agents targeting large bowel

Shigella	Highly contagious. Spread usually faeco-oral but outbreaks can occur related to contaminated milk, ice-cream, or water. Toxigenic phase of fever, pain, diarrhoea starts early after infection.
Campylobacter	Incubation period 24–72 hrs. Usual source is infected animals. Most infections result from improperly cooked chicken (50–70% cases).
Salmonella	See above. Toxic megacolon and perforation due to colitis can occur—commonest when diarrhoea has lasted 10–15 days.
E. coli (EIEC, EHEC)	1–14 d, mean 3 d. See Escherichia coli
Entamoeba histolytica	See amoebiasis
C. difficile	See clostridial infections in GI tract

Investigations

Many attacks of acute diarrhoea are self-limiting. In general, investigation is indicated in the following circumstances:
- Course over 2 weeks;
- Signs of systemic upset including fever;
- Tenesmus or bloody diarrhoea;
- Special circumstances:
  - Outbreaks suggesting food poisoning;
  - Male homosexual;

- Immunocompromised host;
- Ingestion of raw shellfish;
- Antibiotic usage.

Stool culture is often requested but few centres offer tests for all pathogens, mixed infections are common, single stool cultures are insufficient for some pathogens, and results often come back too late to influence management. In practice, apart from the investigation of outbreaks and surveillance, stool culture in uncomplicated cases should be limited to exclusion of those pathogens for which antibiotic treatment is indicated (parasites, *Shigella*, *V. cholerae*) or where there are other possible causes of acute diarrhoea (e.g. inflammatory bowel disease).

Stool microscopy for faecal leucocytes can be very helpful in diagnosing an inflammatory diarrhoea (see box).

Faecal leucocytes in intestinal infections

Present: <u>Shigella</u>, <u>Campylobacter</u>, EIEC, EHEC
Variable: <u>Salmonella</u>, <u>Yersinia</u>, C. difficile
Absent: <u>cholera</u>, ETEC/EPEC, viral diarrhoea, <u>Giardia</u>, <u>amoebiasis</u>.

Identifying microbial antigens ELISA tests for <u>Giardia</u> and serology for <u>amoebiasis</u> are more accurate than stool microscopy and should be ordered given the appropriate history even in the absence of faecal leucocytes. Serology/antibody testing is useful for <u>Yersinia enterocolitica</u>. ELISA kits are available for <u>strongyloides</u> and <u>schistosomiasis</u>.

Abdominal X-ray should be taken if the patient is toxic, to look for evidence of diffuse colitis, ileus, or <u>toxic megacolon</u>.

Treatment

Fluid replacement
- **Oral rehydration** is nearly always the preferred route, but if the patient is vomiting or intravascularly depleted (resting tachycardia with postural drop in blood pressure) **intravenous fluids** may be necessary.
- Unlike the situation in patients with intestinal resection or jejunostomy, where sodium concentration of 90–120 mM provides maximum salt and water absorption, the optimal sodium concentration for rehydration in cases of mild–moderate acute diarrhoea is probably around 50 mM. The substitution of starch from rice or cereal for glucose is associated with less diarrhoea and more rapid resolution.

Diet
Eating during an attack of acute diarrhoea can be uncomfortable because any food can provide an additional stimulus to defecation. There is no benefit to fasting but dairy products should be avoided because of the risk of <u>lactose intolerance</u>. Alcohol, caffeine, and fizzy drinks should be avoided.

Drugs. Antimotility agents can be very useful but should not be used if there is an acute severe colitis because of the risk of precipitating <u>toxic megacolon</u>. <u>LOPERAMIDE</u> is the drug of choice.

Indication for antibiotics
- Pathogens: *Shigella*, <u>*Vibrio cholerae*</u>, <u>*Salmonella typhi*</u>, <u>*Clostridium difficile*</u>.
- Community-acquired diarrhoea: more than 4 stools/day for over 3 days with one or more of pain, fever, vomiting, myalgia, headache. A quinolone such as <u>CIPROFLOXACIN</u> 250–500 mg bd is suggested. Optimal duration is not known; a single dose if given early is very effective.
- Laboratory proven cases of *Giardia intestinalis*.
- Antibiotic treatment of enterohaemorrhagic *E. coli* is controversial and expert advice should be sought (see <u>haemolytic–uraemic syndrome</u>).
- Laboratory proven enteropathogenic *E. coli* infection, especially in the very young or old.
- Traveller's diarrhoea in adults: the duration of diarrhoea is reduced when a quinolone such as <u>CIPROFLOXACIN</u> is used.

Antibiotic therapy of dysentery[*]

	Drug of choice	Alternative
Bacteria *Shigella* spp.	Ampicillin 500 mg qds, 5 days TMP-SMX 2 tabs bd, 5 days Ciprofloxacin[3] 500 mg bd, 5 days	Cefixime[1] 400 mg od 5–7 days Nalidixic acid 1 g qds 5–7 days
Salmonella spp.	Ciprofloxacin[2,3] 500 mg bd 10–14 days	
EIEC	? as *Shigella* spp.	
EHEC	?	
C. jejuni	Erythromycin 250–500 mg qds 7 days	Ciprofloxacin[3] 500 mg bd 5–7 days
Y. enterocolitica	Tetracycline 250 mg qds, 7–10 days	

[*]Adapted from Bloom S (2001). *Practical Gastroenterology: A Comprehensive Guide*. Reprinted with permission from Taylor & Francis Group Ltd.

Contd.

	Drug of choice	Alternative
Y. enterocolitica	Ciprofloxacin[3] 500 mg bd 7–10 days TMP-SMX 2 tabs bd 7–10 days	
C. difficile	Metronidazole tds 400 mg, 7–10 days Vancomycin 125 mg qds 7–10 days	
Protozoa		
E. histolytica	Metronidazole 400 mg tds 5 days Diloxanide furoate 500 mg tds 10 days	Paromomycin 25–35 mg/kg tds 10 days

[1] And other third-generation cephalosporins.
[2] Usually only for bacteraemia.
[3] And other fluoroquinolones such as ofloxacin, norfloxacin, fleroxacin, and cinoxacin.
EIEC; enteroinvasive E.coli.
EHEC; enterohaemorrhagic E.coli.
TMP-SMX;Trimethoprim–sulphamethoxazole.

Diarrhoea in travellers

- 30–50% of travellers to developing countries have an episode of infective diarrhoea.
- Episodes are usually of mild-to-moderate severity and self-limiting.
- Investigation and treatment may be needed for individuals with bloody diarrhoea, when invasive organisms are involved, or when diarrhoea persists after their return home.

Causal organisms

- Enterotoxigenic _E. coli_ (ETEC) is the commonest cause worldwide (also leading bacterial cause of gastroenteritis on cruise ships), but _Shigella_ accounts for increasing proportion, and _Campylobacter_ is important in travellers to Asia.
- Other bacterial pathogens include Aeromonas, Plesiomonas, and Vibrio.
- Viruses (rotavirus, Norwalk virus) are common causes (up to 30% of cases).

- Parasitic causes are uncommon, but *Giardia* is found in 5%. <u>Cyclospora</u> is seen occasionally. <u>Cryptosporidium</u> can be a problem for the immunocompromised.
- Consider <u>amoebiasis</u> caused by *Entamoeba histolytica* in people with bloody stools.
- Geography affects the likely cause. While ETEC and <u>Shigella</u> account for the majority of isolates in Africa and the Middle East, over 50% of people affected in Asia have <u>Campylobacter</u>.

Natural history, mode of infection

- Most cases occur 5–15 days after arrival. Malaise, anorexia, abdominal cramps, watery diarrhoea, and sometimes nausea with vomiting are the hallmarks. Fever occurs in about one-third of cases. Most cases resolve in 6–10 days.
- Gastric hypoacidity and immunosuppression increase the risk. Risk is also increased in patients with <u>ulcerative colitis</u>, <u>Crohn's disease</u>, and <u>coeliac disease</u>.
- Careful selection of food and drink to minimize infection reduces but does not eliminate risk: two other approaches include chemoprophylaxis or dispensing medication to be taken if diarrhoea develops.

Chemoprophylaxis

The Center for Disease Control (CDC; Atlanta, USA) does not recommend routine use of prophylactic antibiotics, because of concerns about side-effects and selection of resistant strains. Two settings where prophylactic antibiotics are used include:

- Short-term travellers (2 weeks or less in an endemic area) whose business or vacation schedule would be severely disrupted by an episode of diarrhoea.
- Patients with an underlying medical condition or the immunocompromised.

Where ETEC, <u>Shigella</u>, or <u>Salmonella</u> predominate a quinolone antibiotic (ciprofloxacin 500 mg od) is the drug of choice. For travellers to Asia, <u>Campylobacter</u> is common and frequently resistant to quinolones: azithromycin 500 mg od should be used.

Self-medication with antibiotics. A single dose of <u>CIPROFLOXACIN</u> 500 mg taken at the first sensation of impending upset can reduce the duration and intensity of infection.

Other aspects of self-treatment. The benefit of adding anti-diarrhoeal agents such as loperamide (see <u>ANTI-DIARRHOEAL AGENTS</u>) to antibiotics is unclear. It is very important to ensure adequate fluid and electrolyte replacement using an oral rehydration solution such as the World Health Organization (WHO) rehydration solution.

Diagnostic approach to diarrhoea in the returning traveller

- Initial approach is the same as that for self-treatment of traveller's diarrhoea (3 days of quinolone or azithromycin, plus loperamide and adequate fluid/electrolyte replacement).
- Diarrhoea can be a prominent symptom of **malaria**. Examine blood film for *Plasmodium* in travellers returning from malarious areas with fever and diarrhoea.
- Watery diarrhoea persisting for longer than 10 days is most commonly due to giardiasis. Send stool to be examined for *Giardia*, *Cryptosporidium*, *Cyclospora*, and *Isospora*.
- Empirical treatment with METRONIDAZOLE or tinidazole for *Giardia* is often reasonable. If this fails to improve the diarrhoea, further investigation with upper GI endoscopy and small bowel biopsy, sigmoidoscopy, and rectal biopsy is required. If symptoms and biopsies are consistent with tropical sprue, tetracycline with folic acid is indicated.

Agitation and confusion in the GI patient

Background

The term 'disturbed consciousness' covers a wide range of clinical states, from mild disorientation and agitation, to drowsiness and coma. The midnight call to the ward to see a confused uncooperative 'liver patient' often represents a diagnostic and management challenge. The range of causes is wide (table), but it is important to make a correct diagnosis, as the treatment for one cause may be detrimental to another. An acute confusional state is usually due to an organic cause, rarely due to mental illness.

Causes of disturbed conciousness in the GI patient

Hepatic encephalopathy	Hypoxia (e.g. pulmonary/fat embolus)
Alcohol withdrawal/delirium tremens	Intracranial bleed (e.g. subdural, extradural, intracerebral)
Wernicke's encephalopathy	Post-ictal/status epilepticus
Sepsis	Zinc deficiency
Illicit drug use/overdose	Psychosis
Encephalitis	Cerebral abscess/tumour
Hypoglycaemia	Acute renal failure

Assessment

- **History** is most usually available from family/friends, and attendant medical/nursing staff. Find out about previous episodes of confusion, head injury, psychiatric disease. Is there a history of alcohol excess? Examine drug chart—any new sedatives/constipating agents? Review observation chart, including temperature. Is the patient in pain (agitation is an important manifestation of pain in patients with dementia or severe cognitive impairment).
- **Full general and neurological examination** is essential. Ensure vital signs stable and airway protected. Specifically look for: signs of sepsis; malnutrition (?Wernicke's encephalopathy); smell breath (?alcohol, fetor hepatis of encephalopathy); jaundice and signs of chronic liver disease or portal hypertension (e.g. splenomegaly, ascites), or a liver flap (?hepatic encephalopathy); needle marks/tracks (?drug overdose, sepsis, including cerebral abscess). Tremulousness, tachycardia, and

sweating may relate to <u>alcohol withdrawal</u> (?stopped alcohol due to admission 48–72 hours previously), sepsis, or hypoglycaemia. Diagnosis of most causes of confusion in GI patients is made on the basis of clinical assessment, with specific investigations only available (and often only possible) after initial empirical treatment.

Immediate investigations

- Do needle prick for glucose BM.
- Pulse oximetry.
- Take blood for:
  - FBC, clotting.
  - U&Es, LFTs, glucose.
  - ESR, CRP.
- Exclude sepsis (CXR, blood cultures, MSU/CSU, ascitic tap).
- Consider CT brain (especially if any history of head injury or focal neurology).
- Blood and urine for alcohol/drug screen.

Management

- If patient agitated or aggressive, remove objects from around bed with which patient may harm themselves or others (e.g. glass vases).
- Nurse in calm, quiet environment, with as few people 'coming and going' as is possible.
- Give thiamine 150 mg IV/PO for 5 days if any risk of <u>Wernicke's encephalopathy</u> (e.g. malnutrition, liver disease).
- Use of haloperidol 5–10 mg IM/PO may be necessary in agitated patient, but should be avoided in patients with <u>hepatic encephalopathy</u> or <u>alcohol withdrawal</u>.
- Specific management will depend on likely diagnosis (see <u>hepatic encephalopathy</u>, <u>alcohol withdrawal</u>, <u>Wernicke's encephalopathy</u> in table on p.10, and A–Z section).

Anaemia and occult GI bleeding

Anaemia (Hb less than 11.5 g/dl in a woman, 12.5 g/dl in a man) is common in GI practice and also a common reason for referral to gastroenterologists by other specialists. Often a gastroenterologist is asked for an opinion on the cause of a macrocytic or microcytic anaemia. Careful testing to confirm the presence of various haematinic deficiencies is crucial (see box opposite). A classification of anaemia related to GI disease is shown in the table.

Classification of anaemia related to GI disease	
GI bleeding	Iron deficiency
Decreased red cell production	**Haematinic deficiency:** vitamin B12 (see cobalamin) and folic acid (deficiency seen in (pregnancy, increased cell turnover, inflammation)
	Marrow failure: aplastic anaemia, red cell aplasia, marrow infiltration
Increased red cell destruction	Congenital (haemoglobinopathies, spherocytosis, red cell enzyme defects)
	Acquired (immune/non-immune)
Abnormal red cell maturation	Sideroblastic anaemia, myelodysplasia
Drug-related anaemia	See text. May be caused by bleeding (NSAIDs, warfarin), drug-induced haemolysis, or marrow aplasia (e.g. mesalazine)
Effect of disease in other organs	Anaemia of chronic disease
	Liver, renal, endocrine disease

Haematinic deficiency

The most important are **iron, folic acid, and vitamin B12**, but **copper and vitamins A, B6, C, E, riboflavin, and nicotinic acid** are also needed for erythropoiesis. Deficiency can arise through inadequate intake, malabsorption, increased need or use, and loss.

Basic tests for haematinic deficiency
- Full blood count (Hb, red cell indices—MCV, MCHC, MCH—white count and differential, platelets)
- Blood film examination
- Reticulocyte count
- Iron, TIBC, ferritin
- B12 and folate (red cell folate)
- U&E
- Liver function tests including albumin and GGT

Causes of haematinic deficiency in GI disease

	Iron	B12	Folate
Nutritional	Rarely sole cause	Vegans	Poor diet—elderly, alcoholics, institutionalized
Malabsorption			
Stomach	Anacidity, atrophic gastritis, gastrectomy	Pernicious anaemia, food—cobalamin malabsorption, atrophic gastritis	Gastrectomy
Small intestine	Coeliac disease, tropical sprue	Stagnant loop with associated bacterial overgrowth, ileal resection, Crohn's, coeliac, sprue, fish tapeworm, selective malabsorption	Gastrectomy, coeliac, tropical sprue, scleroderma, amyloidosis, Giardia, diabetic enteropathy, lymphoma, Whipple's disease
Other		Chronic pancreatitis, liver disease	Alcohol
Increased loss or utilization	Bleeding		Liver disease, Crohn's disease

For details of treatment of haematinic deficiencies and further details of individual causes, see iron deficiency: vitamin B12 (see cobalamin) deficiency: folate deficiency.

Increased red cell destruction: haemolysis

Red cell destruction is mainly extravascular in the liver, spleen, and bone marrow. Haem is metabolized to bilirubin, conjugated in the liver, and excreted in the faeces and urine.

Congenital causes

- Unconjugated hyperbilirubinaemia due to excess haemolysis is seen in the neonate due to:
  - **Congenital spherocytosis** (in the adult spherocytosis indicates antibody-mediated red cell destruction) or
  - **Non-spherocytotic causes** such as inherited red cell enzyme defects (e.g. G6PD deficiency).
- **Haemoglobinopathies**. These include structural haemoglobin variants such as sickle cell disease and disorders of globin chain synthesis (thalassaemias).

Acquired causes

- In adults can be seen in severe liver disease due to abnormal lipid composition of red cells.
- Disseminated cancers (e.g. arising from a gastric or pancreatic primary) can produce disseminated intravascular coagulation and the associated fibrin deposition can produce a microangiopathic haemolytic anaemia.

Diagnosis

Plasma haptoglobins bind to haemoglobin and are reduced in intravascular haemolysis and in liver disease. Haemolysis can result in pigment gallstones that can be the presenting feature of illness.

Drug-related anaemia

Think of:

- Upper GI irritation causing blood loss: NSAIDs and aspirin. The combination of NSAIDs and CORTICOSTEROIDS is associated with high risk of upper GI bleeding.
- Bleeding due to specific drugs, e.g. warfarin, heparin.
- Drug-induced haemolysis—e.g. oxidative haemolysis due to sulphasalazine or dapsone.
- Production impairment, e.g. aplasia secondary to mesalazine.

Anaemia in liver disease

Causes of anaemia in liver disease

Cause	Comment
Dilutional	Increased plasma volume, splenomegaly
Iron deficiency	Bleeding. Iron status can be difficult to establish. Ferritin may be increased as an acute phase protein. Transferrin, accounting for much of TIBC, is often reduced. MCV may be falsely raised due to alcohol
Vitamin B12 and folate	Liver stores B12 and folate. Folate often deficient in alcoholics due to poor nutrition and effect of alcohol in reducing folate absorption
Haemolysis	May be autoimmune in association with <u>autoimmune hepatitis</u>. Red cell lifespan reduced, due to abnormal membrane—if severe can produce 'spur cell' anaemia. Alcohol can cause sideroblastic anaemia. Haemolysis is seen in <u>Wilson's disease</u> (probably due to copper toxicity to red cells). <u>Zieve's syndrome</u>
Aplastic anaemia	Viral hepatitis: parvovirus, <u>hepatitis A, B, C</u>, EBV, CMV. Hepatitis is often mild and marrow aplasia severe: damage may be immune-mediated. Alcohol may have direct marrow toxicity effects

Iron deficiency anaemia presumed due to occult GI blood loss

A common situation in gastroenterological practice and a common reason for referral by non-gastroenterologists. Up to 100 ml blood loss per day can still result in grossly normal looking stools. The source of bleeding is unidentified in about 5% of patients with GI bleeding.

<u>Faecal occult blood testing</u> can be helpful, particularly if menorrhagia is suspected as a cause of anaemia in menstruating women. Iron deficiency is diagnosed either by a low ferritin or by a low transferrin saturation (ratio of <u>iron</u> to TIBC). Beware missing iron deficiency because of a normal TIBC; this reflects mostly transferrin synthesis by the liver, which can be impaired in chronic disease or inflammation.

Diagnosing the cause of iron-deficiency anaemia

History

- Focus on drugs that injure the GI mucosa (e.g. aspirin, nonsteroidals, bisphosphonates, potassium salts).
- Take a careful family history for bleeding disorders.

Examination

Look for cutaneous stigmata of systemic diseases (<u>dermatitis herpetiformis</u>, neurofibromas, lip freckles suggestive of <u>Peutz–Jeghers</u>, mucosal

telangiectasia in <u>hereditary haemorrhagic telangiectasia</u>, osteomas suggestive of <u>Gardner's syndrome</u>).

Investigations

Initial assessment may direct investigations to a particular part of GI tract.
For example:

- Dyspepsia or a clear history of NSAID or other irritant drug ingestion
directs the need for upper GI endoscopy; and a positive family history
of <u>colon cancer</u>, a change of bowel habit, or iron deficiency in an elderly patient with aortic stenosis (suggesting possibility of <u>angiodyspla-
sia</u>) will necessitate colonoscopy.
- In the absence of clear symptoms, upper GI endoscopy and colonoscopy at the same session improves cost effectiveness and results in a
significantly increased diagnostic yield over either investigation alone.
- Always consider duodenal biopsy to exclude villous atrophy (see
<u>coeliac disease</u>) as a cause of unexplained iron deficiency (low iron due
to malabsorption and blood loss).

Investigation of the patient with suspected occult
GI bleeding or definite blood loss but normal upper
GI endoscopy/colonoscopy

This is influenced by the briskness of the bleeding.

- If there is any suggestion of an upper GI lesion, repeat upper GI endoscopy by a senior endoscopist using an enteroscope or paediatric
colonoscope has been shown to identify lesions in a substantial proportion of patients.
- In those with active bleeding, radionuclide scanning with Tc^{99}-labelled
red cells or angiography can reveal the site of bleeding. Tc^{99} scans are
sensitive at confirming GI bleeding, but evidence on their role in
managing patients with GI bleeds is lacking. Angiography is less
sensitive (requires bleeding rate of at least 2 ml/min) but can
accurately locate bleeding point and in skilled hands allows possibility
of therapeutic embolization of bleeding vessel. CT scanning or
<u>Meckel's</u> scans may be helpful.
- Evaluation of possible small intestinal pathology by contrast radiology
gives a very low diagnostic yield and often results in unhelpful exposure of young patients to ionizing radiation. The suggested sequence of
examination is influenced by availability of certain techniques but available evidence favours <u>enteroscopy</u> using either a dedicated enteroscope or, alternatively, a paediatric colonoscope. If this is negative,
video <u>capsule endoscopy</u> is emerging as the diagnostic investigation of
choice to detect lesions of the small bowel providing there are no
symptoms of intestinal obstruction.

Anorectal problems

Anal discomfort or pain and passage of bright blood from the anus are common symptoms often reported with some embarrassment and anxiety by patients. Many people are frightened by the thought of an anorectal examination: a definite diagnosis, with a clear explanation of the condition and available therapies, will make future visits less of an ordeal.

Clinical assessment

- Any bleeding must be carefully defined: spots of fresh blood on the paper suggest a perianal source, while darker blood or blood mixed in with stool suggests pathology higher up the colon.
- In cases of perianal pain, sepsis should always be looked for, but this can be difficult to detect in the clinic.
- While rigid sigmoidoscopy is an essential part of the initial examination, <u>endoanal ultrasound, examination under anaesthetic</u>, and <u>MRI</u> are essential ancillary investigations.

Anal lesions

- Bleeding or prolapse of tissue through the anus is a common presentation of <u>haemorrhoids</u>. The diagnosis can be made on proctoscopy.
- Anal skin tags, fibroepithelial polyps, and thrombosed external piles are all relatively minor conditions that can cause major symptoms: referral to a surgeon for excision may be needed.
- A <u>rectal prolapse</u> can be mistaken for prolapsing haemorrhoids: the diagnosis can usually be made by examining the patient straining to pass stool. Unpleasant as it sounds, it is best to examine the patient sitting in the lavatory rather than in the left lateral position.
- <u>Anal fissures</u> can cause agonizing pain. They may be diagnosed on the history with a careful examination of the anal canal, but sometimes examination under anaesthetic is needed. Treatment of anal fissure is now often medical rather than the traditional lateral sphincterotomy or the discredited anal stretch (see <u>anal fissure</u> for details of medical management).
- <u>Anorectal abscesses</u> usually result from infection of the anal glands along the dentate line. Acute infection may cause an abscess and lead to a chronic fistula. Abscess are classified according to where they extend to and may be perianal, ischiorectal, intersphincteric, or supralevator. Causes and important differential diagnoses are shown in the table.

Causes and differential diagnosis of anorectal fistulae

Causes of anorectal fistulae	Crohn's disease, trauma, TB, foreign bodies, anal surgery
Differential diagnosis	Pilonidal sinus, hidradenitis suppurativa, carcinoma, Bartholin's abscess, lymphoma

- While a perianal abscess may be easy to diagnose, an ischiorectal abscess can be much less obvious. Sepsis higher up the anal canal can present as rectal pain. Abscesses may communicate with the anorectum: this may present as a fistulous tract.
- Assessing anorectal fistulae traditionally involves examination under anaesthetic, but MRI and endoscopic ultrasound (EUS) have a proven role in defining the anatomy. Any discharging area or granulation tissue around the anus should be assumed to communicate with the anorectum until proved otherwise.
- Itching of the perianal area (pruritus ani: the commonest site for intractable itch in the body) has a variety of causes. It is often managed by patients with a variety of creams and lotions that rarely help and may worsen the symptoms.
- The frequency of perianal Crohn's disease varies from about 15% in association with small bowel disease to about 35% in patients with ileocolitis or colitis alone. While management of associated sepsis may involve surgery or radiologically guided drainage, a conservative approach is usually indicated and medical management often provides the best chance of healing, especially with some of the new biological treatments such as anti-TNF monoclonal antibodies (see INFLIXIMAB). Medical approaches include antibiotics (METRONIDAZOLE, CIPROFLOXACIN) and AZATHIOPRINE.
- Several sexually transmitted diseases can have anorectal manifestations—see table.

Sexually transmitted diseases with anorectal manifestations

Organism	Condition
Human papilloma virus	Perianal warts (condylomata accuminata)
Herpes simplex virus	Vesicles can occur around anus or in anal canal
Treponema pallidum (syphilis)	Primary or secondary lesions
Chlamydia	Can cause proctitis or even stricturing
Gonococcus	Can be asymptomatic

Rectal lesions

- Rectal discomfort or dissatisfaction and the passage of blood per rectum are the commonest symptoms of rectal disease. Digital examination and proctoscopy or sigmoidoscopy should allow exclusion of a <u>rectal cancer</u>, inflammation, or <u>solitary rectal ulcer</u>. <u>Rectal prolapse</u> is diagnosed from the history and examining the patient straining to pass stool.
- Outpatient rigid sigmoidoscopy often gives very limited views and many clinicians will proceed straight to flexible sigmoidoscopy to define a cause of rectal bleeding.
- Investigation of rectal discomfort may involve a defecating proctogram (see <u>defecography studies</u>) to define mechanical problems with defecation or a <u>rectocele</u>. Endoanal ultrasound or pelvic MRI are the best tools to define perianal anatomy.
- Injury to the anorectum from radiation therapy is an important cause of symptoms: up to 20% of patients receiving pelvic radiotherapy suffer radiation proctitis (see <u>radiation injury to the GI tract</u>).

Ascites

Causes of fluid within the peritoneal cavity (i.e. ascites)

Mechanism	Causes
<u>Portal hypertension</u>	Parenchymal liver disease (e.g. <u>cirrhosis</u>, <u>alcoholic hepatitis</u>, <u>acute liver failure</u>); right heart failure; constrictive pericarditis; <u>veno-occlusive disease</u>; <u>Budd–Chiari syndrome</u>; <u>portal vein thrombosis</u>
Peritoneal inflammation	<u>Spontaneous bacterial peritonitis</u>; Malignant peritoneal deposits; connective tissue disease (e.g. systemic lupus, <u>sarcoidosis</u>, <u>familial Mediterranean fever</u>), <u>TB</u>; pancreatic ascites
Reduced plasma oncotic pressure	Hypoalbuminaemic states (e.g. nephrotic syndrome, malnutrition, <u>protein-losing enteropathy</u>)
Impaired lymphatic drainage	Lymphatic obstruction (e.g. right heart failure, TB, lymphoproliferative disorders); lymphatic tear (e.g. trauma)

In the developed world, <u>portal hypertension</u> due to cirrhosis accounts for 80%, with intra-abdominal malignancy and heart failure making up most of the rest. Note that ascites rarely occurs due to <u>portal vein thrombosis</u> in isolation, but may develop in setting of systemic sepsis, or low serum albumin.

Assessment of ascites

Always consider

- Is there unequivocal evidence of ascites (hospital admission and intensive investigation of portal hypertension is rarely effective treatment for central obesity!)?
- What is the cause of ascites?
- What is the optimal management?

History

A full history is essential, especially in those with recent-onset ascites. Focus on:

- Symptoms and risk factors for cirrhosis (see <u>Approach to cirrhosis and chronic liver disease</u>), <u>portal hypertension</u>, and cardiac disease.
- Internal malignancy (including recent weight loss and right upper quadrant discomfort in cirrhotics, suggestive of <u>hepatocellular carcinoma</u>).
- Sepsis (including abdominal <u>TB</u> and <u>spontaneous bacterial peritonitis</u>).

Examination

Look for signs of:

- Chronic liver disease (see Approach to GI examination), hepatic encephalopathy (e.g. jaundice, liver flap).
- Portal hypertension (splenomegaly, dilated abdominal veins, caput medusa (superficial veins radiating out from umbilicus)). Ascites due to portal hypertension usually occurs in setting of hyperdynamic circulation (↑HR, peripheral vasodilatation, ↓mean arterial BP).
- Cardiac failure (cardiomegaly, ↑ JVP).

Investigation

- Bloods: FBC, U&Es, LFTs, ESR, CRP, clotting. Full assessment of causes of liver disease as appropriate (see Approach to recent-onset jaundice).
- Imaging. Ultrasound + Doppler or contrast CT scan allow portal vein flow to be assessed, as well as intra-abdominal organs. 'Internal echoes' or 'septae' within ascites may suggest infection or lymphatic cause.
- Diagnostic ascitic tap is essential in all cases, including in patients with known cirrhosis and ascites in hospital (who have a high rate of spontaneous bacterial peritonitis. See paracentesis. 20 ml of fluid should be drawn, and assessed for:
  - **Colour** (see Fig. 1.1). Usually yellow/straw colour. Blood suggests 'blood tap' or malignancy; white/milky suggests chylous ascites.
  - White **cell count**: (normal < 500 white cells/μl, <250 neutrophils/μl).
  - **Ascitic albumin.** This allows calculation of serum to ascites albumin gradient (SAAG), which accurately differentiates ascites due to portal hypertension (SAAG >11 g/l) from non-portal hypertension in > 97% of cases.
  - **Microscopy and culture.** Always inoculate into blood culture bottles. AFB is positive in the fluid of < 20% of cases of peritoneal TB.
  - **Cytology.** In suspected malignancy, providing larger volumes of fluid to the cytopathologist (e.g. > 100 ml) may increase the chance of making a diagnosis.
- Urinalysis +24 hour urine collection if proteinuria.
- Further investigations will be tailored to the results of these tests, and clinical picture (e.g. ECG, CXR, echocardiogram if possible heart failure). Ascitic amylase >2000 IU/l suggests pancreatic ascites (e.g. following pancreatic pseudocyst rupture), and ascitic bilirubin > serum bilirubin supports diagnosis of a biliary leak (e.g. post-cholecystectomy). Microbiological diagnosis of TB ascites varies significantly (10–70% positive cultures). Chylous ascites is diagnosed by a measured ascitic triglyceride (TG) level of > 110 mg/dl (and always with ascitic TG > plasma TG).

See Fig. 1.1 for diagnosis on basis of ascitic fluid analysis.

Management

Vital to treat the underlying cause, not just manage ascites (see <u>Approach to cirrhosis and chronic liver disease</u>).

Portal hypertensive ascites

- **Salt restriction**. No added salt to food should be specified, and low salt diet preferred, but patient compliance with < 1.5 g/day (60 mmol/day) is poor. However, salt restriction alone may lead to resolution of ascites in 20% of patients.
- **Restriction of fluid** to 1.5 l is a standard component of management, but as fluid loss in ascites is directly related to negative Na^+ balance, fluid restriction is rarely effective in absence of salt restriction.
- **Diuretics**. Combination of spironolactone and frusemide usually required. Commence spironolactone 100 mg/day and frusemide 40 mg/day. Increase dosages every 4–5 days, to maximum spironolactone 400 mg/day and frusemide 160 mg/day, titrated against body weight (aim ↓0.5 kg/day) and body weight. Monitor U&Es to exclude renal impairment.
- In 10% of patients this approach does not work, defining them as having 'refractory ascites'. Treatment options then include large volume therapeutic <u>paracentesis</u>, surgical shunting, <u>transjugular intrahepatic portosystemic shunt (TIPSS)</u>, or <u>liver transplantation</u>.
- Surgical portosystemic shunts and peritoneovenous shunts are now rarely used, because of high complication rate and availability of alternatives.
- TIPSS is effective at controlling ascites in most patients, but high occlusion rate (30–50% at one year) and risk of <u>hepatic encephalopathy</u> (up to 30%) raise concern about its long-term role, particularly in those with poor liver synthetic function (i.e. ↑ bilirubin, ↑INR, ↓serum—albumin see Child–Pugh score).
- <u>Liver transplantation</u> is the definitive treatment of patients with cirrhotic ascites, who otherwise have a 5 year survival of 20% with medical therapy alone.

Non-portal hypertensive ascites

Malignant ascites is usually refractory to diuretics, and requires repeated therapeutic <u>paracentesis</u>. It generally indicates a very poor prognosis. Biliary peritonitis requires endoscopic or percutaneous biliary stenting ± surgery, dependent on cause. Similarly, management of pancreatic ascites depends on exact site and cause of pancreatic leak, with approaches including pancreatic rest (e.g. with nasojejunal feeding), percutaneous drainage, endoscopic <u>pancreatic stent</u> insertion, surgical pancreatic resection (e.g. <u>Whipple's procedure</u> or distal pancreatectomy) ± <u>OCTREOTIDE</u> to reduce pancreatic fluid output. TB ascites is treated with appropriate chemotherapy.

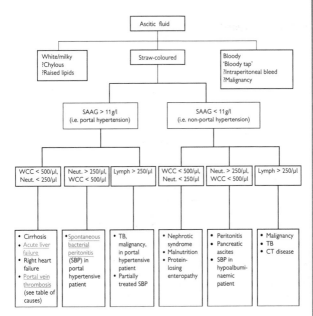

Fig. 1.1 Diagnosis of cause of ascites using serum-ascites albumin gradient (SAAG) and cell count. Although SAAG strongly predicts whether or not ascites is due to portal hypertension, interpretation of WCC results necessitates incorporation of clinical information and other results (e.g. culture, cytology).

Bloating and wind

- Excessive gas production is a common symptom causing patients to seek advice.
- Patients may attribute abdominal cramps, bloating, chest discomfort, audible bowel sounds, belching, and flatulence to gaseousness.

Composition and volume of intestinal gas

The main gases in flatus are oxygen and nitrogen (which come largely from swallowed air) and hydrogen, methane, and carbon dioxide, which come from the intestinal lumen. Hydrogen and methane are largely products of bacterial metabolism: carbon dioxide can be derived from bacterial fermentation of dietary substances.

Excretion of flatus averages 600 ml per day and is no greater in patients complaining of gaseousness, suggesting a heightened sensitivity to intestinal stretch or abnormal motility rather than increased volume, similar to observations in patients with irritable bowel syndrome.

Clinical assessment

History and examination. See box opposite.

Investigation
- FBC, electrolytes, liver function.
- Any blood in the stool should prompt investigation of the colon.
- Plain abdominal X-rays.
- Consider upper and lower GI contrast examinations to exclude intestinal obstruction.

Therapy

- Air swallowing is common: reassurance and stopping gum chewing and smoking can help.
- Belching often results from discomfort due to gastro-oesophageal reflux: acid suppression can be helpful.
- Bacterial overgrowth may contribute and may need treating.
- Excessive flatus may respond to dietary modification (reduction of intake of legumes, beans, fruits, complex carbohydrates).
- Activated charcoal, taken orally before a meal, can reduce breath hydrogen.

- Some patients may have delayed intestinal transit and be constipated. Treatment with increased dietary fibre or non-stimulant osmotic laxatives (not lactulose which is fermented in the gut) can relieve constipation. Promising drugs include new prokinetics for constipation-predominant IBS, e.g tegaserod, a partial 5-HT4 agonist. There is preliminary evidence that some probiotic bacteria (*Bifidobacter infantis*, present in a product called VSL-3) may alleviate the symptom of bloating in patients with irritable bowel syndrome.

Assessment of the gaseous patient
History
- **Diet.** Legumes, beans, apples, prunes, raisins, starches can all be fermented resulting in gas production
- **Medications:** narcotics, analgesics, calcium channel blockers
- **Surgery:** 25–50% of patients get gas bloating after a Nissen fundoplication
- **Psychiatric factors** such as anxiety or depression can be relevant
- **Systemic diseases:** diabetes (gastroparesis due to autonomic neuropathy), scleroderma (altered motility due to neuromuscular dysfunction), neuromuscular disorders such as muscular dystrophy, hypothyroidism

Physical examination
- Examine for signs of weight loss, ascites, air swallowing, anxiety, and peritonitis. Look for a succussion splash

Breaking bad news

- **Effective, empathetic communication** is the cornerstone of good medicine.
- The skill and care with which bad news is broken often defines all further interactions between doctors and their patients/relatives, for good or bad.
- The need to break bad news may cover a wide range of scenarios, including a new diagnosis of cancer, a cancelled procedure, or endoscopic complications. Although the specific approach needed will depend on the individual situation, a number of considerations apply to most cases.
  - **Give thought beforehand** as to what you will say. It is vital that you are as informed as possible about the patient's specific case.
  - Try to see the patient and/or their relatives in a **quiet environment** free of interruptions. Breaking bad news in a private room is always preferable to the open ward or waiting room. Turn off mobile phones/bleeps.
  - Ensure that the patient's **nurse is with you**, so that they may provide further patient support, and are aware of what has been said.
  - Explain things as simply as possible. **Avoid jargon**. Draw simple diagrams where appropriate.
  - **Be honest**. If a mistake or complication has occurred, evasion and dishonesty always compound the already difficult situation.
  - **Record your discussions** in the notes, and ensure that the patient's GP is aware of any important new developments in the patient's case (little is more unsatisfactory for a GP than to see a patient in the community, to discuss their new diagnosis of cancer, about which the GP knows nothing!).
  - Try to be **encouraging and reassuring** but **not falsely optimistic**. For example, whilst a finding of malignancy may be a shock to the patient, confirmation of the diagnosis often allows specific treatment to then be planned.
  - Avoid over-speculation or hypothesis.
  - **Don't worry about expressing emotion**. Maintaining professionalism does not mean displaying a cold, dispassionate approach. In times of grief or upset, patients and relatives appreciate that their doctor understands and empathizes with their distress.
  - **Don't rush**. There are always time pressures, but providing the space for questions to be asked in an unhurried way is important.
  - **Don't delegate** responsibility downwards. If you feel uncomfortable about breaking bad news, ask your senior to do it, and accompany them. By doing so, you may learn vital lessons on how to (and maybe how not to!) approach this vital area of practice. Similarly, if the issue relates to a complication or medical accident, be sure to

discuss the situation with your consultant, who may wish to see the patient/relatives themselves.

- One response to bad news may be anger. Acknowledge this, but never respond in like.
- Don't leave things 'in the air'. Whether the bad news relates to a serious diagnosis, a cancelled admission, or a complication, patients wish to know what the next step entails. Provide information about other sources of support (e.g. hospital patient liaison service, or national support groups).
- Relatives occasionally state that their loved one 'wouldn't want to know' if they had cancer/terminal disease, etc. This may present a difficult situation, requiring sensitive handling. It has been shown that patients want more, not less, information. Sometimes a lack of acceptance by relatives underlies the above statement. Whilst it is essential to keep the family 'on board', the **primary duty is to the patient,** who has the right to know what is going on with his/her body. Scenarios in which relatives, but not the patient, are aware of a serious diagnosis, often develop in a messy and wholly unsatisfactory manner, for all involved. Also see <u>Approach to consent</u>.
- Finally, accept that this is a stressful, often difficult situation. If your approach is to be honest, thoughtful, and compassionate, you won't go far wrong.

Chronic diarrhoea

Definition

Imprecise (if not loose). Acute diarrhoea (less than 14 day's duration) is usually due to infection (see Approach to acute diarrhoea).

A patient's perception of diarrhoea needs to be clarified (increased looseness of stools; increased frequency of stools; urgency; abdominal discomfort; faecal incontinence). Stool weight (> 235 g/day in men, > 175 g/day in women) has been used to define diarrhoea but weighing the stool is unpleasant, disliked by patient, nurse, and laboratory, and in any case stool weight above the upper limit of normal with normal consistency is not necessarily diarrhoea. A working definition of chronic diarrhoea is the abnormal passage of ≥ 3 loose stools per day for over 4 weeks.

Clinical classification into **watery diarrhoea (osmotic or secretory), fatty diarrhoea (steatorrhoea), or inflammatory diarrhoea** is useful, but there is considerable pathophysiological overlap. Investigation of steatorrhoea is described further in Approach to malabsorption and steatorrhoea.

Pathophysiology and causes

Osmotic

Occurs due to presence in the gut of an excess amount of poorly absorbable, osmotically active solutes. Stool water content directly relates to faecal output of solutes exerting an osmotic pressure across the intestinal mucosa. (Electrolyte composition may vary according to the electrical charge on poorly absorbed anions or cations, which is why measuring stool electrolytes is rarely useful. Just as well for junior doctors and lab technicians: but see later for a role in evaluating difficult diarrhoeas.)

This explains two clinical hallmarks of osmotic diarrhoea:
- Diarrhoea stops when the patient fasts or at least stops eating the poorly absorbed solute causing the diarrhoea.
- Stool analysis, if necessary, will reveal an osmotic gap: that is $\{2 \times [Na^+] + [K^+]\}$ (to account for anions) is less than faecal osmolality (usually assumed to be isotonic to plasma, i.e. 290 mOsm/kg).

Secretory

Results from abnormal ion transport by intestinal epithelial cells. Four main categories of disease involved:
- Congenital defect in ion absorption.
- Intestinal resection.
- Diffuse mucosal disease damaging/reduced epithelial cell numbers.

- Abnormal mediators (including neurotransmitters, bacterial toxins, hormones, and cathartics) that can affect intestinal chloride and water secretion through changes in intracellular AMP and GMP.
  Secretory diarrhoea is characterized by two features.
  - Stool osmolality is accounted for by $Na^+ + K^+$, and related anions, so the osmotic gap is small.
  - Diarrhoea usually persists during a 48–72 hour fast.

Inflammatory (exudative)

Inflammation and ulceration may lead to loss of mucus, proteins, pus, or blood into the bowel lumen. Diarrhoea accompanying intestinal inflammation may be due to impairment of normal colonic absorptive function.

Altered motility

Little experimental proof that increased motility causes diarrhoea, but it has been implicated in:

- The diarrhoea of irritable bowel syndrome.
- Post-gastrectomy diarrhoea.
- Diabetic diarrhoea.
- Bile salt induced diarrhoea.
- Diarrhoea associated with hyperthyroidism.
- Drug-related, e.g. erythromycin as a motilin agonist.

Causes of osmotic diarrhoea

Carbohydrate malabsorption

- Congenital
  - Specific (disaccharidase deficiency, glucose–galactose malabsorption, fructose malabsorption)
  - Generalized (abetalipoproteinaemia, congenital lymphangiectasia, enterokinase deficiency, pancreatic insufficiency (e.g. due to cystic fibrosis))
- Acquired
  - Specific (e.g. post-enteritis disaccharidase deficiency)
  - Generalized malabsorption—see Approach to malabsorption and steatorrhoea (pancreatic insufficiency/biliary obstruction, bacterial overgrowth, coeliac disease, parasitic disease, short bowel syndromes, mucosal damage or disease, postmucosal obstruction in lymphangiectasia, previous surgery including gastrectomy or intestinal resection leading to bile acid malabsorption)

Excess ingestion of poorly absorbed carbohydrate

- Lactulose therapy, sorbitol in elixirs or 'sugar-free' sweets, fructose in soft drinks or dried fruits, mannitol in sugar-free products, excess bran or fibre
- Magnesium-induced diarrhoea from antacids and laxatives
- Laxatives containing poorly absorbed anions such as sodium sulphate, phosphate, or citrate

Functional (IBS)

- Consider food hypersensitivity

Causes of secretory diarrhoea

- **Congenital** (microvillus inclusion disease, absent Cl/HCO$_3$ exchanger)
- **Endogenous**
  - Bacterial enterotoxins (cholera, ETEC, *Campylobacter*, *Clostridium*, *Staph. aureus*) or hormones (VIPoma, medullary carcinoma of thyroid (calcitonin, prostaglandins), gastrinoma, villous adenoma, small bowel lymphoma)
  - Stimulant laxatives: phenolphthalein, anthraquinones, castor oil, cascara, senna
  - Drugs: antibiotics, diuretics, theophyllines, thyroxine, anticholinesterases, colchicine, prokinetics, ACE inhibitors, antidepressants (SSRIs), prostaglandins, gold
  - Toxins: plant (*Amanita*), organophosphates, caffeine, monosodium glutamate

Causes of inflammatory diarrhoea

- Infection: bacterial, viral, parasitic
- Inflammatory bowel disease: ulcerative colitis, Crohn's disease, ulcerative jejuno-ileitis, microscopic colitis (often related to NSAIDs)
- Cytostatic agents: chemotherapy, radiotherapy
- Hypersensitivity: eosinophilic gastroenteritis, nematodes, food allergy
- Autoimmune: micoscopic colitis, graft versus host disease
- Diverticular disease/diverticular colitis
- Ischaemia
- Radiation
- Neoplasia (colonic cancer, lymphoma)

Note: some causes of diarrhoea do not fit easily into this classification e.g. ischaemic colitis (see intestinal ischaemia, amyloidosis).

History and examination

Taking a history of diarrhoea

- Clarify what the patient means by diarrhoea (see definition above) and distinguish acute from chronic diarrhoea.
- After this, the aims of the history are:
  - To distinguish organic (e.g. duration < 3 months; weight loss; nocturnal symptoms; continuous symptoms) from functional causes (absence of organic symptoms + long history and presence of positive symptoms as defined by Rome II criteria—see irritable bowel syndrome).
  - To distinguish malabsorptive diarrhoea (bulky, malodorous, difficult to flush, pale stools) from other causes (liquid/loose stools with blood or mucus).

Stool character and associated symptoms
- Consistently large volume diarrhoea is likely to come from small bowel or proximal colon.
- Bloody diarrhoea indicates an infectious, neoplastic, or inflammatory process; accompanying lethargy or anorexia may suggest mucosal cytokine release. Pale, floating stools suggest steatorrhea and are commonly due to pancreatic insufficiency (stools float because of gas content due to carbohydrate fermentation, not fat malabsorption).

Assess for specific causes of diarrhoea
- Family history of inflammatory bowel disease, <u>coeliac disease, colon cancer</u>.
- Previous GI surgery leading to increased transit, <u>bacterial overgrowth</u> or <u>bile salt malabsorption</u> (also see <u>Approach to surgically altered anatomy</u>).
- Systemic disease such as diabetes mellitus, thyroid disease—heat intolerance and palpitations may suggest hyperthyroidism, <u>carcinoid</u> (with associated flushing), systemic sclerosis.
- Drugs (see lists in text/boxes of causes of diarrhoea—alcohol, caffeine, and non-absorbable carbohydrates such as sorbitol are often missed and don't forget surreptitious laxative abuse, as factitious diarrhoea occurs in 4% of those diarrhoea cases in general hospitals, but up to 20% in tertiary referral units).
- Foreign travel, exposure to contaminated water or potential pathogens, e.g. <u>*Salmonella*</u> in food handlers, *Brucella* on farms.
- Evidence of <u>chronic pancreatitis</u>.
- Sexual history is important: anal intercourse is a risk factor for proctitis (causes include *Gonoccocus*, <u>Herpes simplex</u>, *Chlamydia*, <u>amoebiasis</u>).
- Always ask about <u>faecal incontinence</u>: it is common (2% of the population) and not always reported spontaneously. If present, take obstetric history for perineal trauma and possible sphincter damage.
- Ask about diet and stress as aggravating factors. There is a link between physical/sexual abuse and functional bowel disease.
- Ask about illness in companions or family members.

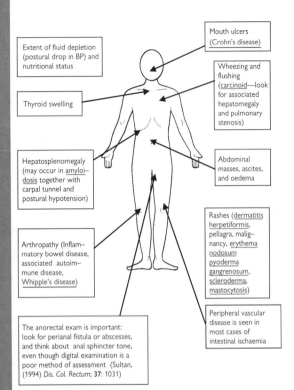

Extent of fluid depletion (postural drop in BP) and nutritional status

Thyroid swelling

Mouth ulcers (Crohn's disease)

Wheezing and flushing (carcinoid—look for associated hepatomegaly and pulmonary stenosis)

Hepatosplenomegaly (may occur in amyloi—dosis together with carpal tunnel and postural hypotension)

Abdominal masses, ascites, and oedema

Arthropathy (Inflam—matory bowel disease, associated autoim—mune disease, Whipple's disease)

Rashes (dermatitis herpetiformis, pellagra, malig—nancy, erythema nodosum pyoderma gangrenosum, scleroderma, mastocytosis)

The anorectal exam is important: look for perianal fistula or abscesses, and think about anal sphincter tone, even though digital examination is a poor method of assessment (Sultan, (1994) Dis. Col. Rectum; **37**: 1031)

Peripheral vascular disease is seen in most cases of intestinal ischaemia

Fig. 1.2 Examining the patient with diarrhoea.

Likely causes of diarrhoea in common clinical categories

- **Acute diarrhoea:** infection (see advice to returning travellers in Approach to acute diarrhoea); drugs/food additives; ischaemic colitis; faecal impaction.
- **Diarrhoea in homosexual HIV-negative men:** amoebiasis, giardiasis, Shigella, Campylobacter, syphillis, gonorrhoea, Chlamydia, Herpes simplex.
- **Diarrhoea in HIV:** Crytosporidium, Microsporidia, Isospora, amoebiasis, Giardia, Herpes, CMV, Adenovirus, MAI, Salmonella, Campylobacter, Cryptococcus, Histoplasma, Candida, lymphoma, AIDS enteropathy (see HIV and the gut).
- **Chronic or recurrent diarrhoea in the patient not previously investigated:** irritable bowel syndrome, Crohn's disease, ulcerative colitis, parasite or fungal infection, malabsorption, drugs or food additives, colonic cancer, diverticulitis, previous surgery, endocrine causes (e.g. thyroid disease), faecal impaction.
- **Chronic diarrhoea in patients previously seen and investigated:** surreptitious laxative abuse, faecal incontinence, microscopic colitis, unrecognized malabsorption, neuroendocrine tumours, food allergy.
- **Nosocomial (hospital-acquired) diarrhoea.** Diarrhoea is among the most common nosocomial illnesses (occurs in 30–50% of patients on ITU) and one-third of patients in chronic care facilities have at least one significant diarrhoeal illness per year. Two classes of patients need particular consideration:
  - **Diarrhoea in patients on ITU:** drugs, especially those containing magnesium and sorbitol, antibiotic-associated diarrhoea (C. difficile but also reduced salvage of carbohydrate by colonic bacteria leading to osmotic diarrhoea—see clostridial infections of the GI tract), enteral feeding, intestinal ischaemia, pseudo-obstruction, faecal impaction, defective anal continence.
  - **Patients with cancer or on chemotherapy.** The incidence of GI toxicity with chemotherapy or radiotherapy can approach 100% with some regimens. Radiotherapy enterocolitis occurs at total body doses of 6 Gy or greater or pelvic irradiation of 3–4 Gy (see radiation damage and the GI tract). Toxic chemotherapeutic agents include cytosine, daunorubicin, 5FU, methotrexate, 6-mercaptopurine, irinotecan, and cisplatin. Some biological treatments such as anti-IL-2 therapy are associated with watery diarrhoea. Typhlitis (neutropenic enterocolitis) is a potent cause of diarrhoea in cancer patients.

Diagnostic tests

Do not accept a diagnosis of diarrhoea without some attempt to examine the stool, even if only on the glove after a rectal exam, to look for blood, mucus, oil, or signs of steatorrhoea.

- 75% of chronic diarrhoeas can be diagnosed by a careful history and examination, coupled with basic haematology and biochemical tests,

stool examination for pathological infection and fat, and sigmoidoscopy
with biopsy.
- Three tests lead to definitive diagnosis in most of the remaining
  patients.
  - Quantitative stool fat.
  - Colonoscopy with biopsies.
  - Response to fasting with measurement of stool volume and
    osmotic gap.
- Indicators of a functional rather than organic aetiology are a long
  history (over 1 year), lack of significant weight loss, absence of
  nocturnal diarrhoea, and straining with defecation. These indicators,
  taken together, are about 70% specific for functional symptoms.

Basic investigations

- Send three stool samples for **culture** (including ova cysts and parasites). Unless there is obvious blood or pus, ask for **stool microscopy**
  as the presence of faecal leucocytes is a hallmark of inflammatory
  diarrhoea. Consider sending stool for *C. difficile* culture and toxin. If
  you suspect factitious diarrhoea or laxative abuse, send the stool and
  urine for a laxative screen.
- **Blood tests**. Full blood count, ESR, CRP, iron, B12, folate, thyroid
  function, glucose, U&Es, calcium, liver function tests including albumin,
  coeliac serology.
- In most cases of diarrhoea where histology helps to make a diagnosis,
  sigmoidoscopy (rigid or flexible depending on what is available) is sufficient rather than full colonoscopy—the exception is when ileal histology is needed, or the changes are patchy throughout the colon.
  Where there is significant weight loss or bleeding to suggest lower GI
  malignancy, full **colonoscopy** is needed.
- **Radiological imaging** may be helpful: a plain abdominal X-ray can show
  faecal impaction, suggest colonic inflammation, pancreatic calcification,
  or intestinal dilatation.

Stool fat

This can be a very useful test but is difficult to get done well (and often
difficult to get done at all).
- Adults absorb about 99% of ingested triglyceride, but only about 90%
  of phospholipid derived from endogenous sources like bile, sloughed
  enterocytes, and bacteria (this is not true for neonates where stool fat
  can exceed 10% of intake).
- About 5–6 g of normal faecal fat excreted per day is unabsorbed
  phospholipid from the endogenous pool, and about 1 g comes from
  the diet. **More than 7 g stool fat per 24 hours is abnormal.**
- Stool fat can be assessed qualitatively or quantitatively. See Approach
  to malabsorption and steatorrhoea.

Response to fasting and stool osmotic gap
- Rarely of practical use in most cases of chronic diarrhoea, but may be useful in difficult cases.
- Steatorrhoeic stools are usually >700 g per 24 h, and stool weight returns to normal on fasting. Inflammatory diarrhoeas respond variably to fasting, but like steatorrhoea stool osmotic gap is usually not helpful.
- Measuring stool electrolytes and osmotic gap may help to classify chronic watery diarrhoeas. Analysis is done on a centrifuged stool sample, so results are possible from spot stool samples or 24–72 h collections.
- Assume that faecal osmolality is the same as plasma (290–mOsm/kg): this is true of freshly passed stool, but with time measured faecal osmolality can become falsely raised due to bacterial degradation of carbohydrate. Large measured deviations below 290 mOsm/kg indicate contamination of stool with urine or water, or a gastrocolic fistula, or hypotonic fluid intake. In principle, stool sodium/potassium is high in secretory diarrhoea (unabsorbed electrolytes retain water in the gut lumen) and low in osmotic diarrhoea (non-electrolytes retain water in the gut lumen). Interpretation of stool osmotic gap and faecal electrolytes is shown in the table.

Stool osmotic gap and faecal electrolytes in the investigation of diarrhoea

Plasma osmolality (approx. 290 mOsm/kg) – 2 × (stool $[Na]^+$ + stool $[K^+]$) =	= Stool osmotic gap
Stool Na > 90 mM and osmotic gap < 50 mM	Secretory diarrhoea: or osmotic diarrhoea caused by sodium sulphate or phosphate ingestion
Stool sodium < 60, osmotic gap > 125 mOsm	Osmotic diarrhoea: if stool volume does not return to normal on fasting, suspect surreptitious magnesium ingestion
Stool sodium > 150 and stool osmolality > 375–400	Suspect contamination with urine
Stool osmolality < 200–250 mOsm	Suspect contamination of stool with dilute urine or water

Other tests used in investigating diarrhoea
Specific tests for malabsorption. (Also see Approach to malabsorption and steatorrhoea.)
- **Small bowel biopsy**. Duodenal biopsy, which may be combined with small bowel aspirate for microbiological analysis, can be useful in diagnosing Crohn's disease (especially in children), coeliac disease, Whipple's disease, giardiasis, lymphoma, eosinophlic gastroenteritis, hypogammaglobulinaemia, amyloidosis, mastocytosis, lymphangiectasia, and various parasitic and fungal infections.
- **Barium studies/small bowel imaging**. These may be useful in fistula, strictures, and previously undetected surgical bypasses.
- Coeliac disease. Serology.

- <u>Pancreatic function tests</u>.
- <u>Schilling test for assessing B12 malabsorption</u>.
- <u>Breath tests</u> for fat, carbohydrate, and bile salt malabsorption, and <u>bacterial overgrowth</u>
- SeHCAT test (see <u>bile acid malabsorption</u>).

Specific tests for watery diarrhoea
Blood and urine hormone levels. Blood levels of certain hormones produced by <u>neuroendocrine tumours</u> such as gastrin, VIP, somatostatin, pancreatic polypeptide, calcitonin, and glucagon may be useful. Urine levels of 5 HIAA can help in diagnosing <u>carcinoid</u>. See <u>gut hormone profile</u>.

Specific tests for inflammatory diarrhoeas
In addition to upper and lower GI endoscopy and small bowel studies, <u>Indium-labelled leucocyte scanning</u> may be useful particularly in children.

Specific tests for enteric protein loss
Faecal α_1-antitrypsin.

Anti-diarrhoeal therapy

These can be divided into those agents useful for mild to moderate diarrhoeas and those useful for secretory or severe diarrhoeas. Most agents in current use work by reducing motility rather than reducing secretion. See <u>ANTI-DIARRHOEAL AGENTS</u> for further details.

Chronic or recurrent abdominal pain

Abdominal pain is a very common cause of patients presenting to doctors. **Acute abdominal pain** usually has an organic cause and is dealt with elsewhere (see emergencies: acute abdominal pain). While there are many pathological causes of **chronic abdominal pain**, most are not due to organic disease, so that the symptom can be a source of worry, frustration, and confusion—to both doctor and patient.

Diagnosis depends on interpreting the patient's experience into a medical model of disease: this can be difficult because of:
- Common innervation of many abdominal organs.
- The low concentration of nerve endings in the viscera.
- The patient's lack of previous experience of pain coming from these organs.
- The non-specific nature of the pain.

Types of abdominal pain

Distinguish:
- **Visceral** pain, originating from noxious stimuli affecting an abdominal viscus and usually felt in the midline.
- **Parietal or somatic** pain arising from stimulation of the parietal peritoneum or abdominal wall and usually located to the site of the lesion.
- **Referred** pain, felt in remote areas supplied by the same neurosegment as the diseased organ because of shared central pathways for afferent neurons from different sites.

Critical features in assessing pain

- The site of the pain, and to where it is referred.
- The **nature** of the pain is important. Ulcers 'gnaw', viscera 'colic', and ruptured aneurysms 'tear'. A long duration of pain tends to correlate with a non-organic cause, especially if not associated with weight loss (see Approach to unintentional weight loss) or other alarm symptoms. Estimating severity of pain is very unreliable.

Factors modifying pain can be very helpful in diagnosis:
- Aggravating foods, or more usually the relationship of pain to eating, may be helpful. Genuine food allergy is rare: food intolerance (e.g. to lactose-containing foods in lactase deficient people) is not. Alcohol can aggravate dyspepsia and intestinal spasm, cause pancreatitis, or worsen lymphoma pain.
- Relief by bowel action or passing flatus suggests a colonic source (see irritable bowel syndrome).
- Pain related to menstruation suggests endometriosis or pelvic inflammatory disease.

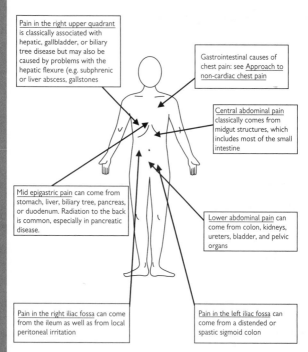

Pain in the right upper quadrant is classically associated with hepatic, gallbladder, or biliary tree disease but may also be caused by problems with the hepatic flexure (e.g. subphrenic or liver abscess, gallstones

Gastrointestinal causes of chest pain: see Approach to non-cardiac chest pain

Central abdominal pain classically comes from midgut structures, which includes most of the small intestine

Mid epigastric pain can come from stomach, liver, biliary tree, pancreas, or duodenum. Radiation to the back is common, especially in pancreatic disease.

Lower abdominal pain can come from colon, kidneys, ureters, bladder, and pelvic organs

Pain in the right iliac fossa can come from the ileum as well as from local peritoneal irritation

Pain in the left iliac fossa can come from a distended or spastic sigmoid colon

Fig. 1.3 Clinical approach to chronic or recurrent abdominal pain.

Physical examination

- **Tachycardia, fever, and sweating** suggest sepsis. Frequent changes of position suggest visceral pain with no or little inflammation.
- **Inspect** for scars, hernias, visible peristalsis.
- **Auscultation** may reveal hyperperistalsis in intestinal obstruction, or <u>ileus</u>, or bruits.
- Do rectal (PR) and if necessary a vaginal (PV) examination (clear prior discussion of the need for internal examination is vital, and the presence of a chaperone is particularly important for the latter). Tenderness on PR or PV examination may not be appreciated by examination of the anterior abdominal wall.
- **Palpate:** rigidity or guarding suggests local peritonism. A palpable mass may result from organ enlargement, inflammation, or a tumour.
- **Percussion** is helpful: tympany suggests excess air, either intraluminal or extraluminal, and light percussion if painful can suggest an area of peritonitis.

Investigations

- Full blood count with MCV (iron studies, B12, and folate if this is abnormal), ESR, and CRP.
- Check renal function and <u>liver function tests</u>.
- Examine urine for pyuria and haematuria, and send sample for microscopy, culture, and sensitivity. If appropriate, check a woman of childbearing age for pregnancy.
- *Do not* use inappropriate radiological tests. An abdominal ultrasound can be highly informative and is non-invasive.
- Other tests depend on the result of the history and examination.

Functional abdominal pain

Functional abdominal disorders account for about half of all patients with abdominal pain seen by doctors and almost all cases with abdominal pain lasting for years. In most cases, a diagnosis of <u>irritable bowel syndrome</u> is possible from the history (see box on Rome criteria for IBS). A small minority of cases have intractable chronic abdominal pain: this may be associated with previous physical or sexual abuse, and the onset may coincide with a bereavement.

The Rome criteria for irritable bowel syndrome

At least 3 months of continuous abdominal pain or discomfort relieved by defecation, or associated with a change in stool frequency, or associated with a change in stool consistency:

Plus two or more of the following, at least 25% of the time:
- Altered stool frequency
- Altered stool form
- Straining, urgency, tenesmus
- Passage of mucus
- Bloating or distension

Causes of chronic or recurrent abdominal pain

Note: some conditions can present acutely!

Generalized parietal pain due to peritonitis
- Bacterial peritonitis (including <u>spontaneous bacterial peritonitis</u>)
- Ruptured cyst
- <u>Familial Mediterranean fever</u>

Localized peritoneal pain
- <u>Appendicitis</u>, <u>cholecystitis</u>, <u>Crohn's disease</u>, endometriosis, chronic pelvic inflammation
- Infiltration due to abdominal neoplasms

Pain from increased tension in viscera
- Intestinal obstruction (mechanical, intussusception, internal herniation)
- Biliary obstruction (<u>choledocholithiasis</u>)
- Ureteric obstruction

Ischaemia
- <u>Intestinal ischaemia</u> (stenosis, embolism, inflammation)

Retroperitoneal causes
- <u>Chronic pancreatitis</u>

Extra-abdominal
- Neurological (neurogenic tumours, spinal degenerative disease, herpes zoster
- Metabolic (diabetic ketoacidosis, acute intermittent <u>porphyria</u>)
- Haematologic (<u>sickle cell anaemia</u>, <u>Henoch–Schönlein purpura</u>)
- Toxic (lead)

Functional causes
- <u>Irritable bowel syndrome</u>
- Non-ulcer dyspepsia
- Biliary pain (<u>sphincter of Oddi dysfunction</u>)

Over-investigation can result from impatience or a lack of clinical knowledge. This tends to sustain the disorder, because the patient recognizes the failure of the doctor to grasp the problem, and gets increasingly frustrated by a succession of normal results. Time, if necessary spread over several visits, may have to be spent exploring emotional factors. The general approach is outlined in the box.

General approach to the patient with functional abdominal pain

Establish rapport and trust
- Acknowledge the symptoms as real
- Maintain a non-judgemental attitude
- Schedule brief but frequent appointments
- Reassure

Avoid temptation to do more diagnostic tests
Set appropriate goals
- Do not expect cure: focus on adjustment
- Emphasize improvement in function
- Emphasize coping and adaptation
- Allow for setbacks

Consider specialized referrals
- Psychiatric, pain clinic, relaxation training

Drug treatment

Analgesics, especially <u>OPIATES</u>, are often not helpful. <u>ANTISPASMODICS</u> can be helpful if targeted to patients with cramping abdominal pain. Start with peppermint tea, oil, or capsules, then consider mebeverine or other similar agents. Low dose antidepressants can be helpful, but patients are often resistant to the idea of taking antidepressants and it is important to emphasize (in layman's terms) that in low doses these drugs have a visceral analgesic effect rather than psychotropic actions.

Cirrhosis and chronic liver disease

Background

- A diagnosis of chronic liver disease is usually made in patients under investigation for abnormal liver function tests (LFTs) or with unexplained jaundice (see Approaches to recent-onset jaundice, and well patient with abnormal liver tests), or in those who present with decompensation (see below).
- The most common causes of chronic liver disease in UK are related to alcoholic liver disease and hepatitis C (see table).
- Cirrhosis is a histological diagnosis characterized by diffuse hepatic fibrosis and nodule formation. Chronic non-cirrhotic liver disease and well-compensated cirrhosis can rarely be differentiated on clinical findings and biochemistry alone (LFTs may be normal, even in established cirrhosis).
- Liver biopsy should be considered in all cases of chronic liver disease. Exceptions may include a patient with clear aetiology of liver disease who has clinically decompensated cirrhosis (e.g. small, irregular liver on imaging, with markedly impaired liver function (↑bilirubin, ↓albumin, ↑prothrombin) and evidence of portal hypertension (e.g. ascites, splenomegaly)).
- A clinical distinction is often made between patients with compensated and those with decompensated cirrhosis. Whilst the distinction may not be absolute, the clinical problems and management of these 2 patterns differ, and so are discussed separately here.
- See also Child–Pugh score.

Causes of cirrhosis and chronic liver disease

Alcoholic liver disease	Haemochromatosis
Hepatitis B	Autoimmune hepatitis
Hepatitis C	Wilson's disease
Primary sclerosing cholangitis	α-1-anti-trypsin deficiency
Primary biliary cirrhosis	Budd–Chiari syndrome
Drugs (e.g. methotrexate)	Secondary biliary cirrhosis
Metabolic liver diseases	Cryptogenic (approximately 15%)
Non-alcoholic fatty liver disease	

Compensated cirrhosis

The patient will have good liver synthetic function (e.g. bilirubin, albumin, prothrombin time may be normal) without ascites or hepatic encephalopathy. The focus of management is to prevent progression of liver disease (decompensation) and avoid complications.

Management

Treat the cause. A nihilistic approach to cirrhosis is not justified. Although the natural course is for progressive fibrosis and liver dysfunction, treatment of the underlying cause has been demonstrated to slow down, and even reverse, clinical progression in patients with established cirrhosis (e.g. haemochromatosis, hepatitis B and C. It is vital to address alcohol dependency. Promising data is emerging on the role of anti-fibrotic therapies in reversing some of the effects of cirrhosis, but no agent approved as yet.

- It is increasingly recognized that osteoporosis is strongly associated with cirrhosis, especially if cholestatic aetiology (e.g. primary biliary cirrhosis) or on immunosuppression. Bone densitometry is indicated, and calcium and vitamin D supplements slow progression of bone loss, and bisphosphonates may be needed (although may cause side-effects, including oesophagitis).
- The complications of portal hypertension may manifest as acute variceal bleeding (see acute upper GI bleeding), ascites, or hepatic encephalopathy (i.e. 'decompensated'—see below). After diagnosing cirrhosis, upper GI endoscopy should be considered, as the finding of gastro-oesophageal varices may merit primary prophylaxis (see portal hypertension).
- The risk of hepatocellular carcinoma (HCC) increases significantly once cirrhosis develops (e.g. yearly incidence of HCC 1–4% in patients with cirrhosis due to hepatitis C). Evidence supports role for 3–6 monthly serum alphafetoprotein (AFP) and ultrasound.
- An additional liver insult may lead to decompensation in patients with cirrhosis. Patients with cirrhosis who are at any risk of hepatitis A or hepatitis B (e.g. frequent travellers to moderate risk areas; drug users; multiple sexual partners) should be tested for immunity, and vaccinated as appropriate.
- Complications of cirrhosis, including ascites, infection, and metabolic bone disease, are more common in malnourished patient. Give thiamine 100 mg od PO, encourage high calorie and protein intake, and refer for nutritional advice as necessary (see Approach to nutritional support). Note that patients with alcoholic liver disease may get high proportion of daily calorie intake from alcohol.
- Prescribing medication in patients with cirrhosis may be complex, as there is a risk of precipitating: bleeding (e.g. NSAIDs); worsening liver function (e.g. statins); hepatic encephalopathy (e.g. OPIATES); or renal impairment (e.g. NSAIDs, aminoglycosides). Also see drug-induced hepatotoxicity.
- Pregnancy may occur in patients who are cirrhotic, although 50% of premenopausal women with cirrhosis have secondary amenorrhea. Close liaison between patient, obstetrician, and hepatologist is essential. See Approach to liver problems in pregnancy.

Decompensated cirrhosis

- This may be indicated by development of jaundice, hepatic encephalopathy, or ascites. Jaundice and encephalopathy are much more commonly due to acutely deteriorating chronic liver disease than acute liver failure.
- Decompensation strongly predicts death, with 1 and 5 year survival in patients with Child–Pugh score C of 42% and 21%, compared with 84% and 44% for Child–Pugh score A disease.

Aetiology of hepatic decompensation

Progressive loss of hepatic function	Dehydration
Additional liver insult (e.g. alcohol, hepatitis A)	Constipation
Acute upper GI bleeding	Renal failure
Hepatocellular carcinoma	Drugs (e.g. opiates)
Infection (e.g. spontaneous bacterial peritonitis)	Non-compliance with treatment
Increased porto-systemic shunt (e.g. transjugular intrahepatic portosystemic shunt (TIPSS))	Vascular impairment (e.g. acute portal vein thrombosis)

Assessment

- Careful history to identify causes of decompensation is vital (see table). Ask about recent binge drinking (see alcohol dependency), any new drugs, infections (common cause, but symptoms and signs of sepsis may be masked in cirrhosis), weight loss or abdominal pain (e.g. hepatocellular carcinoma). Has there been any recent change in bowels (e.g. malaena, constipation) or history of haematemesis?
- As well as looking for signs of chronic liver disease (e.g. spider naevi, gynaecomastia–see Approach to GI examination), are there signs of decompensation (jaundice, liver flap, ascites)? Assess the grade of hepatic encephalopathy. Full general examination to elicit source of possible sepsis (including urine dipstick), and rectal examination to exclude malaena or constipation is necessary.

Investigations

- In all cases blood should be sent for U&Es, LFTs, glucose, FBC, clotting profile. See also Approach to recent-onset jaundice.
- Further investigations will depend on initial results and manifestation of decompensation, but must include a search for a precipitant:
  - Alphafetoprotein (AFP).
  - Abdominal U/S with Doppler of hepatic and portal veins.
  - Culture of blood, urine, sputum.
  - Diagnostic ascitic tap, for cell count and culture (see paracentesis).
  - CXR.

Management

- Directed towards the particular manifestation of hepatic decompensation (e.g. ascites), and treatment of the precipitants. See other sections:
  - Approach to recent-onset jaundice.
  - Approach to agitation and confusion in the GI patient.
  - Approach to ascites.
  - Acute upper GI bleeding (emergencies section)
  - Hepatic encephalopathy.
    - —Hepatocellular carcinoma.
    - —Hepatorenal syndrome.
    - —Paracentesis.
    - —Portal hypertension.
- In patients with acutely decompensated cirrhosis liver support devices, including Molecular Absorbence Recirculation Systems (MARS), may have a role, necessitating transfer to a regional liver unit offering this facility.
- In patients with decompensation due to hepatitis B, LAMIVUDINE therapy may improve liver function and clinical disease.
- In view of the poor long-term prognosis (e.g. 50% 2 year mortality following episode of ascites with spontaneous bacterial peritonitis), liver transplantation assessment should be considered once an episode of decompensation has occurred.

5 point checklist for assessing patient with chronic liver disease

1. Does the patient have cirrhosis, or non-cirrhotic chronic liver disease?
2. What's the aetiology?
3. In the patient with cirrhosis, is it well compensated or decompensated?
4. What interventions may prevent progression to cirrhosis, or to decompensation in the patient with established cirrhosis?
5. What investigations/interventions are needed to avoid/treat the complications of cirrhosis?

Consent for gastroenterological procedures

Never forget that while for the gastroenterologist invasive procedures may be a routine undertaking, for the patient an endoscopy may be a unique experience, engendering fear and anxiety.

- The process of obtaining consent is intended to provide patients with sufficient clear information about the proposed procedure, so that they can make the choice as to whether to proceed. Informed consent is not convincing and coercing the patient to accept an intervention.
- Face-to-face discussion, information leaflets, and the consent form itself should address the following areas.
  - The nature of the proposed procedure.
  - The reason the procedure is being suggested.
  - The benefits of the procedure.
  - The risks and complications of the procedure, including their relative incidence and severity.
  - The alternatives to the procedure, including those that may be more hazardous than the one proposed, and the risks of not having the procedure.
- Most health systems require that consent includes discussion of the substantive risks of the procedure that would influence a reasonable person when making a choice. Every possible <u>endoscopic complication</u> need not be discussed. The British Society of Gastroenterology has suggested that any minor complication with incidence of > 10%, or serious complication of > 0.5% should be discussed (and so specifically recorded in consent form).
- Most complication rates are derived from large multicentre studies, often involving specialist centres. It may be in coming years that consent forms will include the complication rate for the procedure specific to the individual endoscopist or institution, in order to allow truly informed consent.
- Consent should only be obtained by a doctor familiar with all aspects of the procedure (consent is unlikely to be fully informed if the person taking the consent is also not fully informed!).
- Obtaining consent as the patient sits on the endoscopy table prior to the procedure is unsatisfactory. The goal is for this process to occur at least 24 hours beforehand; ideally the process should start when the procedure is first discussed with the patient. There must be time for patients to digest information provided, and then to discuss further as necessary. For outpatients the consent form and appropriate information may be sent to the patient at home, allowing time to read

through and sign their consent. On the day of the procedure the endoscopist discusses any last-minute questions, and countersigns the consent form.

Patients incapable of consenting

- Policies differ between health systems. In the NHS in England and Wales, consent cannot be given or withheld on behalf of a mentally impaired patients (e.g. by next of kin). Nevertheless, it is good practice to discuss the procedure with relatives beforehand. A consent form specific to those unable to give consent is signed by a senior doctor looking after the patient and by the endoscopist involved with the procedure.
- In the case of an emergency no consent is necessary, and the endoscopist takes responsibility on the basis of 'necessity'.

Minors

- Parents/guardians provide consent on behalf of a child up to 16 years. However, a child who is under 16, but of sufficient intelligence to understand the issues involving consent/the procedure should be involved in the whole process (and may in fact give their own consent if the parents refuse).
- In the very unusual event of parental refusal to give consent for a child unable to provide it themselves, and in a situation in which refusal may have serious consequences for the child, legal recourse may be necessary. This should be done with the involvement of senior hospital management and legal department. Going to court to treat a child against a parent's wish is an extremely unpleasant undertaking, and may often be avoidable if parental fears (justified or not) are carefully addressed at an early stage.

Withholding/withdrawal of consent

- Withholding of consent is straightforward. **A patient who is fit to make an informed decision can refuse to consent to any procedure, even if this may lead to their death**. In this event, it is important to record the patient's refusal, and discussion of the implications of this refusal, in the patient's medical records.
- Withdrawal of consent during an endoscopic procedure may be less straightforward. Even with sedation a patient may struggle and find a procedure unpleasant (the amnesic effect of drug may nevertheless result in them having no recall afterwards). If the endoscopist is nearing completion of a procedure they may be inclined to continue for a couple more minutes, but ultimately a **clear demonstration by the patient that they wish the procedure to stop should result in its abandonment**.

Constipation

Definition

Defining constipation is hard. In practice, constipation is defined by reduced frequency of defecation—twice weekly or less. Many patients complaining of constipation have in reality excessive straining at defecation (with or without hard stools), a sensation of incomplete evacuation, or excessive time spent on the toilet, even though frequency may be in the normal range.

Clinical subtypes and related causes (see tables opposite)

Patients may have:

- **Normal transit**, but report hard stools or difficulty in evacuation.
- **Slow colonic transit**, and report a reduced frequency or even absence of the urge to defecate.
- **Incoordination of the rectum, anus, and pelvic floor** present with symptoms of straining, incomplete evacuation, and the need for anal or vaginal digitation in order to empty the rectum.

Evaluation

History

- **Onset**. Constipation from birth suggests congenital cause such as Hirschsprung's or meningocele.
- **Patient age and duration of symptoms**. Constipation may be of recent onset or chronic. A recent change, particularly in adults, needs workup for organic causes. Complaints of several years duration are more likely to be due to functional disorders.
- **Details of bowel habit**. Don't be squeamish. Ask about frequency of defecation, the form of the stool (words like small or hard are subjective; description of stringy or pellet-like stool is more helpful), excessive straining, discomfort, a sense of incomplete evacuation or of 'blockage'. Take note of any pain or bleeding.
- Associated **abdominal pain or bloating** suggest irritable bowel syndrome. Associated genitourinary symptoms may suggest an underlying central or peripheral neurological disorder.
- Evacuatory difficulty. Patients will often only admit this if asked directly about the need to digitate vaginally or rectally or of the need to apply perianal pressure.
- Ask about **laxative use and duration**, and about similar complaints in other family members.
- Ask for or at least make an assessment of potential **affective disorders**. Depression, emotional stress, and the use of mood-altering drugs including antidepressants can affect bowel function.
- Consider the possibility of **sexual abuse**. Somatic reactions to sexual abuse include abdominal pain, constipation, and appetite disturbance.

Clinical subtypes of constipation

Secondary to an organic colonic cause or outlet obstruction	Recent onset or the presence of alarm symptoms indicates need to exclude tumours or stenotic lesions of the colon by endoscopy or radiology
Outlet obstruction	Any painful anal condition (e.g. anal fissure, herpes) or anal cancer can cause difficulty in defecation
Irritable bowel syndrome	Consider when it coexists with bloating and pain in a young person
Constipation with gut dilatation	Causes include idiopathic megacolon or megarectum, Hirschsprung's disease, or chronic pseudo-obstruction
Severe constipation with a normal diameter colon	Chronic, often associated with slow colon transit, and most commonly occurs in young women of reproductive age
Drug-induced constipation	See separate table
Constipation secondary to coexisting systemic illness	See separate table
Psychological	Anorexia nervosa, affective disorder, dementia, childhood physical or sexual abuse, loss of a parent through death or separation, or disturbed toileting behaviour
Constipation due to immobility/age/diet	Elderly or bedridden patients in hospital as well as out may be unable to respond to toileting signals: this can lead to impaction, incontinence, and acute confusional states. Drugs can exacerbate symptoms in this group

Drugs causing constipation

Drug type	Examples
Analgesics	OPIATES
Anticholinergics	Antispasmodics, antidepressants (tricyclics), antipsychotics, antiparkinsonian drugs
Cation-containing agents	Iron, aluminium, calcium, barium, bismuth
Others	Antihypertensives, ganglion blockers, vinca alkaloids, anticonvulsants, calcium channel blockers

Examination

- Examine the abdomen for bowel distension, retained stool, or previous surgery.
- Anorectal and perineal examination is important: look for perineal disease or deformity, wasting of the gluteal muscles, and rectal prolapse. Test for perineal sensation. Digital examination may reveal the pain of an anal fissure, an anal stenosis, or a rectal mass or faecal impaction. Assess the anal tone (even though correlation of this with formal anorectal electrophysiological assessment is poor) and ask the patient to strain as if passing a motion, which can help in the diagnosis of prolapse, a rectocele, or abnormal perineal descent.
- Anismus (a paradoxical increase in anal tone when straining at stool instead of the normal relaxation response) may be seen in victims of rape, incest, or sexual abuse.
- Think of non-gastrointestinal diseases that may cause or exacerbate constipation.
- Do a neurological exam to look for central or peripheral causes; consider testing autonomic function. Check perineal sensation.

Diagnostic approach and investigations

Most chronically constipated patients do not need investigation beyond the history, examination, and exclusion of systemic or gastrointestinal causes.

Structural investigations

These are important to exclude organic disease when accompanied by alarm symptoms (recent onset, weight loss, PR blood, family history of colonic cancer) but are overused in patients with longstanding symptoms.
- **Colonoscopy** has relatively little use unless to exclude a colonic cancer.
- **Flexible sigmoidoscopy** can help in showing stenosing left-sided colonic lesions and also can diagnose laxative abuse via melanosis coli.
- **Radiology** is sometimes useful. A plain abdominal film may indicate stool retention and colonic dilatation in megarectum or megacolon and can help assess the efficacy of laxative treatment if there is clinical uncertainty. Barium studies may show colonic dilatation in Hirschsprung's disease but are not as useful as physiological studies.
- **Rectal biopsies** can be helpful in diagnosing Hirschsprung's disease but a full thickness biopsy is needed.

Functional evaluation (see flow chart)

For the patient with infrequent defecation, a prospective 2 week bowel diary and measurement of colon transit time by colon transit studies (see colonic inertia) is useful and can distinguish normal from slow transit constipation. Delayed colon transit can be due to colonic inertia or outlet obstruction. Colonic inertia produces chronic constipation and often responds poorly to medical treatment. If there is excessive straining, then transit studies are of little use, but studies of anorectal function may be very useful.

Anorectal manometry is useful in patients with suspected Hirschsprung's disease (absent anorectal inhibitory reflex) or in patients with evacuatory difficulty—inability to expel a balloon filled with 50 ml water suggests incoordinated defecation. Normal anorectal function with outlet obstruction suggests withholding behaviour and is common in children.

Defecography or a defecating proctogram may be useful if there is a suspected structural problem influencing defecation, e.g. a rectocele, prolapse, or intussusception, or to assess functional problems in evacuation.

Systemic diseases causing constipation

Type	Examples	Comment
Metabolic/endocrine	Diabetes	Usually mild but common
	Hypothyroidism Hypercalcaemia Hypokalaemia	
	Pregnancy	See Approach to gastrointestinal problems in pregnancy
	Porphyria Phaeochromocytoma Glucagonoma	
Central neurological disorders	Multiple sclerosis Parkinson's disease CVA	
Peripheral neurological disorders	Hirschsprung's Neurofibromatosis	
	Peripheral nerve damage	Transection of parasympathetic supply in the sacral nerves in the rectum or cauda equina (injury to lumbosacral spine, meningomyelocele, low spinal anaesthesia) produces colon dilatation reduced rectal tone and sensation. Constipation may occur with high spinal cord lesions, but the colon reflexes tend to be intact and defecation can be triggered by digitation of the anal canal
	Autonomic neuropathy Chronic intestinal pseudo-obstruction	
Collagen vascular	Scleroderma	
	Amyloidosis	
	Dermatomyositis	
Primary muscle disorders	Myotonic dystrophy	

Treatment considerations

General principles include consideration of dietary fibre supplementation, ensuring adequate toileting arrangements, and avoiding chronic use of stimulant laxatives if possible.

Diet and the role of fibre

Increasing dietary fibre leads to increased stool weight and stool frequency in normal people, and constipation may result from dietary fibre inadequacy in some patients. But there is no evidence that constipated people in general consume less fibre that non-constipated people, and dietary fibre is not usually effective in the management of constipated patients referred to hospital; furthermore it is often poorly tolerated due to bloating and flatulence. Nevertheless, conventional management is to increase dietary fibre to 20–30 g per day.

A top ten list of dietary sources of fibre is shown in the table. The bulking effect of fibre is only partly due to water-retaining capacity; colonic microbial ecology is also important. Fibre can be a substrate for colonic bacteria and increase stool bulk by bacterial proliferation and production of stool gases. This partly explains why fibre can provoke abdominal distension and flatulence in patients with slow transit constipation.

Fibre supplementation is not indicated in patients with <u>megacolon</u> or megarectum, patients confined to bed, or patients with neurological disease.

Drugs

Vast amount of laxatives are consumed, especially by the elderly. A working knowledge of these compounds is essential and the main classes are described in detail in Chapter 3 (see <u>LAXATIVES</u>; see also <u>laxative abuse</u>). For many, laxatives do not provide sustained relief of symptoms.

Drugs to increase colonic transit are an attractive idea but only partially effective: cholinergic agents or anti-cholinesterases have been tried in patients with colonic inertia. <u>PROKINETICS</u> include metaclopramide, which has been used in upper GI motility disorders but does not work in the colon. Currently most interest centres on serotonin (5-HT4) agonists and these are currently under evaluation e.g. tegaserod. Opiate antagonists, possibly given orally, have been suggested as being able to counteract excessive endogenous opioids and these too are under investigation.

Behavioural treatments

Behavioural therapy including <u>biofeedback therapy</u> (teaching the patient to normalize pelvic floor function while watching real time feedback about sphincter function) is an effective treatment for patients with slow transit constipation or impaired evacuation where traditional treatments have failed (about 2/3 of patients benefit). Behavioural treatments include exercises focused on the gut, psychological support, lifestyle/dietary factors and help in stopping laxatives and have been shown to improve symptoms, colonic transit, and psychological well-being and reduce the need for laxatives.

A behavioural approach involving bowel retraining is often tried in children with idiopathic constipation with or without soiling. Details can be found in larger texts (e.g. Yamada MD *et al.* (eds) (2003) *Textbook of Gastroenterology* p.920. Lippincott Williams and Wilkins.)

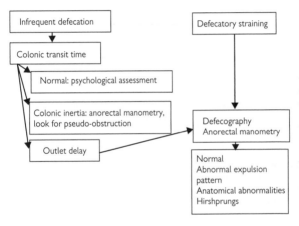

Fig. 1.4 Functional evaluation of chronic constipation.

Food sources of dietary fibre

Food source	Amount of fibre/100 g
Cereals	
All-Bran	26.7
Shredded Wheat	12.3
Cornflakes	11
Whole wheat bread	8.5
Peanuts	9.3
Peanut butter	7.5
Vegetables	
Baked beans	7.3
Peas	6.3
Fruits	
Pear	2.4
Banana	1.7
Apple	1.4

Surgery

Agreed indications

- Hirschsprung's disease.
- Rectocele. About 50% of patients get improvement after repair. Biofeedback is an option in this group.
- Rectal intussusception and prolapse. Surgery is not always curative: intussusception is common in non-constipated people, and its presence in constipated patients is not proof of causation.

Controversial indications

Colonic inertia. The commonest operation is subtotal colectomy with ileo-rectal anastomosis. Segmental resection based on removal of that part of the colon with the greatest hold-up of markers, has not proved effective and there is a high rate of anastomotic leakage. Long-term follow up data indicates a success rate of less than 50%. Antegrade (ACE) procedure, where a stoma is made in the caecum and water instilled distally, is another possibility in patients with slow transit constipation.

Dyspepsia and gastrooesophageal reflux

Definitions and common causes

Current definition of dyspepsia stems from Rome consensus meeting in 1999:
- 'Pain or discomfort in the upper abdomen for at least 12 weeks of the preceding 12 months'. Includes patients with symptoms of gastro-oesophageal, reflux, as well as heartburn, nausea, and vomiting.
- However many other conditions satisfy above definition—e.g. cardiac disease, <u>sphincter of Oddi dysfunction</u>, and pancreatic disease.
- Subdivisions of dyspepsia include 'ulcer-like' (epigastric pain), 'reflux-like' (heartburn and regurgitation), and 'dysmotility-like' (bloating and nausea).

Common causes are:
- Gastro-oesophageal reflux disease.
- <u>Peptic ulceration</u>.
- Non-ulcer dyspepsia.

Most causes of dyspepsia are recurrent and intermittent. Only curative treatments are *Helicobacter pylori* eradication and surgery (including treatment for <u>gallstones</u>).

Epidemiology

- Average prevalence in the community is 39% when patients with mainly reflux symptoms are included, and 23% when they are not.
- 5% of the population consult a GP because of dyspepsia.
- 1% of the population are referred for upper GI endoscopy per year.

When and how to investigate

Alarm symptoms prompting urgent investigation of dyspepsia

- Any sign of chronic gastrointestinal bleeding
- Progressive unintentional weight loss
- Dysphagia
- Persistent vomiting
- Iron-deficient anaemia
- Epigastric mass
- Suspicious barium meal

- Decide if the patient needs urgent referral for investigation (see box: alarm symptoms). If no alarm symptoms, then treat first; investigate later (if necessary).
- Review medications for possible causes of dyspepsia: calcium antagonists, nitrates, theophyllines, bisphosphonates (especially alendronate), steroids, NSAIDs.
- Consider cardiac, biliary, or pancreatic disease in the differential diagnosis.
- Consider simple lifestyle advice (see box).
- In those patients needing investigation, endoscopy is the preferred investigation because it is more sensitive than barium and allows biopsies. Double—contrast barium meal is an acceptable alternative in patients unwilling to undergo endoscopy (see endoscopic complications).

Lifestyle advice for dyspepsia: any use?

All reviews include a section on lifestyle advice but there is almost no evidence it makes any difference—except for **elevating the head of the bed** to decrease nocturnal reflux (not using extra pillows). Other conventional components include:
- Avoiding eating meals within 4 hours of going to bed
- Avoiding late night alcohol and caffeine, which relax the lower oesophageal sphincter
- Weight control, which can reduce symptoms resulting from hiatus hernia

Starting treatment

Initial therapeutic strategies for dyspepsia include:
- Empirical treatment with acid suppressants (patients will often have self-medicated with antacids or alginates).
- PROTON PUMP INHIBITORS are more effective than HISTAMINE RECEPTOR ANTAGONISTS, are safe, and are recommended as first-line treatment.

Testing and treating for _Helicobacter pylori_

Testing and treating for HP increases response rates compared with antacid therapy alone, and testing and treating reduces the need for endoscopy. At present test and treat appears more effective than acid suppression (the costs of these interventions are similar, because HP eradication prevents future development of peptic ulcers as well as ulcer recurrence). 2 weeks off PPIs is necessary before testing for HP using a breath test or a stool antigen test.

Managing gastro-oesophageal reflux disease (GORD)

This includes endoscopically determined <u>oesophagitis</u> and endoscopy-negative reflux disease (where usually a diagnostic course of acid suppression is needed to make the diagnosis). Oesophageal mucosal biopsy does not help in diagnosing reflux disease but does help in diagnosing infection, <u>Barrett's oesophagus</u>, and <u>oesophageal</u> tumours.

In patients who respond poorly or who have chest pain, 24 hour pH monitoring may be needed (see <u>Approach to non-cardiac chest pain</u>).

Treatment of GORD

Most patients are managed with drugs to lower or neutralize gastric acid (see: <u>ANTACIDS</u>, <u>PROTON PUMP INHIBITORS</u>, <u>HISTAMINE RECEPTOR ANTAGONISTS</u>).

- Medical therapy is effective at healing oesophagitis and improving reflux symptoms, but drugs do not restore the normal anti-reflux barrier at the gastro-oesophageal junction and stopping medication often leads to rebound acid hypersecretion, which can precipitate relapse.
- Surgery (see <u>anti-reflux procedures</u>) is often proposed as an alternative and definitive management. Substantial morbidity and frequent need for medical therapy after surgery means that currently surgery is not an ideal solution.
- A variety of endoscopic procedures aimed at improving the barrier function of the lower oesophagus have emerged: these are described elsewhere (see <u>anti-reflux procedures</u>).

Managing peptic ulcer disease

Although the discovery of <u>*H. pylori*</u> as the causative agent of 90% of duodenal ulcers and 75% of gastric ulcers has led to a declining incidence of hospitalization and surgery rates for uncomplicated peptic ulcer, there remains little change in the number of admissions for bleeding <u>peptic ulcer</u>. Overall mortality remains at approximately 6–8% for the last 30 years, partly due to increasing patient age and prevalence of concurrent illness.

Initial diagnosis and follow up

Endoscopy accurately diagnoses gastric and duodenal ulceration and allows biopsy for mitotic change. It also allows diagnosis of many upper GI infections including <u>*H. pylori*</u>.

- In patients with uncomplicated duodenal ulcers whose symptoms resolve on treatment, endoscopic follow up is not necessary.
- All patients with gastric ulcers need follow up endoscopy at 6–8 weeks to confirm ulcer healing. If healing has not occurred, further biopsies are needed, to exclude cancer.
- Failure of gastric ulcers to heal by 6 months is held by many to be an indication for gastric surgery.

Drug therapy with full dose <u>PPI</u> or <u>HISTAMINE RECEPTOR ANTAGONISTS</u> will lead to healing of peptic ulcers in the majority of cases.

Helicobacter and peptic ulceration

Eradicate *Helicobacter* in *HP* positive patients with peptic ulcer disease.

- HP eradication increases DU healing in HP positive patients, with healing of 74% after 4–8 weeks therapy. HP eradication reduces DU recurrence. Recurrent duodenal ulceration after successful eradication of HP is rare and usually the result of HP re-infection.
- Eradication does not increase gastric ulcer healing but reduces gastric ulcer recurrence. See *Helicobacter pylori*.
- Retesting after eradication is not suggested as routine, although this information may be valued by individual patients. In patients with persistent or recurrent symptoms, eradication should be confirmed by a carbon-13 urea breath test **more than 4 weeks after the end of treatment**. A positive breath test requires further courses of eradication treatment. Antibiotic sensitivity by biopsy and culture and patient compliance may need to be checked. **Use of serology after treatment is not helpful** as antibody titres may persist long term. If breath testing is not available, repeat endoscopy may be needed.
- In patients with complicated duodenal ulcer disease, HP eradication should be confirmed: some gastroenterolgists advocate repeat endoscopy to confirm ulcer healing and biopsies to confirm HP eradication.

Gastric ulceration

Most (over 70%) gastric ulcers are HP-associated. Biopsies must always be taken to exclude malignancy: there is some evidence that gastric brushings for cytology increase diagnostic yield.

NSAIDs and peptic ulceration

The risk of <u>peptic ulceration</u> leading to hospitalization associated with NSAID use is about 1 admission per 100 patient years of use in unselected patients. Patients with previous history of peptic ulcer are at higher risk. There is a fivefold increased risk of clinically significant GI bleeding in patients on NSAIDs for musculoskeletal pain and twofold increased risk for patients taking low dose aspirin for secondary prevention of cardiovascular disease. (Also see <u>non-steroidal anti-inflammatory drugs (NSAIDS) and the GI tract</u>.)

- For patients taking NSAIDs with a diagnosed peptic ulcer, stop NSAIDs where possible. Treat with full dose PPI or H2RA and eradicate HP if present.
- In patients using NSAIDs who have a peptic ulcer, eradicating HP does not increase ulcer healing compared with acid suppression therapy. However, eradicating HP reduces the risk of ulcer recurrence
- In patients using NSAIDs who have never had a peptic ulcer, eradicating HP reduces the first incidence of peptic ulceration
- In patients with previous ulcers and in those at high risk, offer gastric protection with PPI/histamine receptor antagonist (a COX-2 selective NSAID may be less ulcerogenic; most clinicians would still combine them with a gastroprotective agent (see <u>COX-2 selective NSAIDs</u>).

- High dose H2RAs or a PPI reduce the incidence of endoscopically detected lesions in patients taking NSAIDs.
- In those on NSAIDs without peptic ulcers, taking a COX-2 selective NSAID is associated with a lower incidence of endoscopically detected lesions. The promotion of healing and prevention of recurrence in those with existing peptic ulcers is not clear.

Non-HP, non-NSAID associated peptic ulcers

Consider the following causes.
- Failure to detect HP due to PPI or recent antibiotic ingestion.
- Surreptitious or inadvertent aspirin or NSAID use.
- Ulcers related to other drugs: potassium chloride, bisphosphonates, immunosuppressive drugs, and more recently SSRIs have all been implicated in GI bleeding.
- Acid hypersecreting states such as Zollinger–Ellison syndrome (especially if associated with diarrhoea, multiple ulcers, weight loss, hypercalcaemia).
- Crohn's disease.
- TB.
- Malignancy.
- CMV in immunocompromised.

Managing non-ulcer dyspepsia

This includes patients in whom endoscopy has excluded peptic ulceration (including erosive duodenitis and gastric erosions, considered part of the spectrum of peptic ulcer disease), malignancy, or oesophagitis. Patients with dominant heartburn or reflux and no oesophagitis on endoscopy are classified as 'endoscopy negative reflux disease'.

There is uncertainty about the cause or best long-term management of this group of patients. Current recommendations include the following.

Eradicate *H. pylori* if present

In a pooled study of 12 RCTs (2900 patients) comparing HP eradication compared with placebo in reducing dyspeptic symptoms in NUD, the response in the control group averaged 36% and eradication increased this by 7%, with a number needed to treat for one patient to benefit of 14.

If symptoms continue or recur, PPI or H2RA may be taken on an 'on demand' basis at the lowest dose needed to control symptoms.

Prokinetic drugs

These have been advocated particularly for the dysmotility-predominant group of patients. Although a meta-analysis of 14 trials involving over 1000 patients shows a beneficial effect of prokinetics compared with placebo at reducing dyspepsia in short-term (2 to 8 week) courses, caution has been expressed over the validity of this result because of heterogeneity of patient inclusion (many trials not excluding patients with reflux) and the inclusion in many studies of the drug cisapride, which has been withdrawn from the UK market. Further studies are needed of the effectiveness of DOPAMINE RECEPTOR ANTAGONISTS (e.g. METACLOPRAMIDE and DOMPERIDONE).

The role of *Helicobacter* testing and eradication in managing dyspepsia

Initial testing for HP can include serology, faecal antigen testing, carbon-13 urea breath testing, or endoscopic biopsy. Retesting should always use a carbon-13 urea breath test.

HP eradication is appropriate for peptic ulcer disease, non-ulcer dyspepsia, and as part of a HP test and treat strategy in uninvestigated dyspepsia. A number of eradication therapies are effective (see *Helicobacter pylori*).

Guidelines for management

Guidelines from the UK National Institute for Clinical Excellence (NICE) published in 2004 focus on primary care and are mainly concerned with managing symptoms.

Even in patients referred for endoscopy, where the prevalence of significant disease is presumed to be greater than in unselected patients in primary care, correlation between symptoms and endoscopic diagnosis is poor. Management in those referred to hospital is based around diagnosis.

The 2004 NICE guidelines emphasize two key points:
1. Urgent specialist referral or endoscopy is indicated in patients with dyspepsia of any age when presenting with 'alarm symptoms'.
2. Patients > 55 years with dyspepsia and no alarm symptoms **do not** require routine referral for endoscopy (represents a change from previous guidelines). However, endoscopy may be considered if symptoms persist despite HP eradication, a course of proton pump inhibitor therapy, or where there is risk of gastric cancer or anxiety about cancer is heightened (e.g. previous gastric ulcer/gastric surgery, pernicious anaemia, or in those using NSAIDs, as well as patients with jaundice or an upper abdominal mass).

Why no threshold age for endoscopy in the NICE guidelines?

Previous recommendations for endoscopy recognized that cancer is very rarely found in patients under 55 without alarm symptoms (Gillen, D and McCall, KEL (1999). *Am. J. Gastroenterol.* **94**: 75). Recent data suggest that an age threshold alone in the absence of alarm symptoms is of little use in predicting cancer (NICE guidelines, p. 80).

Faecal incontinence

- A common problem (up to 2% people are faecally incontinent once a week: Kamm, MA (1998), *Br. Med. J.* **316**: 528) but often difficult for patients to discuss with doctors or close relatives.
- Direct questioning of the patient is often necessary, as is an understanding of continence mechanisms (see box).
- Continence depends on the sphincter muscles (see box), stool consistency, and cognitive factors.

Continence mechanisms

- Spongy vascular tissues within the anal canal play a minor role in continence by assisting with anal closure. Minor degrees of seepage may be seen after partial excision of this tissue at haemorrhoidectomy.
- The major mechanisms of continence depend on the anal sphincters. The internal sphincter is the continuation of the circular muscle layer and is under autonomic control. It contributes 70% of resting anal tone. The external sphincter is striated, supplied by sacral nerves S2–4. Tonic neural activation contributes 30% of resting tone, but voluntary squeeze of the external sphincter at times of distension can double normal resting tone.

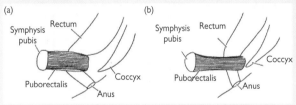

(a) Symphysis pubis   Rectum   Puborectalis   Coccyx   Anus

(b) Symphysis pubis   Rectum   Puborectalis   Coccyx   Anus

Fig. 1.5 Reproduced from Feldman M, Friedman LS, and Sleisenger MH (2003). *Sleisenger and Fordtran's Gastrointestinal and Liver Disease, p165*, with permission from Elsevier

- The puborectalis muscle wraps around the anorectal junction, forming a sharp angle between the rectum and anal canal (a). Relaxation of puborectalis allows straightening of the recto-anal angle for defecation (b).
- The anal canal is very sensitive to touch, pain, and temperature and this allows for discrimination of solid, liquid, and gas contents, which can allow selective passage of these materials.
- Rectal sensation and compliance is important in maintaining continence. Neuropathies can impair sensation and compliance may be reduced by radiation, colitis, or ischaemia.

Clinical evaluation

History Ask about passive incontinence and urge incontinence. Ask also about duration and severity (solid, liquid, or gas? a slight stain on underpants or the whole stool?). Ask about coincident urinary incontinence.

Ask about potential causes: obstetric history (maximum birth weight, instrumentation, tears/episiotomies, presentation of baby, e.g. occipito-posterior); previous anal surgery; other systemic/neurological diseases.

Examination Routine examination including perianal examination, rectal exam (look for faecal impaction), and sigmoidoscopy (rectal inflammation, mucus-secreting polyp such as villous adenoma) is essential. It's important to assess anal tone and squeeze pressure but digital examination correlates poorly with operative and histological findings.

Investigations include anorectal physiology and endoanal ultrasound. See the table for causes of incontinence.

Causes of faecal incontinence

Internal anal sphincter degeneration	Most common cause—elderly
Obstetric trauma	One-third of primiparous women have some damage to the anal sphincter after their first delivery. Forceps delivery, a large baby, and occipito-posterior position are further risk factors
Surgical damage	Surgically induced sphincter damage can occur after lateral sphincterotomy or major colonic resection
Anal dilatation	Incontinence may complicate manual dilatation of the anus (which used to be performed for anal fissures) or anal fistulae passing through the sphincter muscles. Receptive anal intercourse is also a risk factor
Rectal prolapse	Incontinence in 30–80%. EUS can help in the diagnosis
Congenital	Half of all patients with spina bifida soil regularly. One-third of children operated on for Hirschsprung's are incontinent at age 4. Soiling may complicate surgery for sacral tumours
Spinal injury	Soiling occurs in 30% patients with multiple sclerosis
Radiation injury (see radiation damage to the GI tract)	Radiation to the anorectum combined with proctitis and reduction in compliance can produce incontinence
Systemic disease	Diabetics can have somatic and autonomic neuropathy. In scleroderma, internal sphincter muscle atrophy, acquired megacolon, and bacterial overgrowth can all occur

Treatment

Conservative

Conservative treatments include <u>ANTI-DIARRHOEAL AGENTS</u>, e.g. loperamide tablets or syrup titrated to achieve beneficial effect, mechanical barriers, or behavioural treatments including <u>biofeedback</u>, which is effective even in patients with structural sphincter damage.

Surgical

As a minimally invasive surgical approach, sacral nerve stimulators may help and have the benefit that a temporary wire can initially be tried to assess for efficacy. Surgery should be reserved for patients with major faecal incontinence in whom conservative methods have failed. The external sphincter can sometimes be repaired after obstetric disruption with an overlap repair. The internal sphincter is not amenable to surgical repair. Repair of a prolapse may be possible by rectopexy. Other surgical treatments undergoing evaluation include dynamic gracialoplasty and the artificial bowel sphincter. Colostomy remains an alternative that can return the patient to a near normal lifestyle.

Gastrointestinal examination

Overview

- Clinical examination remains important even as non-invasive imaging becomes ever more revealing.
  - It allows the differential diagnosis to be honed down.
  - It allows focused investigations to be arranged.
  - This leads to more speedy and cost-effective diagnosis/management.
- The GI examination is in essence an expansion of the general examination (see *OHCM* p.52), as disease in most systems may cause symptoms and signs in the GI tract (e.g. right heart failure leading to hepatomegaly and ascites).
- A full examination is rarely possible in a busy outpatients' clinic, and the examination may be directed to a particular anatomical area or disease spectrum (e.g. GI and extraintestinal signs of inflammatory bowel disease).
- Clinical experience and the likely problem based on the patient's history may allow the examination to be tailored, but a systematic approach should be used for all patients.

Initial inspection

First impressions count! Be sure to explain that you wish to examine the patient, and try to put them at their ease (it is particularly difficult to elicit abdominal signs in the tense patient). Does the patient look well or sick? Is the patient thin and malnourished (prominent cheek bones, obviously loosely fitting clothes—see Approaches to unintentional weight loss and obesity. On studying the skin, note should be made of colour change (jaundice, pigmented in haemochromatosis), excoriations (? biliary obstruction), and rashes (erythema nodosum, pyoderma gangrenosum).

Hands

Start with the hands, as this may be the first point of physical contact with a handshake, and patients find this less intrusive than heading straight for the abdomen. Look for the following.

- **Temperature**: cold hands in the patient with a GI bleed usually suggests peripheral vasoconstriction due to a significant bleed.
- **Leuconychia**: white patches in the nails: may be a marker of low albumin or cirrhosis.

- **Koilonychia:** spoon-shaped nail sometimes seen in iron-deficiency anaemic
- **Clubbing:** loss of angle between nail and adjacent nail bed, often with lateral and longitudinal curvature of the nails. Associated with wide range of diseases, including chronic liver disease and inflammatory bowel disease.
- **Dupuytren's contracture:** flexure deformity of fingers (usually 4th or 5th) due to palmar fascial thickening. Reported association with alcoholic liver disease.
- **Arthropathy.**
- **Palmar erythema:** redness of thenar and hypothenar eminences linked to chronic liver disease, thyrotoxicosis, pregnancy.
- **Liver flap:** this is *not* a resting tremor (which may be present in the patient with alcohol withdrawal) but a transient reduction in muscle tone. Ask the patient to 'stop the traffic' (arms extended at elbows, wrists and fingers extended): look for a coarse jerky flap at wrist and fingers. Indicates hepatic encephalopathy.
- **Radial pulse.** Hyperdynamic, bounding pulse found in cirrhosis; weak pulse with tachycardia in GI bleeding.
- **Blood pressure:** lying and standing/sitting BP essential in patients with GI bleeding to assess for a postural drop. See comments in Acute upper gastrointestinal bleeding

Face

- Look for anaemia by examining the lachrymal surface of the lower eye lid, and at sclerae for jaundice at the same time. Absence of malar fat pads suggests malnutrition/cancer cachexia; 'moon face' is associated with prolonged high dose steroids, Cushing's syndrome, or pseudo-Cushings related to alcohol dependency and parotid enlargement. Yellowish deposits around eyes (xanthelasma) suggests primary biliary cirrhosis. Episcleritis in IBD. Kayser–Fleischer rings.
- Examination of the mouth may show oral ulceration (inflammatory bowel disease, coeliac disease), angular stomatitis (rarely seen in association with iron or vitamin deficiency). Brown macules on the lips suggests Peutz–Jeghers syndrome, which should not be confused with the multiple telangiectasia on lips and tongue seen with hereditary haemorrhagic telangiectasia (Osler–Weber–Rendu syndrome). See plate section. Poor dentition and gum hypertrophy may be linked with malnutrition/alcohol excess.
- With the patient at 45 degrees, examine for raised jugular venous pressure.
- Sit the patient forward, and from behind palpate for cervical and supraclavicular nodes (?Virchow's node in gastric cancer). With patient sitting forward, check for scars due to nephrectomy (classic exam 'catch out'!)
- Examine the chest, looking for spider naevi (central arteriole feeding multiple draining capillaries), and in the male loss of axillary hair and palpable breast tissue (gynaecomastia), suggestive of chronic liver disease.

Abdomen

The patient should be lying flat, with abdomen fully exposed, and arms by sides.

- **Inspect** for:
  - Scars of previous surgery.
  - Distension (ascites/ileus/mass/pregnancy), abdominal striae (common after pregnancy, but also seen due to rapid increases in abdominal girth due to obesity or ascites).
  - Bruising around flanks (Grey Turner's sign) may relate to retroperitoneal bleeding, and periumbilical bruising ('Cullen's sign') from intraperitoneal bleeding, both associated with severe <u>acute pancreatitis</u>.
  - Dilated superficial abdominal veins running longitudinally should be checked for direction of flow (put forefingers of both hands together on vein, then separate along vein by 6 cm, keeping vein compressed. On removing most inferior finger, vein will rapidly refill if there is underlying portal hypertension or inferior vena cava obstruction). Very rarely superficial veins radiate out from umbilicus, due to <u>portal hypertension</u> and portosystemic shunting in presence of patent umbilical vein ('caput medusa').
- Before **palpating** the abdomen, ask about areas of tenderness. Starting in right iliac fossa, initially palpate lightly in all 4 quadrants.
- Examine for **hepatomegaly**. Palpate gradually towards right subcostal margin, in 3 cm steps, from right iliac fossa, with the patient taking slow deep breaths. An enlarged liver is usually felt at least 2 cm below the right costal margin (see table), although a prominent Reidel's lobe may lead to this being falsely diagnosed. Although hepatomegaly may be a feature of all forms of chronic liver disease, advanced cirrhosis classically does not cause a big liver, due to extensive fibrosis and liver volume loss. (Note the texture of the lower border of the liver: irregular and firm may suggest <u>cirrhosis</u> or <u>hepatocellular carcinoma</u>; smooth and tender may point towards acute <u>hepatitis</u>.) It is logical to percuss immediately after palpation for hepatomegaly, not after all other areas have been palpated. A depressed diaphragm, for example in emphysema, may push down the liver, giving the impression of hepatomegaly: always percuss the upper border of the liver (a 12 cm span in the mid-clavicular line is the upper limit of normal).
- To elicit **splenomegaly**, deep palpation again begins in the right iliac fossa, advancing towards the left subcostal margin in stepwise movements. The spleen is usually double its normal size before it is palpable.

Features that differentiate spleen from left kidney:

- Cannot 'get above it'.
- It moves with respiration.
- A splenic 'notch' may be palpable.
- It is not ballotable like the kidneys.
- Dullness to percussion over the splenic bed (9th intercostals space, mid-axillary line) may sometimes be found in patients with splenomegaly (see table opposite).

- To examine for enlarged **kidneys**, one hand is placed firmly in the left or right hypochondrium, and the other in the corresponding flank. The hand under the patient is pressed firmly upwards, towards the other hand, and if the kidney is large it may be 'ballotable'.
- To look for **ascites**, initially percuss in the left flank. If this is clearly resonant there is no need to examine further for ascites. If dull, percuss back towards the midline, where it should become resonant. Ask the patient to roll over towards you, into right lateral position, wait 30 seconds, and then percuss back towards left flank from midline, looking for 'shifting dullness'. Whilst the patient is in this position, palpation again under the left costal margin may allow splenomegaly to be elicited (this is much more effective than trying to 'lift up' the spleen with the left hand placed under posterior ribs, which is sometimes advocated).
- **Deep palpation** of the abdomen separately from examining liver, spleen, and kidneys is important, including in the iliac fossae, epigastrium, and periumbilical areas. The sigmoid colon is easy to feel in slim people.
- The hernial orifices should be examined, and a rectal examination may be necessary (see box). In a young man with central abdominal pain, examine the testes so as not to miss a torted testicle.
- **Auscultation** is essential in the patient with acute constipation or abdominal pain, to look for signs of obstruction ('tinkling' bowel sounds) or ileus (absent bowel sounds), and very occasionally in the clinic auscultation results in renal artery bruits, or a hepatic bruit related to hepatocellular carcinoma, being identified.

Causes of hepatomegaly

All causes of **chronic liver disease/cirrhosis** (see Approaches to cirrhosis and chronic liver disease)	**Acute inflammation:** viral hepatitis, alcoholic hepatitis, drug-induced hepatotoxicity (e.g. paracetamol overdose)
Venous congestion: congestive cardiac failure, tricuspid regurgitation, constrictive pericarditis, Budd–Chiari syndrome	**Mass lesions:** polycystic disease, simple cyst, adenoma, hepatocellular carcinoma, metastases, amoebiasis and pyogenic/liver abscess, haemangioma, hydatid disease
Storage diseases: Gaucher's disease, histiocytosis X, amyloidosis	**Fatty liver:** alcoholic liver disease and non-alcoholic fatty liver disease (NAFLD)
Blood disorders: sickle cell anaemia (sequestration), thallassaemia major (extramedullary haemopoiesis), myelo-pro-liferative disorders, malaria.	Granulomatous hepatitis (see hepatic granulomas)

Causes of splenomegaly

Portal hypertension*	Myeloproliferative disorders: myelofibrosis*, chronic myeloid leukaemia*
Leukaemias*, lymphomas*	Haemoglobinopathies: sickle cell anaemia* (in children, prior to autoinfarction), thallassaemia major*
Tropical splenomegaly syndrome	Storage diseases: Gaucher's disease*, amyloidosis*
Infection: Epstein–Barr virus (EBV) *, malaria, leishmaniasis, schistosomiasis*	

* May cause hepatosplenomegaly

Rectal examination

'If you don't put your finger in it, you put your foot in it'
(Old English medical saying, unattributed)

Traditionalists may argue that the PR is as central to a proper general examination as measuring BP. But just as tumour markers are a poor screening test in the absence of clinical indication, the yield from 'speculative' PR is very low, and is found unpleasant by many patients. Nevertheless, it should not be avoided because of embarrassment (on behalf of doctor or patient), or where there is a possibility of pathology being found (e.g. unexplained weight loss, anaemia). It may require a chaperone (see Approach to consent for gastroenterological procedures) and needs to be performed correctly:

- Patient lying on left side ('left lateral').
- Press posteriorly on the anal skin with the pulp of the gloved lubricated second finger of the right hand. This allows relaxation of anal tone and easy passage of the finger.
- Do not simply stick in the finger at right angles to the anus: this causes reflex contraction of the anus and surprise if not pain to the patient.
- Also look for perianal pathology—skin tags (associated with Crohn's disease), fistulae, abscesses.

Gastrointestinal problems in pregnancy

Gastrointestinal symptoms are common in pregnancy and they can be difficult to investigate and treat. They result from:
• Changes in gut motility and tone.
• Effects of the gravid uterus.
Abnormal liver function in pregnancy is discussed separately (see Approach to liver problems in pregnancy).

Nausea and vomiting

Nausea occurs in 50–90% of pregnant women during pregnancy (often during weeks 6–8), and 25–55% experience vomiting. It is often termed 'morning sickness', although many mothers dream that it would last only until midday! **Risk factors** include young maternal age, smoking, 1st pregnancy, and multiparity. In most cases it is self-limiting, with no need for specific investigation, but careful assessment is necessary to exclude other causes (e.g. UTI).

Mild symptoms may respond to reassurance and dietary change (small, regular meals). Anti-emetics, including DOPAMINE ANTAGONISTS (e.g. metoclopramide) and ANTIHISTAMINES (e.g. cyclizine) may be used in severe cases. Alternative therapies, such as pyridoxine and ginger, have been shown to be beneficial.

Hyperemesis gravidarum

This is characterized by intractable vomiting, and occurs in 0.1% of pregnancies, with onset usually in weeks 6–8. Dehydration, hypovolaemia, and metabolic disturbance (ketosis, metabolic alkalosis, $\downarrow Na^+$, $\downarrow K^+$) may result, and it is occasionally life-threatening.

Management includes:
• Admission to hospital. This, and addressing possible psychosocial problems, may improve symptoms.
• Take blood for FBC, clotting, U&E, LFTs, Glu, Ca^{2+}, Mg^{2+}, bicarbonate.
• IV rehydration with 0.9% N saline ± K+ supplements. Avoid rapid correction of $\downarrow Na^+$, which may result in central pontine myelinolysis.
• Give thiamine 150 mg PO od, or 100 mg IV weekly) to prevent Wernicke's encephalopathy.
• Anti-emetics are usually used, including metoclopramide 10 mg PO/IV/IM tds or cyclizine 50 mg IV tds.
• If vomiting continues, total parenteral nutrition may sometimes be needed. See Approach to nutritional support.

- Acid suppression can help.
- Steroids have been shown to be beneficial in uncontrolled trials. If commenced they should probably be slowly reduced, but not stopped, until after delivery.

Despite its symptomatic severity, the outcome of pregnancy complicated by hyperemesis gravidarum is no different from that of the general population.

Heartburn and reflux symptoms

Symptoms of gastro-oesophageal reflux disease (GORD) occur in more than 50% of pregnant women, probably due to the combined effects of reduced gastric emptying, relaxation of lower oesophageal sphincter, and, in 3rd trimester, increased abdominal pressure due to the gravid uterus.

- Endoscopy and investigation for disorders of oesophageal motility are almost never necessary.
- Antacids may be liberally used (as they are not systemically absorbed), with lifestyle advice to eat small regular meals, and to elevate the head of the bed being of some use.
- H2 ANTAGONISTS are the next line of treatment (ranitidine 150 mg PO bd), and have been shown to be effective in randomized trials.
- Whilst PROTON PUMP INHIBITORS appear safe in pregnancy, experience of their use is less than that of H2 ANTAGONISTS. They are not licensed for this indication, and so should not be used as first- or second-line treatment of GORD in pregnancy. Also see Approach to dyspepsia and gastro-oesophageal reflux.

Abdominal pain

- Acute abdominal pain in pregnancy may represent a particular diagnostic and management challenge, due to several factors:
  - Clinical confusion with pregnancy associated symptoms due to episodic uterine contraction ('Brackston–Hicks'), true labour, or pressure effects from the gravid uterus.
  - Atypical presentation of GI disease in pregnancy.
  - Reluctance to use invasive investigation (e.g. endoscopy) or X-rays (e.g. CT scanning) in pregnancy.
- Gallbladder sludge can be shown in 30% of pregnancies, and asymptomatic GALLSTONES in up to 11%. CHOLECYSTITIS develops in 0.1%, and biliary obstruction and gallstone PANCREATITIS may occur. CHOLECYSTECTOMY may occasionally be necessary, and is the second most common non-obstetric indication for surgery during pregnancy (behind appendectomy—see appendix and appendicitis). Surgery is probably safest in the 2nd trimester.
- Endoscopic retrograde cholangiopancreatography (ERCP) may be necessary for biliary obstruction. It should only be performed if absolutely necessary, but appears safe in pregnancy. In view of risks of radiation exposure, screening time should be kept to a minimum, lead protection for the fetus is essential, and the procedure should ideally be avoided in the 1st trimester.

- Symptoms of ectopic pregnancy, including rupture, usually develop in weeks 5–8, with localized pain, peritonitis, and shock secondary to haemorrhage. It may represent a surgical emergency.
- <u>Peptic ulceration</u> may present in pregnancy, but appears to be less common than in the non-pregnant population.

Constipation

Affects more than 30% of pregnant women, probably due to combination of reduced motility and water reabsorption. Increasing fibre and fluid usually helps, but osmotic laxatives (e.g. movicol) and bulking agents often effective. Castor oil should not be used.

Diarrhoea

No increased incidence of infectious diarrhoea, compared to non-pregnant population, but consequences may be more serious. It is vital to send stool cultures in any pregnant women with new-onset diarrhoea, as *Salmonella* and *Campylobacter* infections have been associated with both fetal and maternal mortality, and may indicate a role for early antibiotics (see <u>Approach to acute diarrhoea</u>). *Listeria monocytogenes* infection may arise from eating unpasteurized dairy products (e.g. soft cheese), and is an important cause of fetal death. As well as diarrhoea it may present with early labour and flu-like symptoms. After sending blood and stool samples, empirical antibiotic treatment should be given (e.g. amoxycillin 500 mg PO qds).

Inflammatory bowel disease

Patients with symptoms suggestive of undiagnosed inflammatory bowel disease (IBD) (see <u>ulcerative colitis</u>, <u>Crohn's disease</u>) during pregnancy (e.g. chronic bloody diarrhoea) require appropriate investigation (including colonoscopy, which may be performed if essential) as active IBD is linked to fetal loss. The great majority of patients with well-controlled disease have a normal pregnancy. In patients with known IBD, steroids and 5-ASA preparations are safe. Although azathioprine should not be started in pregnancy, there is no strong evidence for its risks during pregnancy, and most clinicians advise continuation after discussion with the patient. The risk of pregnancy complications is certainly higher in those patients who reactivate IBD after precipitous cessation of immunosuppression. Methotrexate is contraindicated in pregnancy.

Rectal bleeding

The most common cause in pregnancy is <u>haemorrhoids</u>, which may develop due to increased abdominal pressure related to the gravid uterus and be exacerbated by constipation. Bleeding may also occur due to anal fissure or inflammatory bowel disease.

Imaging the GI tract

GI imaging modalities

In the era of advanced endoscopy it is important to remember that many other imaging modalities retain a vital role in diagnosis and therapy of common GI diseases.

Note: endoscopic techniques are described elsewhere (see colonoscopy, endoscopic retrograde cholangiopancreatography (ERCP), endoscopic complications, endoscopic ultrasound, enteroclysis, enteroscopy)

- **Plain and contrast radiology.** Plain films are simple to obtain, and the ability to show air/tissue boundaries can be very helpful in evaluating patients with abdominal pain, distension, or clinical sign of an acute abdomen. But CT is much more sensitive for diagnosing patients with acute abdominal symptoms. See barium studies.
- **Ultrasound (U/S).** Transabdominal and endoscopic probes can both give very valuable information (see endoscopic ultrasound (EUS)). The great and unique strength of ultrasound lies in its ability to image flow and soft tissues in real time without the use of ionizing radiation.
- **Computed tomography (CT) scanning.** CT relies on radiographic attenuation to provide image contrast: the vascularity of structures can be inferred by the changes imparted by IV contrast agents.
- **Magnetic resonance imaging (MRI)** has certain advantages over CT. MRI has several parameters that can distinguish abnormal tissue (T1, T2, lipid content, magnetic susceptibility imparted by metal ions such as iron in the liver) and characteristics of flowing blood. MRI avoids the use of ionizing radiation, and the only patients at risk are those with certain types of implanted devices such as cochlear implants, cerebral aneurysm clips, or cardiac pacemakers. The risks of anaphylaxis to available contrast agents (gadolinium) is low. See MRI in A–Z section.
- **Radionuclide imaging** depends on administration of a radiolabelled compound that localizes to a specific organ system or the location of an ongoing physiological process. Common applications include the detection of heterotopic gastric mucosa associated with Meckel's diverticula using Tc^{99} (see Meckel's diverticulum); the detection of a site of bleeding from the GI tract by labelled red blood cells; the labelling of test meals to study the rate of gastric emptying; and white cell scanning to investigate inflammatory processes involving the bowel.
- **Positron emission tomography (PET) scanning** is an imaging modality that reflects physiological function rather than anatomical structure. A wide variety of substrates can be labelled by positron emitting isotopes allowing assessment of perfusion and, substrate metabolism and the study of chemical recognition systems such as enzymes and hormone receptors. Currently PET scanning is of proven utility particularly when combined with CT scanning in assessing colorectal cancer spread.

- **Angiography**. Diagnostic angiography has a role in the diagnosis of mesenteric vascular disease and localizing GI bleeding as well as helping to assess certain tumours such as hepatocellular carcinoma. Traditional techniques of visceral angiography using selective cannulation have an important role particularly where transcatheter embolization of bleeding vessels can be life-saving; tumour embolization and arterial administration of chemotherapy to selective vascular beds are frequently used. Angiographic information can also be obtained by triple phase CT scanning and MR angiography.
- **Laparoscopy and laparotomy**. Diagnostic laparotomy can improve diagnostic accuracy and is occasionally useful in making diagnoses beyond the resolution of non-invasive imaging techniques (e.g. detecting peritoneal seeding of tumour or tuberculosis). Laparoscopy allows directed biopsy of lesions and produces less postoperative pain and intestinal ileus than laparotomy. Disadvantages include the need for the patient to be fit for anaesthetic, and the difficulty of the technique in the face of multiple abdominal adhesions.

Choosing the right test and some common clinical scenarios

With a wide array of possible tests, the clinical question is which to choose, and when. Decision may be influenced by range of factors, including local provision/access to test; comparative risks/invasiveness of techniques; sensitivity/specificity of test for particular conditions; and local expertise and performing/interpreting test.

Investigating dysphagia

The traditional view that barium swallow should always precede endoscopy in patients with dysphagia is now challenged by many. Careful intubation and endoscope advancement, and prior awareness of possibility of oesophageal stricture, makes perforation at diagnostic endoscopy very unusual (see endoscopic complications). Endoscopy also allows biopsy for histology and endoscopic dilatation, as necessary. See also oesophageal obstruction.

Suspected bile duct stones (BDS)/biliary obstruction

See also choledocholithiasis. Transabdominal U/S has high yield for identifying gallstones and biliary dilatation, but less good for BDS. Magnetic resonance cholangiopancreatography (MRCP) is accurate, non-invasive, and virtually risk free (see MRI), and is indicated when suspicion of BDS is low–moderate (e.g. abnormal LFTs, no jaundice, no biliary dilatation on U/S, but does not allow intervention. MRCP very useful in defining site and complexity of obstruction in biliary obstruction due to cholangiocarcinoma. EUS is not widely available in UK, but in expert hands is comparable with MRCP at identifying BDS. ERCP is invasive and carries risks, but is indicated where probability of BDS ± biliary obstruction is high (e.g. jaundice, dilated bile duct on U/S), and may be performed in conjunction with EUS. ERCP also allows endoscopic stenting to relieve jaundice, brush cytology, endoluminal biopsy.

Pancreatic disease

Different imaging modalities provide complementary information. Pancreatic <u>CT</u> provides excellent detail on pancreatic anatomy and local vascula-
ture. <u>ERCP</u> remains 'gold standard' for pancreatic duct abnormalities, and
allows advanced diagnostics (see <u>sphincter of Oddi dysfunction</u>) and intervention. MRCP may provide comparable information, with information
gained following secretin injection on pancreatic juice output and obstruction to flow. Criteria for <u>chronic pancreatitis</u> on EUS have been defined,
and EUS has important role in investigation of <u>pancreatic cystic tumours</u>.
Transabdominal U/S is widely used, but may give poor views of pancreas.

Suspected terminal ileal disease (e.g. Crohn's disease)

- Traditional contrast techniques of small bowel follow-through (barium
  taken by mouth) and small bowel enema/barium enteroclysis (barium
  enters small bowel from naso-enteral tube sited in stomach/
  duodenum—more invasive but may allow better small bowel
  definition) are still widely used to investigate distal small bowel.
  Disadvantages include duration of test, high X-ray exposure, and
  identification of intraluminal change only after extensive damage
  (although separation of loops may indicate wall thickening).
- U/S increasingly used, providing accurate information on extent of
  terminal ileal disease, with high diagnostic sensitivity and specificity for
  both strictures and fistulae in some studies. Fistulae, particularly those
  in the pelvis, are best shown with MRI.
- Fistulae, particularly those in the pelvis, are best shown on MRI.
- Ileal intubation at colonoscopy should always be attempted, as it
  allows histology. Success should be over 90% in expert hands: this
  author advises buscopan 20 mg IV as an aid to get through the
  ileocaecal valve.

Radiology versus colonoscopy for investigating the colon

- Colonosopy is more accurate than radiology in demonstrating mucosal
  abnormalities in the colon and allows biopsy of any suspicious areas. It is
  not the ideal primary investigation when symptoms suggest an intramural or extrinsic lesion affecting the bowel. In this situation contrast radiology, probably using a <u>CT pneumocolon</u> technique, is advised.
- Barium enema now used rarely by many units, as patients find it
  unpleasant, and it misses more polyps than colonoscopy (identifies
  <50% of polyps > 1 cm); (Winawer, S J et al. (2000) New Eng. J. Med.
  342 (24): 1766).
- For polyp detection, colonoscopy remains 'gold standard', although
  there is a substantial miss rate in the detection of small polyps, even by
  expert colonoscopists (Rex, DK et al. (1997) Gastroenterology **112**; 24.).
  Recent data on comparative efficacy of CT pneumocolon ('virtual
  colonoscopy') is contradictory, but this technique is likely to get better
  over next few years, and carries virtually no risk, in contrast to colonoscopy (see <u>endoscopic complications</u>).
- Colonoscopy is still advocated for surveillance of patients with
  conditions known to predispose to cancer of the colon.

Diverticular disease

This makes interpretation of double contrast radiological studies difficult, and many radiologists find a single contrast technique easier to interpret. In the presence of diverticulits with perforation and a peri-colic abcess, extravasation of barium is undesirable and water soluble contrast media are often used. The technique of <u>CT pneumocolon</u> with IV contrast is becoming increasingly used in this situation.

Focal liver lesions

Several tests can provide complementary information. Transabdominal U/S is very useful in differentiating small cysts from < 1 cm masses (e.g. metastases). CT detects > 90% focal liver lesions, as small as 5–6 mm. IV contrast injection allows assessment of arterial phase (e.g. hypervascular <u>hepatocellular carcinoma</u> or <u>neuroendocrine tumours</u>) and portal venous phase (hypovascular <u>colonic cancer</u> metastases). Delayed films often needed to diagnose <u>haemangioma</u>. <u>MRI</u> has few advantages over CT for focal liver lesions, but is excellent at defining ductal anatomy, and helps differentiate haemangioma from other lesions. <u>PET scanning</u> is finding increasing use in investigating possible liver metastases from colorectal cancer or <u>pancreatic endocrine tumours</u>/<u>carcinoid</u>.

Liver problems in pregnancy

- Changes in <u>liver function tests</u> (LFTs) during pregnancy are common.
- Depending on the pattern of derangement and clinical scenario, these changes may range from reflecting a normal physiological response to pregnancy, to a potentially fatal complication of pregnancy necessitating expeditious delivery.
- Normal pregnancy may be associated with the development of palmar erythema and spider naevi (in up to 60%), and laboratory abnormalities including ↓ serum albumin (mean 31 g/l in 3rd trimester), and up to x5 ULN ↑ serum ALP. Other LFTs, including bilirubin and transaminases, fall or remain normal.

Clinical assessment

- When assessing liver abnormalities in pregnant women ask:
  - Why now?
  - Whether the abnormalities are independent of, or related to, the pregnancy.
- The duration of pregnancy and presence of clinical features of liver disease may provide vital clues.
  - Have results been abnormal in the past (check with GP, pathology records)?
  - Are there risk factors/clinical features to suggest pre-existing liver disease?
- Mild LFT abnormalities in the asymptomatic women may be an incidental finding during 1st trimester antenatal assessment (including <u>hepatitis B</u> serology), and may represent the first health care contact at which an underlying liver disease is identified. Further assessment and management will depend on pattern of LFTs and associated features (see <u>Approach to well patients with abnormal liver tests</u>). It is important to make a diagnosis, because of possible changes in the activity of chronic liver disease during pregnancy or fetal risks (e.g. viral transmission).
- LFT derangement may occur in 50% of women with hyperemesis gravidarum (see <u>Approach to GI problems in pregnancy</u>), often during 1st and 2nd trimester, with mild increases in bilirubin (rarely jaundice) and liver enzymes, and usually resolves with adequate nutrition.
- Acute viral hepatitis (especially <u>hepatitis A, B, E</u>) is the commonest cause of jaundice during pregnancy worldwide. It is associated with a higher rate of morbidity and mortality in pregnant, compared with non-pregnant, women (see <u>hepatitis E</u>), and is an important cause of fetal loss. Jaundice may occur in pregnancy due to any cause, and so requires active investigation (see <u>Approach to recent-onset jaundice</u>).

Effects of chronic liver disease on pregnancy

Immunological changes during pregnancy have been implicated as the cause of both deterioration (with associated clinical presentation) and improvements in liver function due to <u>autoimmune hepatitis</u>, <u>primary biliary cirrhosis</u>, and <u>primary sclerosing cholangitis</u>. Non-cirrhotic chronic viral hepatitis rarely causes problems during pregnancy, with management mainly related to prevention of neonatal infection. Perinatal vaccination is highly effective at reducing the risk of chronic HBV infection (see <u>hepatitis B</u>). Neonatal acquisition of <u>hepatitis C</u> from an infected mother is approximately 5%, but no vaccine is presently available, and there is no convincing evidence that mode of delivery (vaginal versus caesarean) effects transmission. Although nucleoside analogues (e.g. <u>LAMIVUDINE</u>— see drugs) may be safely given for <u>hepatitis B</u> during pregnancy, the use of ribavirin for <u>hepatitis C</u> is absolutely contraindicated, because of teratogenicity.

<u>Cirrhosis</u> often leads to infertility, but where pregnancy does occur, variceal bleeding due to <u>portal hypertension</u> is a particular risk in the 2nd and 3rd trimesters. Prophylaxis with β-blockers should not be stopped because of pregnancy. Although pregnancy may be successful post-<u>liver transplantation</u>, there is an increased risk of complications.

Pregnancy-related liver disease

A range of hepatobiliary conditions may present or be exacerbated by pregnancy, as discussed above (and see <u>Approach to GI problems in pregnancy</u>). Several others are peculiar to pregnancy, and may have life-threatening consequences. It is vital to consider these in all pregnant patients with symptomatic disease and LFT abnormalities, particularly in the 3rd trimester. These include <u>acute fatty liver of pregnancy</u> (AFLP), <u>HELLP syndrome</u>, and <u>obstetric cholestasis</u>. Prompt diagnosis of these conditions is crucial, as delay in delivery in AFLP and HELLP syndrome is associated with high maternal and fetal mortality.

Investigations

- Bloods: All patients will require FBC, clotting, U&Es, LFTs, Glu. Other bloods will be tailored to the specific clinical scenario, as discussed above (and see <u>Approaches to well patients with abnormal liver tests, recent-onset jaundice</u>).
- Ultrasound is vital, to look for evidence of biliary obstruction, chronic liver disease with <u>portal hypertension,</u> fatty liver, liver haematoma, <u>gallstones</u>.
- Liver biopsy is rarely necessary, although it remains the 'gold standard' for diagnosing AFLP and diagnosing cirrhosis in those with chronic liver disease.

Management

- Depends entirely on the diagnosis.
- Expert obstetric and hepatology advice should be sought for most cases, particularly for pregnancy-related liver disease (e.g. AFLP, HELLP), or in any patient with significant liver disease for whom intervention may be required during pregnancy (e.g. chronic <u>hepatitis B</u>).

Malabsorption and steatorrhoea

Definitions

Malabsorption refers to defective uptake or transport of digested nutrients from the small bowel mucosa (e.g. coeliac disease).

Maldigestion refers to impaired breakdown of food in the gut lumen (e.g. due to pancreatic insufficiency in chronic pancreatitis, or inadequate bile in primary biliary cirrhosis).

In practice, the term malabsorption is usually used to cover both maldigestion and malabsorption. There are many causes of malabsorption (see box).

Steatorrhoea is the passage of bulky, pale, foul-smelling stools that float and are difficult to flush away (in fact, most stools float due to gas, not fat content). A greasy film or even droplets of oil may be seen in the toilet pan.

Causes of malabsorption

- Pancreatic insufficiency
- Bacterial overgrowth
- Bile acid malabsorption
- Whipple's disease
- Post-gastrectomy
- Extensive small bowel resection
- Coeliac disease
- Tropical sprue
- Giardiasis
- Lactase deficiency
- Small bowel Crohn's disease
- Lymphoma
- Eosinophilic gastroenteritis
- Lymphangiectasia
- Radiation damage (small bowel)
- Systemic mastocytosis
- Diabetic enteropathy
- Thyroid disease

Assessment

Clinical clues

- Chronic diarrhoea is a common feature in patients with malabsorption (see Approach to chronic diarrhoea).
- A history of pale, bulky, terribly smelly stools that are difficult to flush suggests steatorrhoea.
- Abdominal discomfort, bloating, and flatulence is common.
- Ask about symptoms related to fat-soluble vitamin (A, D, E, K) deficiency:
  - Bleeding, easy bruising, night blindness, metabolic bone disease), low calcium, magnesium, phosphate (e.g. tetany, muscle weakness), iron (microcytic anaemia), vitamin B12 (macrocytic anaemia, glossitis, angular stomatitis).
- Is there a history of weight loss, failure to thrive (in children), or primary/secondary amenorrhoea?
- Does patient have a clinical problem known to predispose to malabsorption (e.g. chronic pancreatitis, coeliac disease, small bowel Crohn's disease)?

Confirming malabsorption

- **Bloods:** FBC, ESR, CRP, Glucose, U&Es, LFTs, Ca^{2+}, PO^{4-}, Mg^{2+}, clotting, vitamins A, D, E, B12, folate, coeliac antibodies, anti-mitochondrial antibodies.
- **Stool analysis:**
  - **Sudan III stain.** This qualitative test of faecal fat is positive in > 80% of patients with true steatorrhoea, provided they are ingesting 75–100 g of fat/day).
  - **3 day faecal fat** is the 'gold standard' to confirm steatorrhoea, with >7 g stool fat/24 hours abnormal. However, test is unpleasant for all involved, and requesting a 3 day faecal fat on every patient with chronic diarrhoea is a good way to alienate your nursing and laboratory colleagues.
  - **Faecal fat concentration.** Gut mucosal disease usually leads to malabsorption of water and electrolytes, and so fat is relatively diluted within stool. This is in contrast to maldigestion (e.g. in pancreatic insufficiency), when faecal fat concentration > 9.5 g/100 g stool is characteristically seen.

Identifying aetiology

- Clues to the aetiology in history and initial results will lead to tests being tailored to each case. A basic approach to excluding luminal and pancreatic disease are shown in the algorithm. The aim should be to organize non-invasive tests early in assessment (e.g. don't wait until all endoscopies and barium studies have been performed to send a stool sample for faecal elastase!).
- **Endoscopy.** Upper GI endoscopy with distal duodenal biopsies is indicated in all patients with suspected malabsorption, unless other obvious cause. Take four duodenal biopsies to give your pathologist the best chance of a well oriented specimen to allow proper assessment of crypt and villous architecture. Terminal ileal biopsies at ileo-colonoscopy may be useful.

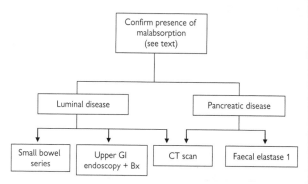

Fig. 1.6 Initial approach to defining aetiology of malabsorption.

- **Imaging.** Abdominal X-ray may show pancreatic calcification. A barium follow through can give useful information (e.g. strictures due to <u>Crohn's disease</u>, large diverticulae in scleroderma, <u>lymphoma of GI tract</u>). CT scanning may demonstrate thickened bowel loops and lymphadenopathy, and accurately defines pancreatic anatomy (but remember that pancreatic anatomy is not synonymous with function). MRI/MRCP with secretin may provide some additional indication of pancreatic juice output (see <u>pancreatic function tests</u>).
- **Other tests:**
  - Stool microscopy: culture and microscopy (ova, cysts, parasites—e.g. *Giardia*).
  - Faecal elastase 1: simple and reliable test of <u>pancreatic insufficiency</u> (except in patients with watery diarrhoea). See <u>pancreatic function tests</u>.
  - <u>Schilling test</u>: findings may help not only to confirm malabsorption of vitamin B12, but possible aetiology.
  - SeHCAT test (see <u>bile acid malabsorption</u>).
  - Stool osmotic gap (see <u>Approach to chronic diarrhoea</u>).
  - Hydrogen <u>breath tests</u> can help with the diagnosis of <u>bacterial overgrowth</u>.

Management

- Exact treatment depends on making a specific diagnosis, and treating specific disease (see relevant A–Z section).
- Where the aetiology of malabsorption is difficult to establish, therapeutic trials may direct clinician to the aetiology, e.g.:
    - PANCREATIC ENZYME SUPPLEMENTS in suspected pancreatic insufficiency may lead to rapid improvement in steatorrhea.
    - Antibiotics may improve bacterial overgrowth.
    - Bile acid sequesters (e.g. CHOLESTYRAMINE) may improve diarrhoea/steatorrhoea related to bile acid malabsorption.
- Vitamins, micronutrients, and haematinics need replacing if deficient.
- Consider effects of bone loss (see osteoporosis), so arrange bone densitometry, and provide fracture prophylaxis as necessary.
- Bacterial overgrowth may improve with surgical resection of large small bowel diverticulum or strictures, but always risks exacerbating the problem with further adhesions.

Mouth and swallowing problems

Problems with the mouth

Causes of a sore tongue

- Geographic tongue may be normal variant, but associated with atopy. Can be asymptomatic or cause a sore tongue. Increased frequency in Reiter's syndrome and psoriasis (see Colour Plate 1).
- Glossitis can be caused by iron, vitamin B12 or folate deficiency and acute candidial or herpetic infection (see Colour Plate 2).
- Radiotherapy and <u>graft versus host disease</u> are important causes of a mucositis that can affect the mouth.
- Rare causes of a painful tongue include diabetes and drugs (captopril).

Painful mouth ulcers

- Traumatic ulcers.
- <u>Aphthous ulcers</u>: 20% have associated iron, B12, or folate deficiency. Often associated with systemic diseases.
- Malignant ulcers.

Painless mouth ulcers

These are frequently innocuous and caused by dentures or cheek biting. However, remember:

- Lichen planus.
- Leukoplakia.
- Oral candida.
- Oral telangiectasia seen as part of <u>hereditary haemorrhagic telangiectasia</u> (see Colour Plate 13).
- Other pigmented lesions (Addison's disease, Kaposi's sarcoma, black tongue in patients on tetracyclines or bismuth).
- Blisters can be caused by pemphigus, pemphigoid, or drugs. Other so-called blistering disorders like epidermolysis bullosa and erythema multiforme tend to cause mouth ulcers rather than blisters.

Halitosis

Common causes are:
- Dental or tonsillar abcesses.
- Gingivitis/stomatitis.
- Any cause of dry mouth (drugs, fever, dehydration, Sjögren's syndrome, radiotherapy).
- Some foods (ethanol, garlic, dimethyl sulphoxide).
- Diseases outside the oropharynx include chronic lung pathology (bronchiectasis, lung abscess), liver failure, uraemia, and diabetic ketoacidosis.

Evaluation and management. Ask about diet, medication, and non-oral disease. Emphasize importance of oral hygiene and dental hygiene. Routine tongue brushing can help. Antiseptic mouthwashes can be useful, as can artificial saliva in patients with xerostomia.

Mucocutaneous features of HIV (see HIV and the gut)

- Over 90% of HIV infected patients have at least one oral manifestation.
- The commonest HIV-associated mouth infection is candida (see candidiasis). Most viral causes are secondary to herpes viruses (herpes simplex, cytomegalovirus, varicella zoster virus. Oral hairy leukoplakia is seen in 40% of HIV patients and is associated with Epstein–Barr viral infection.
- Bacterial infection leading to periodontal disease is common and may progress to severe necrotizing stomatitis.
- Neoplasms. Kaposi's sarcoma and lymphoma are important in HIV disease.

Problems with swallowing

Do not confuse **dysphagia** (a difficulty with the act of swallowing or of food proceeding into the stomach) with **globus** (the sensation of a lump or something in the throat). Although globus is often functional, it can be caused by lesions in the neck, pharynx, or larynx. The old term globus hystericus is not appropriate: hysterical or histrionic features are nearly always absent. There is little evidence that a high pressure upper oesophageal sphincter is associated with globus sensation. Globus is a common somatization symptom (Othmer, E and De Souza C. (1985) *Am. J. Psychiatry* **142**: 1146.

Odynophagia means pain on swallowing. This suggests oesophageal inflammation or ulceration. Two common causes are medications and infections—odynophagia rarely occurs with reflux disease. Pill-induced oesophagitis usually has an acute history and a careful history of medication will usually suggest the diagnosis. Infections are becoming more common in immuno-compromised patients: symptoms are non-specific but certain infections are more common in HIV (candida) or transplant patients (herpes or CMV).

MOUTH AND SWALLOWING PROBLEMS

Oral manifestations of disease

Disease	Oral manifestation
Vascular disorders	
Hereditary haemorrhagic telangiectasia	Telangiectasia on lips and mouth
Blue rubber bleb naevus syndrome	Dark blue soft compressible nodules
Bullous eruptions	
Epidermolysis bullosa	Mouth involvement most common in the scarring (dystrophic) form
Pemphigus/pemphigoid	Oral lesions are common in pemphigoid and almost universal in pemphigus
Rheumatologic disorders	
SLE	Oral ulcers
Scleroderma	Telangiectasia, microstomia
Behçet's	Oral ulcers
Miscellaneous	
Amyloidosis	Small waxy amber papules on face and lips
Fabry's disease	Angiokeratomas on lips and mouth
Kaposi's	Blue-red macules on oral mucosa
Porphyria	Photosensitivity
Pernicious anaemia	Glossitis
Crohn's	Aphthous ulceration
Coeliac disease	Aphthous ulceration

Dysphagia: oropharyngeal and oesophageal

Difficulty with initiating swallowing is called **oropharyngeal dysphagia**. There are many local, neurological, and muscular causes; the dysphagia is usually part of a wider disease process and diagnosis is usually straightforward (see box opposite). Difficulty with the passage of swallowed substances down the oesophagus into the stomach is referred to as **oesophageal dysphagia**. The causes include motility problems or mechanical lesions (intrinsic or extrinsic to the oesophagus) and are listed in the box.

Clinical evaluation

History and examination

Trouble starting a swallow or transferring the food from the mouth into the oesophagus suggests oropharyngeal dysphagia. Associated symptoms include nasal regurgitation, dysarthria, and nasal speech. There may be cranial nerve abnormalities. There may be signs of weakness caused by muscular disease or a stroke: careful examination of the pharynx and larynx is important.

In oesophageal dysphagia, 3 questions in the history are important.
- What kind of food (solid or liquid) produces the symptoms?
  - Motility disorders tend to result in slowly progressive dysphagia for solids and liquids, while in mechanical obstruction the dysphagia is worse for solids.
- Is dysphagia intermittent or progressive?
  - Classic causes of intermittent dysphagia are a Schatzki ring or some motility disorders like diffuse oesophageal spasm.
- Is there associated heartburn?

The site of localization is of limited value: in particular dysphagia localized to the neck is often referred from below.

Presenting features of clinical conditions

The various clinical conditions causing dysphagia are listed in the A to Z section.

Causes of oropharyngeal dysphagia

Neuromuscular diseases

CNS
- Brainstem CVA
- Parkinson's disease
- <u>Wilson's disease</u>
- Multiple sclerosis
- Amyotrophic lateral sclerosis
- Tabes dorsalis

PNS
- Bulbar polio
- Peripheral neuropathies (diphtheria, botulism, rabies, diabetes)

Motor end plate
- Myasthenia gravis
- Muscular dystrophy
- Metabolic disease (thyrotoxicosis, steroid myopathy)
- Amyloidosis, SLE

Local structural causes
- Inflammatory (abscess, TB, syphilis)
- Neoplastic
- <u>Web</u>
- <u>Plummer–Vinsen</u> syndrome
- Extrinsic compression
- Surgical resection

Disorders of the upper oesophageal sphincter
- Hyper- or hypotensive upper oesophageal sphincter

Causes of oesophageal dysphagia

Motility disorders
- <u>Achalasia</u>, <u>scleroderma</u>, diffuse oesophageal spasm, secondary motility dorders (collagen vascular diseases, Chagas' disease)

Mechanical, intrinsic
- Peptic stricture
- <u>Oesophageal ring</u>
- <u>Oesophageal cancer</u>
- Rare causes include webs, diverticula, benign tumours, oesophageal haematoma, foreign bodies (e.g. food bolus)

Mechanical, extrinsic
- Vascular compression, cervical osteoarthritis, mediastinal abnormalities

Assessment

Although modern endoscopy with intubation under direct vision is safe in most cases, there is a risk of intubating an oesophageal pouch, which is one traditional reason for suggesting barium swallow as the initial investigation. More importantly, endoscopy is a crude and inappropriate tool for assessing the dynamic process of swallowing. For oropharyngeal dysphagia, a video barium swallow with a solid or semi-solid bolus such as a marshmallow is the best test. If there is any evidence of an obstructing lesion, an endoscopy should be performed, with biopsy of any lesion. If endoscopy is negative or suggests a motility disorder, oesophageal manometry should be done.

Therapeutic considerations

- Oropharyngeal dysphagia caused by Parkinson's, hypothyroidism, myositis, and myasthenia is treatable, emphasizing the importance of making a specific diagnosis.
- Dysphagia resulting from degenerative neurological disease can often be helped by a rehabilitation programme organized by a speech and language therapist.
- Treatment of mechanical obstruction depends on the cause but may involve surgery, dilatation, or stenting (see oesophageal obstruction: treatment).
- Motility disorders are treated medically and sometimes surgically.

Nausea and vomiting

Definitions and neurophysiology

The **vomiting centre** lies in the medulla, close to centres controlling respiration and salivation (hence associated hyperventilation and salivation). It receives signals from the chemoreceptor trigger zone (located in the fourth ventricle, also known as the area postrema, with blood supply from posterior inferior cerebellar artery and no blood–brain barrier). This area is the site of action of certain drugs causing vomiting (see box) but also receives afferent fibres from stomach, intestines, gallbladder, peritoneum, and heart.

- Nausea is probably mediated by similar pathways, which overlap with those mediating satiety: anorexia therefore usually accompanies nausea.
- Distinguish vomiting from regurgitation (latter usually effortless without the muscular activity involved in vomiting, it is associated with a sour or bitter taste, and not associated with nausea).

Clues in reaching a diagnosis

Timing. Early morning vomiting may be associated with pregnancy, but hyperemesis gravidarum is more serious (see Approach to GI problems in pregnancy). Vomiting associated with raised intracranial pressure, uraemia, or post-gastrectomy often occurs in the morning. Vomiting during or soon after a meal is often due to psychogenic causes, while vomiting one to several hours after a meal is more associated with gastric stasis (pyloric stenosis, upper small intestinal obstruction, or functional stasis in diabetic gastroparesis (see Diabetes and GI tract), scleroderma, or coeliac disease).

Pain. Think of non-GI causes: severe pain such as renal colic can cause nausea and vomiting, and may be the only sign of a urinary infection. Same may be true of pneumonia, especially in elderly. Pain of peptic ulceration (epigastric, meal-related, causing night-time waking, not periumbilical or diffuse) is often relieved by vomiting. Vomiting associated with severe back pain can be caused by posterior duodenal ulcer, pancreatitis, or pancreatic cancer. Central colicky pain associated with gurgling and profuse vomiting of bile-stained fluid suggests small bowel obstruction. Vomiting with large bowel obstruction usually occurs late, accompanied by distension and absolute constipation.

Systemic symptoms and signs. Normal appetite should raise suspicion of a psychogenic cause, although can be associated with mechanical obstruction. Weight gain suggests an absence of serious organic disease, but patients with <u>peptic ulcers</u> may put on weight due to eating relieving their symptoms.

Nature of vomitus. Recognizable food suggests gastric stasis. Vomiting that smells feculent suggests small bowel obstruction, <u>ileus</u>, gastro-colic fistula, or <u>bacterial overgrowth</u>. Blood in the vomit is potentially serious and may require management as for <u>acute upper GI bleeding</u> although 'coffee-ground vomiting' is non-specific, representing the appearance of many different kinds of vomited particulate matter. Blood first appearing after several vomits may be due to damage around the oesophagogastric junction (see <u>Mallory–Weiss syndrome</u>).

Past medical history. Details of previous surgery are important. Information on childhood health may be relevant, and <u>gallstones</u>, inflammatory bowel disease, and <u>coeliac disease</u> can be familial.

Social factors. Information about home, marriage, job, children, and sexual problems or abuse may be relevant, particularly if no cause can be identified, and if questions in these areas elicit anxiety or emotion.

Approach to investigation

- Blood tests are usually simple and based on the history and examination.
  - FBC may reveal anaemia; iron deficiency may suggest peptic or malignant ulceration, or disease of the small bowel.
  - ↑ MCV may suggest alcohol excess, <u>vitamin B12</u> or folate deficiency.
  - U & Es may be abnormal secondary to vomiting (e.g. $\downarrow K^+$, $\downarrow Na^+$ hyperchloraemic metabolic alkalosis), or may reflect underlying primary renal dysfunction: check calcium level and also <u>liver function tests</u>. Send <u>amylase</u> in acute presentation to exclude <u>acute pancreatitis</u>.
- Upper GI endoscopy may help, particularly to exclude peptic ulcer or other mucosal abnormality, and bile reflux. However, endoscopy is a poor test of function and barium studies may be better in assessment of upper GI stasis and obstruction.

Management

- Central goal is to identify cause (see box), as this determines treatment.
- Where psychogenic factors appear important, specialist psychological input may be beneficial.
- Lifestyle advice, including abstinence from alcohol, may help.
- A wide range of drugs is available for nausea and vomiting, which should be used in a step-wise manner, with the knowledge that all carry the risk of side-effects (see <u>ANTI-EMETICS</u>).

Drugs causing nausea and vomiting

- Via chemoreceptor trigger zone: opiates, digoxin, L-dopa, ipecacuanha, cytotoxic drugs
- Antibiotics (tetracyclines, <u>METRONIDAZOLE</u>, <u>ERYTHROMYCIN</u>)
- Sulphonamides (including salazopyrine)
- <u>ASPIRIN</u>, <u>NSAIDS</u> damage the gastric mucosa and may stimulate the vomiting centre via ascending afferents
- <u>Alcohol</u> acts directly on the chemoreceptor trigger zone and via gastric mucosal damage.

Causes of nausea and vomiting

See boxes for painless causes of vomiting and causes of vomiting without nausea.

Painless causes of vomiting

Infective

- Viral gastroenteritis
- Food poisoning, possibly infection associated with *Helicobacter pylori*. Infections elsewhere such as UTI or pneumonia in the elderly
- Viral labyrinthitis.

Mechanical obstruction

- Pyloric stenosis, or duodenal obstruction due to gastric or pancreatic cancer
- Oesophageal cancer
- Biliary reflux, particularly if there has been previous gastric surgery or a gastro-enterostomy.

Alcoholic gastritis

- Often causes early morning retching, usually small volumes, often blood stained.

<u>*Acute liver failure*</u>

E.g. <u>paracetamol</u> overdose, <u>acute fatty liver of pregnancy</u>

Metabolic causes

- Addison's disease (look for postural hypotension, mucosal pigmentation—↑ or normal K^+ particularly important, since ↓K^+ more expected after vomiting)
- Also consider hypercalcaemia, uraemia, and hyperthyroidism
- Up to 30% of diabetic patients may have intermittent nausea or vomiting—see <u>Diabetes and the GI tract</u>.

Causes of vomiting without nausea

- **Intracranial tumours**
  - Ask about headache, double vision; examine for gait disturbances
- **Raised intracranial pressure**
  - Look for nystagmus, papilloedema, cranial nerve abnormalities
- **Encephalitis**
- **Meningitis**
- **Migraine**
- **Cyclical vomiting**
  - Usually occurs in 2–3 month cycles, in children, teenagers, or young adults. It may accompany migraine and may respond to beta blockers.

Non-cardiac chest pain

- Up to 30% of patients undergoing coronary angiography for acute or recurring chest pain have normal coronary arteries: a substantial proportion of these are referred to gastroenterologists for an opinion.
- Major non-cardiac causes of chest pain include musculoskeletal problems, psychological or psychiatric problems, and oesophageal disorders.
- Oesophageal distension or acid perfusion of the oesophagus can produce pains mimicking angina pectoris.

Characteristics and causes of oesophageal pain

- The pain can be similar to anginal type pain and may be exercise-related. It may be triggered by hot or cold food or drink. Other oesophageal symptoms are usually present (heartburn, reflux, dysphagia). Meal-related pain or pain relieved by antacids is suggestive.
- Specific mechanisms are not well understood. See table for causes, and see oesophageal motility disorders.

Evaluating the patient with non-cardiac chest pain

- Rule out cardiac disease first. In young patients, a negative ECG during pain with a normal echo and stress test is sufficient: in the older patient or where diagnostic uncertainty remains, coronary angiography remains the gold standard.
- Consider musculoskeletal causes (look for point tenderness) and psychological or psychiatric causes.
- For possible oesophageal causes, do upper GI endoscopy (but see below) or barium studies. If normal, try high dose PPI for 6–8 weeks in twice daily dosage. 24 h pH testing and oesophageal manometry may be useful.

Reflux as a cause of non-cardiac chest pain

Significant reflux occurs in 50% patients with normal coronary arteries on angiography and chest pain, with episodes of pain coinciding with reflux on the pH record. Since most patients do not have oesophagitis, **upper**

GI endoscopy is not a useful diagnostic test. Barium studies can be more useful in assessing possible motility problems. Trial of high dose PPI or 24 hour ambulatory pH testing are the two most useful tests.

Cause of oesophageal pain	Comments
Reflux of gastric contents	Causes heartburn—but same symptoms are elicited by alkaline reflux of bile salts and experimental balloon dilatation of the oesophagus. Correlation between episodes of reflux and symptoms is poor. 30% of patients with Barrett's are acid-insensitive
Oesophageal motility disorders	Patients with non-cardiac chest pain often have motility disorders on manometry: high ampli-tude contractions or frequent simultaneous contractions
Change in temperature or luminal distension	Hot or cold liquids or food bolus impaction can produce chest pain. A low pain threshold or visceral hypersensitivity may contribute

Treatment of oesophageal chest pain

Reassurance based on diagnostic tests can sometimes help (although many patients continue to believe cardiac disease is still present). Opti-mal acid suppression may involve night-time HISTAMINE RECEPTOR ANTAGONISTS as well as high dose PPIs: identifying reflux is important because many drugs used in an attempt to relieve pain due to motility disorders (nitrates, calcium antagonists) can aggravate reflux. Low dose tricyclic antidepressants have been effective in clinical trials but should be taken for at least 2 months before maximal benefit is shown: they may work by altering visceral pain thresholds.

Nutritional support

Principles of nutritional assessment

- There is a high prevalence (20–40%) of undernutrition in patients admitted to hospital that tends to worsen during admission.
- There is no gold standard for determining nutrtional status: all approaches have been validated by assessing outcome rather than nutrition-specific parameters.
- The best simple assessment is the body mass index(BMI).
- Serum albumin is a good predictor of surgical outcome but correlates poorly with overall nutritional status, because like many indicators of nutritional status it is influenced by illness or injury.

Clinicians need to recognize, assess, and treat patients with protein–energy malnutrition as well as those with specific nutrient deficiencies.

Indications for nutritional support

Sick people eat more if they are given assistance at mealtimes and the opportunity to eat what they like. They should be allowed to eat food bought in by friends and family if desired.

Indications for supplemental feeding
- Weight loss of more than 10% within 1 month.
- A body mass index of less than 20 kg/m^2.
- Inability to eat for more than 5 days.

Use the enteral route where possible
- Some nutrients are not available via the parenteral route (e.g. short chain fatty acids for colonic mucosa provided by bacterial degradation of fibre or carbohydrate).
- Intestinal mucosal atrophy found in animals on parenteral nutrition.
- Parenteral nutrition is associated with complications related to line sepsis.

Indications for parenteral feeding
- Inadequate length of absorptive intestine: short bowel syndrome (less than 100 cm small intestine, or less than 50 cm small intestine if in contiunuity with colon).
- Intestinal obstruction (but endoscopically placed enteral feeding tubes can be used to bypass oesophageal or duodenal partial obstruction).
- Severe mucositis (e.g. complicating chemotherapy).
- Severe sepsis producing ileus.
- High output enterocutaneous fistula in those patients where reduced enteral intake reduces fistula output.
- Very rarely, patients with chronic intestinal pseudo-obstruction.

Techniques for delivering nutritional support

Enteral

Supplemental or sip feeding

There are a variety of <u>oral rehydration therapies</u> that have benefit in patients with severe fluid loss, high output enterostomies, and short bowel syndromes.

Defined '<u>**formula foods**</u>' can be.

- Single nutrients (e.g. protein, carbohydrate, or fat).
- Elemental (monomeric).
- Polymeric.
- Disease-specific.

Tube feeding and enterostomy feeding

This approach is useful where patients have a functioning GI tract but cannot or will not eat adequately. Many different approaches are possible (e.g. nasogastric, nasojejunal, gastrostomy, jejunostomy): choice of route depends on physician experience, prognosis, estimated duration of feeding, and of course patient preference.

Soft bore nasogastric tubes can stay in place for several weeks and allow eating. However, if feeding is required for longer than 4–6 weeks, a <u>percutaneous endoscopic gastrostomy</u> (PEG) is appropriate. Nasojejunal feeding can be useful in patients with gastroparesis or <u>pancreatitis</u>, but this mode of feeding does not necessarily decrease the risk of aspiration or dislodgement. Generally, continuous drip feeding is better than bolus feeding (can lead to reflux or diarrhoea) and if a dietician is not available starting at a rate of 30 ml/hour is appropriate (unless risk of refeeding).

Feeding enterostomies are usually inserted using the technique of <u>PEG</u>, although surgical or radiological placement is not uncommon. Jejunal feeding tube placement is possible by threading a tube through an existing gastrostomy or a surgical approach.

The routine use of endoscopic gastrostomy tube insertion has revolutionized the management of patients debilitated by progressive neuromuscular diseases including stroke. A common indication is inability to eat satisfactorily 2 weeks after the initiating event. There is a significant incidence of complications, which requires informed management.

Parenteral feeding

Peripheral or central venous access

Parenteral feeding is associated with life–threatening complications unless managed optimally.

- With modern feeds, **peripheral catheters** can be used short term (up to 2 weeks). Thrombophlebitis is related to the duration of feeding and to the osmolarity of the feed and can be minimized by careful insertion, aseptic technique, and GTN patches. **Peripherally inserted central catheters** (PICC lines) are inserted via the basilic vein at the antecubital fossa (avoid the cephalic vein as it joins the axillary vein at a sharp angle that can make advancement beyond this point difficult).

- **Central venous catheters** are placed via a subcutaneous tunnel from a point on the chest wall distant from the point of entry of the catheter into the vein. Insertion is via the infraclavicular or low jugular routes. The tip of the catheter should be proximal to the reflection of the pericardium on to the SVC, in order to avoid the small risk of tamponade consequent on erosion of the catheter through the heart or lower SVC wall (this can be done by checking the tip is no lower than 2 cm below a line joining the lower borders of the medial ends of the clavicles on a PA chest X-ray and is true for any central venous catheter). **Always** check the catheter is in the lumen before commencing feed. Central catheters must be used only for feeding and not for giving drugs or taking blood. In the case of a fever in a patient with a central catheter, blood cultures should be taken both peripherally and centrally.

Calculating the requirements and choosing the feed

Calculate energy requirements

Calculate the **basal metabolic rate**. Energy requirements depend on weight, activity level, and underlying disease. Historically this was done using Schofield charts (Schofield, WN (1985). *Hum. Nutr. Clin. Nutr,* **39c:** 5.) but there are a variety of websites available with on-line calculators (e.g. www.room42.com, www.motionworksfitness.com).
- Add 10% for each degree centigrade increase in temperature.
- Adjust for patients mobility:
  - On ventilator: –15%.
  - Unconscious: BMR.
  - Bedbound and awake: = +10%.
  - Sitting in a chair = +20%.
  - Mobile on ward= +30%.
- Add up to 600 kcal per day if weight gain is required.

Protein

The mean requirement for protein measured in grams of nitrogen (g N) per day is:
- 9 g N per day for men
- 7.5 g N per day for women
- 8.5 g N per day for pregnant women

Often in disease requirements are increased: if patients are burnt, septic, or otherwise catabolic increase the nitrogen to a usual maximum of 1 g N per 100 kcal. This can be checked by monitoring nitrogen loss via urinary urea excretion. In general:
- In low catabolic states, N requirements are 0.16 g/kg/24 hours.
- In intermediate catabolic states, N requirements are 0.2–0.3 g/kg/ 24 hours.
- In high catabolic states, N requirements are 0.25–0.35 g/kg/24 hours.

Carbohydrate

Glucose is the usual predominant energy source and is the required fuel for blood cells, bone marrow, and renal medulla, and the preferred fuel for the brain. Usually the infusion rate is kept below 4 ml/kg per min.

Fat

Lipid emulsions provide energy and are a source of essential fatty acids as well as linoleic and lenolenic acids. The optimal percentage of calories that should be infused as fat is not known; at least 5% of total calories should be given as lipids to prevent fatty acid deficiency. Most complications of lipid infusion (pulmonary dysfunction, pancreatitis, hypersensitivity) occur with over 1 kcal/kg/h: in practice this translates to a maximum of 500–1500 ml of a 10% emulsion over 24 hr.

Electrolyte requirements

- Sodium: provide patient's weight in kg as mM sodium as a baseline. Add calculated losses.
- Potassium: provide weight in kg as mmol/24 hr as a baseline, add losses.
- Calcium: 5–10 mmol per day.
- Magnesium: 5–10 mmol per day.
- Phosphate: 10–30 mmol per day.
- Vitamins and trace elements (see Elia, M. (1995) Lancet, **345**: 1279).

Approximately 9 litres of fluid pass through the duodenum per day, of which only 1.5 litres reach the colon.

Contents of intestinal fluids

	Volume (ml/24 h)	Na (mM/l)	K (mM/l)	HCO₃ (mM/l)
Saliva	500–1500	20	14	14
Gastric juice	2–3000	50–60	8–14	
Bile	600	146–149	5	25–30
Pancreatic juice	700–2500	125	8	10–45

Monitoring nutritional support

Refeeding syndrome

Refeeding syndrome is a complication of too rapid reintroduction of feed after prolonged starvation. Can occur in patients who have starved for > 7 days; lost > 20% body weight in 3 months; chronic alcoholics; anorexia nervosa.

Daily weight: In the presence of ascites or oedema, there may be initial weight loss as the expanded extracellular space diminishes.

Blood sugar: Stressed patients may be insulin resistant: monitor blood or urine glucose daily.

Temperature: Take blood from the feeding line and a peripheral vein if there is a spike of fever. If there is clinical suspicion of a line infection, stop the feed until the result of cultures is known.

Bloods: check renal function, as well as calcium, phosphate, magnesium, liver function at regular intervals.

Clinical applications of nutritional support

Perioperative nutritional support

Routine perioperative nutrition support should be limited to early use of sip feed supplements as oral fluids become allowed. There is some evidence that this leads to a reduction in postoperative complications and length of hospital stay. Parenteral feeding is advised in malnourished patients or in those with an unusually prolonged postoperative course.

Short bowel syndrome

A small group of patients who have lost large amounts of intestine need supplemental intravenous fluids and/or nutrition.

- Patients with a jejunostomy and < 100 cm residual jejunum are likely to need long-term parenteral fluid and electrolytes.
- Patients with a jenunostomy and < 75 cm residual jejunum are likely to need long-term parenteral nutrition, fluid, and electrolytes.
- Patients with a short bowel joined to colon are likely to need long-term parenteral nutrition if < 50 cm jejunum remains.
- The above refers to adapted bowel—intravenous support may be necessary during the adaptation phase with a jejunostomy and < 200 cm of remaining bowel.
- Additionally the quality of the remaining bowel is important—if diseased as in extensive Crohn's disease, longer lengths of bowel are needed.

Patients with <u>short bowel syndrome</u> often have negative sodium balance and large GI fluid losses and need an oral rehydration solution (ORS) with a higher sodium concentration than usual ORS.

The patient on ITU

The difficulty in maintaining lean body mass during critical illness means that artifical feeding should not be delayed. If the patient has lost 10% or more of their body weight (or if their BMI is less than 20 even if they have not lost weight) and will not be able to eat adequately within 2 days, immediate feeding is indicated. The enteral route is preferred wherever possible. Special attention must be given to those nutrients most likely to need hour to hour manipulation. In patients with respiratory failure, the excess carbon dioxide accompanying lipogenesis underlies the advice not to provide excess energy in the feed—especially not as glucose—if the patient is retaining carbon dioxide.

Liver disease

The most important principle is to avoid giving too much sodium, which will aggravate fluid retention and ascites. Protein may rarely need to be restricted in patients with <u>hepatic encephalopathy</u>, although normal protein intakes are often tolerated if infused slowly over 24 hours. Glucose infusion is needed in liver failure because of the failure of gluconeogenesis.

Inflammatory bowel disease

Ulcerative colitis

Apart from avoiding lactose-containing foods because of the risk of lactose intolerance in colitis, there is no evidence to support bowel rest in severe disease. Foods that may worsen diarrhoea such as caffeine-containing drinks should be avoided. A low fibre diet may be better tolerated by patients, even if there is proximal faecal loading above distal colitis.

Parenteral nutrition has no value as primary therapy (unlike in <u>Crohn's disease</u>). The indications for perioperative parenteral feeding in patients with IBD are no different than in other patients undergoing surgery.

Crohn's disease

Enteral nutrition as primary therapy

There is considerable data from prospective randomized trials showing that enteral feeding has higher efficacy than placebo as sole primary therapy. Meta-analyses fail to show equivalence with steroids as primary therapy (overall remission 58% compared to 80%) although enteral feeding may have some role in reducing steroid requirements or facilitating weaning off steroids.

Polymeric feeds are as effective as elemental feeds and tend to be more palatable. Input from dieticians is needed to enhance compliance, which is the main problem with using nutrition as a sole therapy. Enteral feeding is more costly and compliance is poorer than with pharmacotherapy. Enteral feeding may have a particular role in managing Crohn's disease in childhood because of the desirability to avoid steroids and minimize growth failure due to inadequate dietary intake.

Parenteral nutrition in Crohn's

Parenteral nutrion is indicated if there is intestinal failure due to obstruction, fistulating disease, or extensive resection. This has proven efficacy as primary therapy, especially in patients with small bowel disease, but there is a high relapse rate (60% at 2 years).

Acute pancreatitis

There is current interest in the correct way to feed patients with moderate to severe <u>acute pancreatitis</u>. In the past it has been assumed that a nil by mouth regimen was important to reduce pancreatic enzyme secretion, implying a need for TPN. However this has the effect of increasing mucosal permeability and prolonging endotoxaemia. Infusing enteral feeds (nasojejunally, and may be even nasogastrally) has little effect on pancreatic secretion and may reduce the systemic inflammatory response. There is some controlled evidence to support this approach (Kalfarentzos, F et al. (1997) Br. J. Surg. **84**: 1665).

Obesity

- Defined as a <u>body mass index</u> (BMI) of 30 or more, where BMI is weight (kg)/height squared (in metres). 'Overweight' is a BMI of 25–29.9.
- In 2000, 21% of the UK population were obese. 55% of the adult population were overweight or obese.
- Obesity is well known to cause or contribute to a large number of health problems:
  - Cardiovascular: hypertension, coronary heart disease.
  - Central nervous system: stroke, intracranial hypertension.
  - GI: cholelithiasis, non-alcoholic steatohepatitis, reflux oesophagitis.
  - Respiratory: obstructive sleep apnoea.
  - Metabolic: insulin resistance, type 2 diabetes, dyslipidaemia.
  - Reproductive: polycystic ovaries.

Recent developments in understanding obesity

- Recognition of a syndrome of insulin resistance (the 'metabolic syndrome') that is important in the pathophysiology of non-alcoholic steatohepatitis (NASH) (see <u>Non-alcholic fatty liver disease</u>). This syndrome includes:
  - Abdominal obesity.
  - Hypertriglyceridaemia and reduced levels of HDL.
  - Raised insulin levels.
  - Glucose intolerance.
  - Hypertension.
  - Elevated apo-B and raised plasminogen activator inhibitor 1.
- Considerable progress has been made in understanding the neuronal and peripheral signals mediating control of appetite and eating.

Taking a history

- Include a dietary history and assessment of activity.
- Screen for depression.
- Eating disorders occur in 30% of obese patients: ask about binging, purging, lack of satiety.
- Consider comorbidities, and think about rare causes of secondary obesity: hypothyroidism, Cushing's, insulinoma, hypothalamic disorders, polycystic ovarian syndrome, genetic syndromes such as Prader–Willi, oral contraceptive use, medication-related (see table).
- Ask about a family history.

Drugs associated with obesity

Drug	Mechanism
Phenothiazines	
Valproate	Increased appetite
Tricyclics	Increased appetite
Lithium	
Steroids	
Sulphonylureas	

Blood tests

- Full lipid panel (minimum fasting cholesterol, triglycerides, HDL, LDL).
- Liver function tests.
- Thyroid function.
- 24 h urinary free cortisol.
- Fasting glucose.

Managing obesity

There are many ways to induce negative energy balance and short-term weight loss, but effective management involves maintaining lowered weight and minimizing risk of related chronic diseases.

Lifestyle modifications

- Weight-reducing diets (see <u>slimming diets</u>).
- Increasing physical activity.
- Behavioural management.

Drug therapy of obesity

- Pancreatic lipase inhibitors (<u>ORLISTAT</u>), which produce a dose-dependent reduction in dietary fat absorption, inducing iatrogenic steatorrhoea. Supplementation of fat soluble vitamins may be needed.
- Centrally acting anti-obesity drugs include sibutramine (inhibits serotonin and noradrenaline reuptake).
- Potential future drugs: leptin initially gave hopes of a therapeutic breakthrough but in fact most obese patients are leptin resistant. Peptide YY when given IV acts as an appetite suppressant but current data are preliminary.

Surgery for obesity

There are three forms of <u>obesity surgery</u>: gastric resection, gastric by-pass, and biliopancreatic diversion. Prospective follow up shows significant weight loss maintained in surgically treated patients compared to medically treated controls, with a reduced prevalence of diabetes but no difference in blood pressure or lipid profiles.

For a review, see Kopelman, PG and Grace, C (2004). *Gut* **53**: 1044.

Recent onset jaundice

Background

- Jaundice is a yellow pigmentation of the sclerae due to subcutaneous deposition of bilirubin (Bn). Usually detectable when Bn > 60 μmol/l. It arises due to either increased Bn production, or decreased hepatobiliary excretion. See bilirubin metabolism.
- In assessment of patients with recent onset of jaundice 4 questions need to be answered.
    - What type of jaundice is present?
    - What is the causative agent or process?
    - If due to liver damage, is jaundice a result of acute or acute-on-chronic liver disease?
    - Is there evidence of liver failure?

Type of jaundice

(On the basis of history, examination, and routine biochemical tests (see clinical algorithm), it is usually possible to categorize the jaundiced patient into one of 3 disease groups. Within each group there are a wide range of causes (see table).

Disorders of bilirubin production/metabolism ('pre-hepatic')
Usually asymptomatic hyperbilirubinaemia, with few physical findings, and normal transaminases (ALT/AST) and cholestatic liver tests (ALP/GGT).

Liver disease ('hepatic')
- In chronic liver disease jaundice may present with other evidence of decompensation (e.g. ascites, variceal bleeding, hepatic encephalopathy). Acute liver injury more commonly presents with abdominal discomfort and clinical hepatomegaly.
- Wide variability of LFTs seen, depending on cause of liver injury. Serum ALT > 1000 U/l is unusual for alcoholic liver disease (even alcoholic hepatitis) or autoimmune liver disease (e.g. autoimmune hepatitis), and suggests acute liver injury due to viruses (e.g. hepatitis A, B), ischaemia (? recent hypotension), or drugs (e.g. paracetamol).
- In absence of cause for new-onset jaundice it may be clinically difficult to distinguish acute from acute-on-chronic disease. Poor/failing hepatic function is not indicated by elevation of liver enzymes, but most reliably by ↑ bilirubin, ↓ albumin, ↑ prothrombin time. ↑ ALP/GGT, in absence of biliary dilatation suggests intrahepatic cholestasis, due to a range of causes (e.g. primary biliary cirrhosis, drugs, TB, lymphoma).

Biliary obstruction ('post-hepatic')

- Jaundice is often associated with pruritis because subcutaneous deposition of bile acids is extremely irritant. Abdominal pain and nausea associated with bile duct stones, and progressive, painless jaundice with malignant obstruction, but history often imprecise.
- Elevation of ALP/GGT classically seen in patients with <u>biliary stricture</u>, but associated marked elevation of transaminases characteristically may occur with biliary obstruction due to stones (<u>choledocholithiasis</u>).

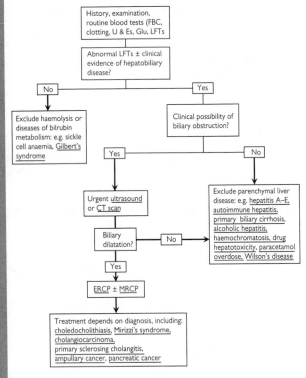

Fig. 1.7 Clinical approach to recent-onset jaundice.

Causes of jaundice

Disorders of bilirubin metabolism	Liver disease	Biliary obstruction
Hereditary haemolysis: e.g. sickle cell anaemia	Viral hepatitis A–E	Bile duct stones (choledocholithiasis)
Acquired haemolysis: e.g. transfusion reaction	Alcohol	Primary sclerosing cholangitis (PSC)
Defective conjugation e.g. Gilbert's syndrome, Crigler–Najjar	Drugs (see drug-induced hepatotoxicity)	Intrinsic biliary stricture (e.g. ischaemia, or trauma)
Impaired Bn excretion: e.g. Dubin–Johnson syndrome	Ischaemia (hypotension, venous/arterial thrombosis)	Cholangiocarcinoma
	Wilson's disease	Extrinsic biliary compression (e.g. aneurysm, hilar nodes)
	Haemochromatosis	Pancreatic carcinoma
	α1-Antitrypsin deficiency	Acute or chronic pancreatitis (and pancreatic pseudocyst)
	Autoimmune hepatitis	HIV cholangiopathy
	Primary biliary cirrhosis (PBC)	Biliary infestation, e.g. Clonorchis
	Non-alcoholic fatty liver disease (NAFLD)	
	Graft versus host disease	
	Pregnancy-related liver disease (see Approach to liver problems in pregnancy)	
	Granulomatous liver disease (see hepatic granulomas)	
	Budd–Chiari syndrome, veno-occlusive disease	
	Malignant infiltration	
	Bacterial sepsis	
	Viral infection: e.g. EBV, CMV, HSV	
	Leptospirosis	

Clinical assessment

History

Determine the onset of jaundice, and associated symptoms (prodrome, abdominal pain, weight loss?); previous illnesses (autoimmunity?); alcohol intake (amount, type, duration, pattern of drinking); needle exposure (IV drugs, tattoo, transfusions?); drug history (recreational, prescription, over-the-counter, herbal remedies, drug chart?); travel and vaccination history; occupational risks (e.g. health staff, publican?); sexual history; observation charts (hypotension?); family history.

Examination

Look for:

- Hints to cause of jaundice: smells of alcohol, needle marks, self-harm scars.
- Evidence of chronic liver disease: clubbing, Dupuytren's contracture, leukonychia, xanthelasma, Kayser–Fleischer rings, gynaecomastia, multiple spider naevi, testicular atrophy, splenomegaly, dilated superficial veins on abdomen.
- Evidence of <u>acute liver failure</u> or <u>hepatic encephalopathy</u>: liver flap, confusion/drowsiness/coma, bruising, ascites and dependent oedema.
- Observation chart—low BP?

Investigations

Blood tests

May be tailored according to the clinical setting, but are likely to include tests for:

- **Viruses.** <u>hepatitis A</u> (α-HAV IgM, IgG), <u>hepatitis B</u> (HBsAg, α-HBc IgM, IgG, HBeAg, α-HBe, and HBV DNA if HBsAg +ve), <u>hepatitis C</u> (α-HCV, HCV RNA), Epstein–Barr virus (α-EBV IgM, IgG), <u>cytomegalovirus</u> (α-CMV IgM, IgG), <u>herpes simplex virus</u> (α-HSV IgM, IgG).
- **Metabolic diseases.** <u>Haemochromatosis</u> (serum iron, TIBC, ferritin), <u>Wilson's disease</u> (serum copper, caeruloplasmin), α_1-<u>antitrypsin deficiency</u> (α_1-antitrypsin).
- **Drug toxicity** (including random blood alcohol level, <u>paracetamol</u> levels, and urine for toxins).
- **Autoimmune liver disease.** <u>Autoimmune hepatitis</u>, <u>primary biliary cirrhosis</u> (immunoglobulins, α-smooth muscle Ab, α-mitochondrial Ab, α-nuclear Ab, α-LKM1 Ab).
- Initial screen for disorders of <u>bilirubin metabolism</u> may include measurement of conjugated and unconjugated bilirubin. Although unconjugated hyperbilirubinaemia classically seen in <u>Gilbert's syndrome</u>, mixed conjugated/unconjugated usually seen, and measurement is useful only on occasions.
- Haemolysis is assessed by FBC + film, reticulocyte count, and haptoglobins.
- Culture of blood, urine, and ascites may be relevant, as may *Leptospira* serology for suspected <u>leptospirosis</u>.

- Tests to define degree of liver function impairment and associate disease include: FBC + film, clotting profile (PT, INR, APPT), U&Es, venous bicarbonate (± arterial blood gases), LFT screen, glucose.
- Markers of impaired synthetic liver function, as mentioned, and which may be seen in liver failure include ↑ serum bilirubin, ↓albumin, ↑PT/INR, ↓bicarbonate/arterial pH.

Imaging

Indicated in all cases.

- Abdominal <u>ultrasound</u> is easily available, with 91% sensitivity, and 95% specificity for biliary obstruction, and allows identification of mass lesions, exclusion of <u>portal vein thrombosis</u>, hepatic vein thrombosis (<u>Budd–Chiari syndrome</u>) and hepatic arterial impairment (if has Doppler facility), evidence of <u>portal hypertension</u>, demonstration of liver texture (?cirrhotic, fatty infiltration), ascites, and splenomegaly.
- CT is of comparable use, but may be less available, and intravenous contrast to define vessels may be nephrotoxic, particularly in patients with associated renal injury (e.g. <u>hepatorenal syndrome</u>).

<u>Liver biopsy</u>

Rarely required in the initial assessment of recent-onset jaundice. Its 2 roles are as an aid to diagnosis where no cause for jaundice secondary to parenchymal liver injury can be found, and in patients with a proven cause in whom the grade (degree of inflammation) and stage (degree of fibrosis) of liver injury histologically will affect management (e.g. alcoholic hepatitis in patient with established cirrhosis). In the patient with coagulopathy (e.g. INR > 1.3, platelet count < 80×10^9/l) a transjugular liver biopsy may be required.

Management

- Effective management is wholly dependent on the prompt identification of the cause of jaundice, and of the severity of any liver disease, as specific treatment will depend on the type of jaundice and its aetiology and the presence or absence of liver failure (see <u>Acute liver failure</u> and <u>A–Z entries</u>).
- In patients with evidence of biliary disease on initial assessment and imaging, non-invasive modalities should be used for further investigation (e.g. MRI/MRCP), unless there is a high clinical suspicion of large duct obstruction (e.g. biliary stricture, common bile duct stones), in which case ERCP should be planned.

Screening and surveillance of GI cancers

- **Screening** is the one-time application of a test that allows detection of disease at a stage when intervention may significantly improve the natural course and outcome.
- **Surveillance** is the repeated application of such a test over time.

The GI tract, including the hollow organ of the gut, liver, pancreas, and biliary trees, is the site of more cancers and of people dying of cancers than any other organ system. While there is no simple common cause of GI tumours, and a wide variability of tumour incidence between countries, common principles of screening are:

- High risk groups can be identified for several cancers.
- Morbidity and mortality decreased by early diagnosis, ideally in asymptomatic individuals.

Surveillance involves monitoring those people known to have previous GI neoplasia or those with premalignant conditions with the objective of preventing cancer. Some GI tract cancers are so common that screening of the general population at average risk of cancer is being considered. The paradigm is screening for colon cancer (see <u>colon cancer screening</u>).

People at increased risk of digestive tract cancer

- Those with a positive family or personal history of neoplasia. This is best established for colorectal cancer.
- Individuals affected by genetic syndromes predisposing to cancer.
- Patients with other conditions of the GI tract associated with an increased risk of cancer, e.g. inflammatory bowel disease.
- Patients with other diseases associated with an increased risk, e.g. acromegaly.

Colon cancer

For details, see <u>screening for colon cancer</u>.

High-risk individuals

- Those affected by highly penetrant autosomal dominant syndromes such as <u>familial adenomatous polyposis</u>, <u>hereditary non-polyposis colorectal cancer</u>, and the rarer hamartomatous polyposis syndromes <u>Peutz–Jeghers</u>, <u>juvenile polyposis</u>, <u>Cowden's disease</u>).

- those with longstanding inflammatory bowel disease of the colon (see ulcerative colitis and Crohn's disease, surveillance for patients with pancolitis for 8 years and left-sided colitis for 15 years from the onset of symptoms or patients with IBD and primary sclerosing cholangitis (PSC) starting at the time of diagnosis of PSC.
- Those with certain other conditions predisposing to colon cancer, e.g. acromegaly.

Moderate-risk individuals

People with a family history of cancer: indirect evidence suggests marginal benefit for colon surveillance in people with one first-degree relative with colon cancer aged < 45 years or with two affected first-degree relatives, and colonoscopy is recommended either at consultation about family history or between the ages of 35 and 40 years, whichever is later. If initial colonoscopy is clear then repeat at 55 years old.

Other hollow organ GI tract cancers

Oesophageal cancer

Screening for squamous cell cancer is effective in high-incidence areas such as northern China, where 5 year survival approaches 90% for cancers detected through screening. Surveillance of Barrett's mucosa is controversial although widely practised (see Barrett's oesophagus).

Stomach cancer

Screening has been used successfully in Japan where double contrast radiography of the general population picks up 12 cases for every 10 000 screening exams. Most of these undergo surgery: the 5 and 10 year survival is about 90%. There is no evidence of any difference in tumour biology in Japan compared to Europe.

Although retrospective autopsy studies show that post-gastrectomy patients are at 2–4-fold increased risk of gastric cancer, prospective surveillance studies do not provide a strong case for annual screening.

Liver cancer

Rationale

- Patients with cirrhosis are screened for hepatocellular carcinoma because the annual incidence of developing HCC in this group is 1–6% and the vast majority of patients with liver cancer have underlying cirrhosis. Dysplasia on liver biopsy in cirrhotics identified those at high risk of progression to cancer. In hepatitis C related cirrhosis, necroinflammatory activity is an important predictive factor.
- Liver cancer is often diagnosed in previously unknown cirrhotics, and many programmes extend screening to include cirrhotic patients with hepatitis C and those seropositive for hepatitis B virus.

Mechanism of screening

Most screening and surveillance programmes combine measurement of serum alpha fetoprotein and hepatic ultrasound.

- A raised AFP is sensitive for large (over 3 cm) HCC but only found in 35% of tumours of less than 2 cm diameter.
- Sensitivity of ultrasound for tumours over 1 cm is 95%.
- Surveillance intervals vary but 6 monthly is reasonable, given an average tumour doubling time of 4–6 months.

Pancreatic cancer

<u>Pancreatic adenocarcinoma</u> is a common malignancy with a poor 5 year survival. Genetic alterations favouring unrestrained growth are beginning to be defined and some may be hereditary, with an autosomal dominance pattern. Genetic disorders predisposing to pancreatic cancer include <u>multiple endocrine neoplasia</u>, <u>hereditary non–polyposis colorectal cancer</u>, <u>familial adenomatous polyposis</u>, and <u>von Hippel–Lindau syndrome</u>. However, hereditary genetic factors appear to play a role in only about 5% of newly diagnosed cases of pancreatic cancer. There is no evidence relating to screening or surveillance for pancreatic cancer, with the possible exception of screening cases of <u>hereditary pancreatitis</u>, where there is a 40% lifetime risk of developing pancreatic carcinoma.

Cancer of the biliary tract

Cholangiocarcinoma

Sporadic occurrence is uncommon. The tumour usually arises in association with parasitic infestations in localized populations, or with lower frequency but in more global conditions such as <u>primary sclerosing cholangitis</u>. There is no evidence supporting routine screening or surveillance.

Surgically revised anatomy and stomas

Oesophagectomy

Surgical resection is the principal curative treatment for oesophageal cancer. The Ivor-Lewis operation uses a combined abdominal/right thoracic approach; a transhiatal approach can also be used to avoid the need for thoracotomy. Complication rates and outcomes are similar. Early complications include anastomotic leak (0–13%); pulmonary problems including pneumonia and PE (6–50%); recurrent laryngeal nerve injury (1–13%); and cardiac complications (2–25%). Mortality ranges from 1 to 13% with 5 year survival of 1 to 35%.

Usually the stomach is used for oesophageal replacement but the left colon can also be used.

Partial gastrectomy

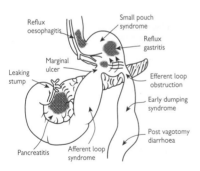

Fig. 1.8 Reproduced from Feldman M, Friedman LS, and Sleisenger MH (2003). *Sleisenger and Fordtran's Gastrointestinal and Liver Disease*, p 804, with permission from Elseiver.

Early complications

Apart from immediate surgical complications such as postoperative haemorrhage and leakage from anastomoses with abscess formation, early satiety and pain 30–60 minutes after meals are the commonest problems. Frequent small meals are needed to minimize these symptoms, which usually improve over 6–12 weeks.

Late complications

Disorders associated with delayed gastric emptying or gastric stasis

- Recurrent or marginal ulcers. Probably related to reduced resistance to acid digestion of jejunal tissue or to partial obstruction due to scarring or oedema. Incomplete vagotomy, persistent hypersecretion of acid (?Zollinger–Ellison syndrome), and continued use of NSAIDs are also possible causes.
- Gastroparesis. Can result from truncal vagotomy and in diabetics. Prokinetics may help but can be very difficult to treat.
- Afferent loop syndrome.

Bile reflux

Gastric cancer

Gastrectomy is associated with twofold risk of gastric cancer at 15 years. This may relate to chronic reflux of intestinal contents into the gastric remnant.

Syndromes associated with rapid gastric emptying

- Post-vagotomy diarrhoea. Incidence is 5–50%. Pathogenesis poorly understood; loperamide and codeine phosphate can help.
- Dumping syndrome, early and late.

Nutritional

- **Weight loss**. Mostly mechanical relating to the degree of resection and the difficulty in eating large meals. A decrease in small bowel transit time may be contributory.
- **Anaemia** is common. Iron deficiency is caused by less absorbable ferric iron in an alkaline medium, and bypass of the duodenum which is a major site of iron absorption. Intrinsic factor is lost after total gastrectomy and contributes to macrocytic anaemia: hypochlorhydria reduces B12 binding to food. B12 absorption may be reduced by bacterial overgrowth in afferent loop.
- **Bone disease**. Calcium loss may result in osteopenia.

Ileostomies

There are three common varieties: the Brooke (non-continent) ileostomy, the Koch (continent) reservoir, and ileal pouches anastomosed to the anus.

- The **Brooke ileostomy** is not continent and involves suturing the mucosal surface of the small intestine to the skin (see diagram): this is necessary because ileal contents are very irritant to the serosa.
- The continent ileostomy was first reported in 1969 by Nils Koch. It is a reservoir made from terminal ileum with a nipple valve providing continence in 90% in the best series. However the price is additional operations and this operation is now rarely performed.

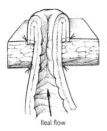

Fig.1.9 Brooke ileostomy*

Ileal flow

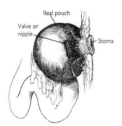

Fig.1.10 Koach (continent) ileostomy*

Ileal pouch
Valve or nipple
Stoma

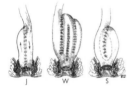

J   W   S

Fig 1.11 Ileal pouch–anal anastomosis*
*Reproduced from Feldman M, Friedman LS, and Sleisenger MH (2003). *Sleisenger and Fordtran's Gastrointestinal and Liver Disease*, with permission from Elseiver.

- The <u>ileal pouch–anal anastomosis</u> is now the procedure of choice for patients with UC or FAP. An ileal reservoir is constructed and the ileal mucosa attached to the midanal canal. Different designs for the pouch exist; the simplest is the J pouch and results are no worse than for other types. Average day-time stool frequency is 6 times a day and once at night. Night-time incontinence is common. 30% of patients wear a pad for protection. Pouch failure rates are 6–10%.

Physiology and functional implications of ileostomy

- **Loss of the absorptive capacity of the colon** means that all three types of ileostomy should discharge 300–800 g material daily: 90% is water, and the small bowel is less good than the colon at conserving sodium in conditions of low salt intake or high salt loss; patients with ileostomies have obligatory sodium losses of 30–40 mEq/day. The increased water loss in stools contributes to relative oliguria and urolithiasis (around 5%, usually urate of calcium stones).
- **Resection of terminal ileum** (often necessary in <u>Crohn's disease</u> but not in UC or FAP) can lead to reduced bile acid reabsorption (secondary bile acids disappear from bile after ileostomy: no important metabolic consequences have been recognized) and malabsorption of vitamin B12.

Complications of ileal pouches

Overall morbidity is still around 25–30%; main complications include:
- Early postoperative **pelvic sepsis** (5% of patients with UC). Commonly due to anastomotic leakage. Image with CT; treat conservatively or by CT-guided drainage.
- **Abdominal sepsis** or peritonitis (incidence 5%) is more ominous with a higher chance of ultimate pouch failure.
- **Stricturing** of the ileoanal anastomosis is common; small bowel obstruction occurs in 15% of cases.
- <u>Pouchitis</u> **(10–15%)**
- **Sexual dysfunction.** Impotence develops in 1.5% of men. Dyspareunia develops in 7% of women.
- **Reduced fertility in women.**

Ileo-rectal anastomosis

This is sometimes done for ulcerative colitis and frequently done for Crohn's colitis if the rectum is relatively spared from disease.

The aim is to remove most of the diseased colon and reduce many of the complications of colitis while retaining continence.

Advantages
- Avoids permanent stoma.
- Avoids risk of damage to pelvic nerves.
- Easy to perform.

Disadvantages
- Subsequent proctectomy required in up to 35% of patients.
- Risk of cancer 15% at 25 years.

<u>Pouchitis</u>

See A to Z section.

<u>Short bowel syndrome</u>

See A to Z section.

Unintentional weight loss

Background

- Unexplained, unintentional weight loss is a common reason for referral to the gastroenterology clinic. This often provides an interesting diagnostic challenge, not least because of the huge range of causes (see table), and the need for a careful history and examination.
- Weight loss is not the same as low weight; a patient whose <u>body mass index</u> (BMI) has unintentionally fallen from 30 to 20 in 2 months requires as intensive investigation as the patient who is obviously malnourished.

Causes of unintentional weight loss

Occult malignancy (e.g. especially <u>pancreatic cancer</u>, <u>gastric cancer</u>)	Chronic inflammatory disease (e.g. <u>Crohn's disease</u>)
Hyperthyroidism	Clinical depression
Severe cardiorespiratory disease (e.g. 'cardiac cachexia')	Chronic infection (e.g. <u>TB</u>, abdominal abscess, subacute bacterial endocarditis (SBE))
Malabsorption (e.g. <u>chronic pancreatitis</u>, <u>Whipple's disease</u>, <u>coeliac disease</u>)	Autoimmune disease (e.g. systemic lupus erythematosus, rheumatoid)
Swallowing difficulties (e.g. oesophageal stricture)	Endocrine disease (e.g. Addison's) Diabetes mellitus
<u>Anorexia nervosa</u>	Neuromuscular disease/dementia
Chronic liver disease (especially in alcoholics with malnutrition)	Starvation/malnutrition
<u>HIV disease</u>	

History

A careful history may make the diagnosis. **How much weight** has been lost, and over what period of time? Is there **evidence** for this (e.g. weight chart, photos, change in dress size)? Clarify that the patient has not been intending to lose weight, and take a dietary history. Is there a problem with perceived **body image** suggesting <u>anorexia nervosa</u> (patients with this will rarely seek out help to gain weight, but may well be encouraged to attend by concerned relatives, and the psychiatric nature of this condition often results in significant deception surrounding eating habits)? Is the appetite good, or is the patient anorexic ('off their food'—often seen in malignancy)? Is the patient depressed (explore recent life changes, e.g. bereavement, social isolation, redundancy)? Have other clinical problems recently worsened, explaining weight loss (e.g. severe chronic obstructive airway disease)? Ask about swallowing (see <u>Approach to mouth and swallowing</u>), and chest symptoms (? TB, lung cancer). Is there any history of fever? Are there any areas of pain or discomfort? What about their bowels (change in bowel habit may suggest <u>colon cancer</u> or <u>Crohn's disease;</u> steatorrhoea suggests malabsorption (e.g. <u>chronic pancreatitis</u>)). Are there any risk factors for <u>HIV</u>, or history of AIDS-defining illnesses (HIV-wasting disease was historically known as 'slim's disease' in Africa).

Examination

A careful examination is essential (see <u>Approach to GI examination</u>). Does the patient look thin and unwell? Dishevelled patient with poor dentition may have malnutrition (e.g. associated with <u>alcohol dependency</u>). Are their clothes obviously loose-fitting (change in belt notch is good clue)? Look for signs of hyperthyroidism (agitated, warm palms, palma erythema, fine tremor, tachycardia, goitre). Splinter haemorrhages suggest SBE; fine, lanugo hair on face may suggest <u>anorexia nervosa</u>. Look for lymphadenopathy, and carefully exclude a heart murmur. Exclude abdominal masses (but abdominal imaging will be necessary, as certain organs, such as pancreas, are poorly identified on examination). Perform a rectal examination (? large prostate, low rectal lesion). Test the urine for blood, glucose, and white cells. Don't forget to **weigh the patient** (surprising how often this is forgotten, but it provides invaluable evidence for subsequent review). Calculate the <u>BMI</u>.

Investigations

Focused tests will be guided by findings on history and examination. In patients with significant weight loss, but no obvious cause, non-invasive investigations may give clues to aetiology:

- Bloods: FBC, ESR, CRP, U&Es, LFTs, glucose, autoantibodies (e.g. rheumatoid factor, antinuclear antibodies), iron studies, vitamin B12 levels, folate, coeliac antibodies, thyroid function tests. Serum tumour markers rarely of use in absence of any specific clues, but consider prostatic-specific antigen (PSA) in elderly male with weight loss.
- CXR.
- Abdominal ultrasound/CT scan.
- Invasive tests (e.g. endoscopy, colonoscopy) may be needed where there is a high clinical suspicion of upper or lower GI malignancy (e.g. iron deficiency in setting of weight loss), but are rarely indicated as first-line investigations, in absence of other indicators.
- Associated pyrexia of unknown origin (PUO) requires multiple blood cultures from different sites, urine culture (including x3 early morning urines for TB), and echocardiogram (even in absence of a murmur).

Management

- Entirely dependent on making a diagnosis as to cause of weight loss.
- In patient with no obvious cause, and normal initial investigations, reassessment and reweighing in 4–6 weeks is a very useful strategy. It is not uncommon for no ongoing weight loss to be demonstrated, despite the patient's perception to the contrary. This hard evidence may allow further invasive tests to be avoided, reassurance to be given, and other patient issues to be addressed. Conversely, documented ongoing weight loss necessitates more intensive investigations.

Well patients with abnormal liver tests

The wide availability of automated biochemical analysis of blood has resulted in the increasing identification of abnormal liver function tests (LFTs) in the otherwise well patient. For example, 50% of patients with primary biliary cirrhosis are now identified whilst asymptomatic.

The clinical skill is in:
- Identifying the cause without employing an analysis of all possible aetiologies of liver injury.
- Defining the extent of underlying liver disease.
- Identifying those who need to be exposed to the risk of liver biopsy.
- Deciding who needs long-term follow-up or treatment.

Virtually any cause of liver disease or biliary obstruction (see Approach to recent-onset jaundice) may present in the asymptomatic phase, and so the usual rules of making a diagnosis apply.

History

Alcohol; drugs (recreational, prescription, over-the-counter, herbal remedies, review the drug chart. Can derangement of LFTs be correlated with their introduction?); risks for viral hepatitis (blood transfusions, IV drug misuse, sexual contacts); autoimmune diseases (e.g. thyroid disease, inflammatory bowel disease); family history; other medical problems (e.g. diabetes mellitus).

Examination

The patient may be asymptomatic, but full examination is essential. Is there hepatomegaly? Are there signs of chronic liver disease (see Approach to gastrointestinal examination), e.g. palmar erythema, clubbing, spider naevi, and of extent of liver injury, e.g. splenomegaly, ascites? Are there hints to aetiology (e.g. obesity, needle marks, tattoos, xanthelasma)?

Investigation and management approach

What is the pattern of LFT derangement?
- A hepatitic picture (i.e. raised ALT/AST) may suggest chronic hepatitis B or C, non-alcoholic fatty liver disease (NAFLD), alcohol liver disease,

or <u>autoimmune hepatitis</u>. ALT > AST suggests NAFLD or viral hepatitis, AST > ALT is more characteristic of <u>alcoholic liver disease</u> (especially if GGT, MCV elevated). Remember to consider other sources of AST (e.g. striated muscle—suggested by raised creatine kinase).

- A cholestatic picture (i.e. raised ALP/GGT) may point towards <u>primary biliary cirrhosis</u> (PBC) or <u>primary sclerosing cholangitis</u> (PSC), <u>hepatic granulomas</u>. A cholestatic pattern also necessitates exclusion of large duct biliary obstruction (e.g. <u>biliary stricture</u>, <u>pancreatic cancer</u>) and liver metastases. Consider an extrahepatic source of ALP, such as bone (especially if isolated rise and GGT normal).

- Isolated raised GGT is a frequent finding with automated blood analysis. May occur due to alcohol excess (? ↑ AST, MCV), drugs (e.g. steroids, anticonvulsants, statins), fatty liver. Invasive, extensive investigation rarely yields significant pathology. Patients should have tests repeated a few months later, and investigated further only if additional biochemical abnormalities, significantly increasing GGT, or new clinical problem.

- Abdominal <u>ultrasound</u> should be performed in all cases. Heterogeneous fatty infiltration is consistent with NAFLD, a common finding in this setting.

- Further imaging (e.g. CT, ERCP, MRCP) may be necessary, depending on ultrasound findings.

- <u>Liver biopsy</u> should be considered if no cause is identified and LFTs remain abnormal over 6–12 months (e.g. > ×2 ULN), and despite initial interventions. It may also be needed in order to define the degree of liver injury where a cause is identified (e.g. viral hepatitis, <u>alcoholic liver disease</u>).

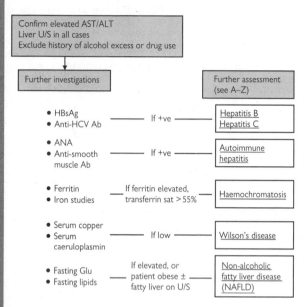

Confirm elevated AST/ALT
Liver U/S in all cases
Exclude history of alcohol excess or drug use

Further investigations

Further assessment
(see A–Z)

- HBsAg
- Anti-HCV Ab —————— If +ve —————— Hepatitis B / Hepatitis C

- ANA
- Anti-smooth
  muscle Ab —————— If +ve —————— Autoimmune hepatitis

- Ferritin
- Iron studies —— If ferritin elevated, transferrin sat > 55% —— Haemochromatosis

- Serum copper
- Serum
  caeruloplasmin —————— If low —————— Wilson's disease

- Fasting Glu
- Fasting lipids —— If elevated, or patient obese ± fatty liver on U/S —— Non-alcoholic fatty liver disease (NAFLD)

Fig. 1.12 Approach to investigation of raised transaminases.

If all the above tests are negative, and LFT derangement persists, consider: undeclared alcohol excess and alcoholic liver disease (especially if AST > ALT, raised GGT, and elevated MCV, coeliac disease, glycogen storage disease, Addison's disease, and α-antitrypsin deficiency.

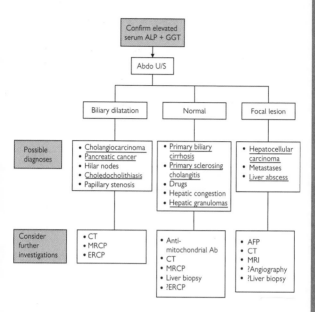

Fig. 1.15 Approach to investigation of raised cholestatic LFTs.

Treatment

Depends on diagnosis. If no clear cause is identified, however, and the patient presents with a hepatitic pattern of LFT derangement, initial approaches include advising about losing weight, cutting alcohol intake, and stopping all possible medications.

Section 2: An A to Z of gastroenterology and hepatology

A

Abetalipoproteinaemia

Autosomal recessive disorder of lipid metabolism resulting from mutation in the gene for a microsomal triglyceride transfer protein. There is
steatorrhoea and malabsorption of fat soluble vitamins A, D, E, K,
ataxia, retinitis pigmentosa, acanthocytic erythrocytes. Reduced synthesis
of apolipoprotein B leads to absence of chylomicrons, LDL, VLDL. Small
intestinal biopsy shows lipid droplets in intestinal epithelial cells. Treatment involves substituting medium chain triglycerides for long chain
triglycerides.

Acetaminophen

See: paracetamol overdose.

Achalasia

Disorder characterized by failure of relaxation of lower oesophageal
sphincter and aperistalsis of oesophageal body, leading to functional obstruction at lower end of the oesophagus, food stasis, and oesophageal
dilatation. Increased risk of **squamous cell cancer** (see oesophageal
tumours), presumed due to stasis of food and mucosal irritation.

Aetiology. Ganglion cells of myenteric plexus are reduced but cause is
unknown: viruses and autoimmune mechanisms have been proposed. The
so-called 'non-adrenergic, non-cholinergic' inhibitory innervation (mostly
nitric oxide mediated) is impaired, which mediates sphincter relaxation.

Clinical features. Usual symptomatic onset age 30–50 years, with
dysphagia, which is often intermittent. Non-bilious, non-acid reflux is
common feature, as is chest pain, which may relate to oesophageal
spasm. Heartburn sometimes reported, but true reflux is (predictably)
rare.

Investigation. Diagnosis made on basis of history, radiological,
endoscopic, and manometric findings. Chest X-ray may show an air fluid
level in a dilated oesophagus (see figure). Barium swallow shows dilated
oesophagus with reduced peristalsis. Endoscopy essential in all patients
to exclude mucosal pathology and pseudoachalsia.
Oesophageal manometry shows raised lower oesophageal sphincter
pressure and incomplete or absent sphincter relaxation. Differential
diagnosis of achalasia includes oesophageal spasm, trypanosomiasis
(Chagas' disease), and pseudoachalasia.

Management. Options include drugs, endoscopy, and surgery.
- Drugs do not work well: nitrates and calcium channel blockers
  provide, at best, short-lived effects on lower oesophageal sphincter
  pressure and have side effects. BOTULINUM TOXIN injected into the
  sphincter does reduce sphincter pressure and relieve symptoms, but
  the effects are short-lived and repeated injections are necessary
  every 6–12 months.

- Endoscopic dilatation performed using 30, 35, or 40 mm balloons passed over a guide wire. The balloon is inflated for 1–2 min. Response is good in 60–70% patients but many patients need more than 1 procedure. <u>Endoscopic complications</u> include perforation (1–5%, commoner with larger balloons) and reflux (about 10%).
- Surgical myotomy effective in 90% but causes reflux in 10%: an anti-reflux procedure is often done at the same time (see <u>anti-reflux procedures</u>). Laparoscopic myotomy is becoming more available and for some patients is the treatment of choice. Practical approach to treatment is to start with balloon dilatation since many patients will do well with this: if there is rapid relapse a myotomy can be offered.

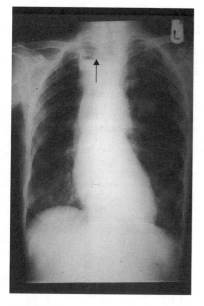

Fig. 2.1 CXR in patient with achalasia, showing air–fluid level (arrowed) within dilated oesophagus.

Achlorhydria

Defined as failure of intragastric pH to fall below 4 under stimulation with pentagastrin. In absence of gastric acid, negative feedback control of gastrin is lost and hypergastrinaemia is seen (see box).

<u>Gastrinoma</u> (Zollinger–Ellinson syndrome) may be suspected and acid secretory studies may be necessary. Atrophic gastritis may be associated with reduced intrinsic factor secretion (see <u>pernicious anaemia</u>).

Acquired immune deficiency syndrome

See: <u>HIV and the gut</u> and <u>HIV and the liver</u>.

Acromegaly and GI tract

- Increased risk of <u>colonic polyps</u> and <u>colon cancer</u> in acromegaly: precise extent of risk unclear. British Society of Gastroenterology guidelines recommend initial screening by colonoscopy at age 40, repeated every 5 years (3 years if increased risk—adenoma at first colonoscopy or increased IGF-1 levels). Evidence for this based on single centre experience showing 13–14 times increased risk of colon cancer, particularly right-sided (Jenkins, PJ and Fairclough, PD. (2001). *Clin. Endocrinol.* **55:** 727). Larger studies suggest × 2–3 risk over controls.
- Colonoscopy often difficult due to long redundant colon. Conventional <u>bowel preparation</u> is less effective in acromegalics, and double quantities, preferably of osmotically active polyethylene glycol-based solutions (e.g. Kleenprep), are suggested.
- Clinical enlargement of spleen, liver, or kidneys is unusual and warrants further investigation. Other GI complications include macroglossia and those relating to the use of the somatostation analogue <u>OCTREOTIDE</u> (used because it suppresses growth hormone secretion and can shrink a proportion of pituitary tumours because of their high somatostatin receptor density).

Causes of achlorhydria

- <u>Atrophic gastritis</u>, either autoimmune such as <u>pernicious anaemia</u> or environmental such as *Helicobacter pylori*
- Mucolipidosis type 4 (crippled parietal cells due to absent protein needed for vacuolar trafficking)
- Previous <u>gastrectomy</u> or vagotomy
- Rare tumours that produce hormones inhibiting acid secretion (e.g. somatostatinoma—see <u>pancreatic endocrine tumours</u>)
- Severe hypocalcaemia impairs parietal cell acid secretion
- Acid secretion is also reduced in AIDS

Actinomycosis

Subacute or chronic inflammatory disease caused by a variety of fermentative actinomycetes causing multiple abscesses and draining tracts. Requirements for active tissue invasion in humans include a prior break in epithelium (e.g. post-surgery), tissue ischaemia, or prior infection by other organisms. Most cases involve the face or neck. Abdominal involvement is rare and is usually associated with perforating/fistulating GI conditions (appendicitis, diverticulitis, surgery, foreign bodies—such as fish bones). May present as slowly growing tumours. Classically, sinus tracts contain sulphur granules. Diagnosis made by culture and microscopy. Antibiotic treatment includes augmentin + metronidazole possibly with an aminoglycoside (e.g. gentamicin).

Acute fatty liver of pregnancy (AFLP)

Background

- Rare disease, characterized by mitochondrial cytopathy, with incidence 1:14 000 pregnancies in USA.
- Unlike other liver conditions specifically related to pregnancy (HELLP syndrome and obstetric cholestasis), AFLP frequently associated with acute liver failure.
- Pathogenesis unclear, but associated with inherited long chain 3-hydroxyacyl coenzyme A dehydrogenase (LCHAD) deficiency, first pregnancies, and in those carrying male fetuses or twins.

Clinical features

- Usual presentation at 34–37 weeks of pregnancy, only rarely before 20 weeks or after delivery.
- Characteristic presentation with nausea, vomiting, abdominal pain, and confusion, with pre-eclampsia (thirst, headache, blurred vision, proteinuria, hypertension, peripheral oedema).
- Jaundice common (in contrast to HELLP syndrome), with additional features of acute liver failure (hypoglycaemia, bleeding, hepatic encephalopathy). Pruritus may be an initial symptom, and clinical overlap with obstetric cholestasis rarely seen. Diabetes insipidus reported.

Investigations

See also Approach to liver problems in pregnancy.

- Blood results may show ↑ WCC, ↑ AST/ALT (but usually < 750 U/l), ↑ bilirubin x6–8 ULN (i.e. approximately 100µmol/l). ↑ PT suggests significant liver impairment, and ↑ uric acid, urea, and creatinine also common.
- Imaging with ultrasound should be performed, in part to exclude other conditions (e.g. biliary obstruction, subcapsular haematoma), but no diagnostic features of AFLP.
- Liver biopsy classically shows microvesicular fat. Rarely performed during pregnancy if delivery to be expedited. May be performed by transjugular route, if coagulopathy present.

Management

- Intensive care setting, with specialist hepatology and obstetric input essential. Prompt delivery is cornerstone of treatment, with management of <u>acute liver failure</u> and <u>hepatic encephalopathy</u> as necessary.
- DDAVP may be required for diabetes insipidus.
- <u>Liver transplantation</u> has been successful, but is rarely required unless delivery is delayed.
- Maternal mortality < 1% with specialist care, and perinatal mortality 7%.
- Mother, infant, and father should be tested for the G1528C mutation in LCHAD.

Acute intermittent porphyria

See: porphyrias.

Acute pancreatitis (AP)

Background

Incidence varies (5–25 per 100 000). Alcohol dependency and gallstones account for most cases (see first table). Evidence of acute pancreatic inflammation (sometimes with other organ involvement) differentiates AP from chronic pancreatitis, but clinical distinction may be difficult. Activation of trypsinogen, leading to pancreatic autodigestion, occurs early, but role of primary pancreatic duct obstruction remains uncertain.

Clinical features

Severe, unremitting epigastric pain radiating to the back, with nausea and vomiting. Signs of shock may be present. Bruising in flanks ('Grey–Turner sign') or umbilical area ('Cullen's sign') seen in 1%, and indicates haemorrhagic pancreatitis with poor prognosis. Ileus is common.

Complications

Local complications: inflammatory mass, infected necrosis, pancreatic pseudocyst formation, pseudoaneurysm, obstructive jaundice, gastric outflow obstruction, portal vein thrombosis.
Systemic complications: sepsis, acute respiratory distress syndrome, acute renal failure, disseminated intravascular coagulation.

- Severe AP usually associated with pancreatic necrosis, which occurs in 20–30% of cases of AP. Infected necrosis occurs in 30–70% of cases of pancreatic necrosis, and accounts for > 80% of deaths.
- 5–10% overall mortality, with first episode of AP x10 more likely to lead to organ failure than recurrent episodes. Obesity is linked with more severe course. Half of deaths occur in first 14 days.

Investigation and assessment of severity

- Serum amylase makes the diagnosis (> 1000 U/l in appropriate clinical setting), but poor correlation with disease severity.
- FBC, U&E, LFT, Glu, Ca, CRP, Bicarb essential in all (see Glasgow criteria table). Serum ALT/AST > 150U/l is > 95% specific for gallstones as cause of AP, rather than alcohol.
- Difficult to predict course/prognosis at onset, but various scoring systems have been verified (e.g. Ransom/Glasgow/APACHE II). No criteria 100% reliable, and may be hampered by need for assessment at 48 hours. Best at predicting patients with mild disease, rather than those at risk of severe attack. High serum CRP (e.g. > 210mg/l at 48–72 hours) appears highly sensitive for necrotizing pancreatitis. Other indicators of poor prognosis include clinical impression of severe disease at 24 hours, obesity (body mass index > 30), > 2 Glasgow criteria (see table), and organ failure.

- Abdominal <u>ultrasound</u> excludes stones in gallbladder and biliary dilatation, but often poor views of pancreas.
- Plain AXR may show 'sentinel loop' due to local small bowel ileus. Pleural effusion on CXR correlated with severe disease.
- Contrast-enhanced CT scan should be performed 48 hours after clinical onset, unless pancreatitis clinically mild, as necrosis predicts prolonged course and potential mortality (see third table). CT also defines peri-pancreatic inflammation, and evidence of chronic pancreatitis (e.g. calcification). MRI/MRCP may also define pancreatic duct disruption.

Causes of acute pancreatitis

<u>Gallstones</u>/sludge (35%)	Drugs (e.g. HAART for HIV, azathioprine, NSAIDs, valproate)
Alcohol (30%)	
Hypertriglyceridaemia	<u>Pancreas divisum</u>
Post-<u>ERCP</u>	<u>Hereditary pancreatitis</u>
Ampullary disease (e.g. stenosis, <u>sphincter of Oddi dysfunction</u>)	Infection (e.g. mumps, coxsackie, *Ascaris*, *Chlonorchis*, scorpion bites)
Hypercalcaemia	Trauma
<u>Pancreatic cancer</u>	Cause unknown/idiopathic (30%)

Modified Glasgow criteria

WBC > 15 × 10⁹/l	Urea > 16 mmol/l
Glucose >10 mmol/l	Ca^{2+}< 2 mmol/l
LDH > 600 IU/l	Albumin < 32 g/l
AST > 200 IU/l	PaO_2 < 8 kPa

More factors, worse the prognosis.

Correlation of pancreatic necrosis with outcome in AP

CT finding	Morbidity	Mortality
Necrosis	82%	23%
No necrosis	6%	0%

Management
- Mortality low with prompt intensive care for those who need it; 20% if specialist referral delayed.
- Expert supportive therapy paramount.
- Intravascular volume expansion (colloid/crystalloid) vital, as large losses due to ileus, 'third spacing' in peri-pancreatic tissue. Consider central line insertion to monitor fluids.
- Analgesia (OPIATES usually required).
- Enteral feeding (naso-jejunal tube) may reduce bacterial translocation, so preferable to TPN (but ensure ileus resolved). Start within 72 hours.
- Prophylactic antibiotics for severe AP remains controversial, but recent evidence suggests no reduction in mortality. If clinical suspicion of sepsis, take cultures urgently (including aspiration of necrotic collections) and give high dose IV antibiotics (e.g. imipenem, 3rd generation CEPHALOSPORIN + METRONIDAZOLE), guided by microbiology. Surgery in pancreatic necrosis only rarely needed.
- Urgent ERCP + sphincterotomy for presumed gallstone pancreatitis only clearly indicated if Bn > 70 mmol/l (and not settling at 48 hours), or definite cholangitis. ERCP in cases of gallstone pancreatitis not advised, as may worsen pancreatitis further, and stones already passed in 80% of cases. In gallstone pancreatitis, cholecystectomy should be performed as soon as AP settled (prior to discharge).

Adenoma-to-carcinoma hypothesis

There is good epidemiological, clinical, pathological, and molecular evidence that most colon cancers arise within previously benign adenomas. Cancer cells in a malignant polyp share the same molecular alterations as in surrounding adenoma cells, but have additional mutations that are critical for malignant behaviour.

There are two general stages in colon carcinogenesis. **Tumour initiation** involves the formation of an adenoma. All adenomas are thought to arise from an initial loss of APC gene function. Sporadic adenomas arise through acquired somatic mutations of both alleles; this takes years to occur so these polyps occur late in life and are relatively uncommon. In familial adenomatous polyposis, one APC allele is inherited in a mutated form, the second mutation takes much less time to acquire, so polyps occur at a younger age—FAP is a disorder of tumour initiation. The progression to cancer is a consequence of number of polyps rather than increased malignant potential of individual adenomas.

The second step involves progresson from adenomas to carcinoma and is termed **tumour promotion**. It involves mutations or deletions in tumour suppressor genes located on chromosomes 17 (p53) and 18 (Deleted in colon cancer or DCC gene). Hereditary non-polyposis cancer (HNPCC) is marked by an accelerated tumour promotion stage: adenomas progress more rapidly to cancer, which is why surveillance intervals in HNPCC need to be shortened.

Adenovirus

- Serotypes 40 and 41 of subgroup F of this large family of DNA viruses are known as enteric adenoviruses because of an association with acute watery diarrhoea in infants and children (incidence 4–10% in developed countries, second in importance to rotavirus as viral cause of infectious diarrhoea). Non-enteric adenovirus types have been found in AIDS patients with diarrhoea.
- Symptoms include watery diarrhoea and vomiting, with respiratory symptoms and low grade fever. Diagnosis requires immune electron microscopy. Incubation period 7 days; virus shed in stool for 10–14 days.

No specific treatment: goals of therapy are to prevent dehydration and maintain nutritional intake. Complications can include lactose intolerance and malabsorption. See also Approach to acute diarrhoea.

Afferent loop syndrome

- One of a number of <u>post-gastrectomy syndromes</u>, usually associated with <u>Billroth</u> II (polya) <u>gastrectomy</u> (see <u>Approach to surgically revised anatomy and stomas</u> and <u>dumping</u>). The afferent loop (the segment of small intestine leading to the stomach) can fill with bile, particularly when the gallbladder contracts after a meal. This causes upper abdominal pain after meals, often relieved by vomiting bilious fluid. Obstruction may be caused by stenosis of the anastomosis, adhesions, twisting of the intestinal loop, and rarely by tumour, stones, or enteroliths.
- Diagnosis made by showing dilatation of the afferent loop and the site of obstruction. This is possible with barium studies, scintigraphy (HIDA scanning), CT, or MRI.
- The term is sometimes confused with small bowel <u>bacterial overgrowth</u> (incidence 50% in Billroth II gastrectomy) producing classical symptoms of weight loss, diarrhoea, steatorrhoea, and deficiency of B12 and fat soluble vitamins.

Alagille's syndrome

A familial term of intrahepatic cholestasis. Autosomal dominant condition (1:100 000 live births) characterized by multisystem abnormalities (hepatic, renal, cardiac, facial, skeletal, ocular). May present with persistent cholestasis, pruritis, hepatomegaly, and failure to thrive (the latter due to severe gastro-oesophageal reflux (see <u>Approach to dyspepsia and gastro-oesophageal reflux</u>) and malabsorption due to <u>pancreatic insufficiency</u>). Treatment involves intensive nutritional support and, although normal liver function regained in 50% by adolescence, others require <u>liver transplantation</u>.

Albumin (use in liver disease)

> 'You like potato and I like potahto ... let's call the whole thing off'. Sung by Fred Astaire 1937.

- Few issues cause greater disagreement in hepatology than use of human albumin solutions (e.g. 20% HAS) in patients with cirrhosis, ascites, and hypoalbuminaemia. Problem arises due to absence of well designed randomized controlled studies.
- Supporters (usually hepatologists) argue that HAS has been used for years with few problems, helps to maintain intravascular volume and thus renal perfusion (with recent data suggesting significant benefit with HAS + <u>TERLIPRESSIN</u> in <u>hepatorenal syndrome</u> (Ortega, R *et al.* (2002) Hepatology; **36**: 941)).

- Opponents point to data (SAFE Study Investigators (2004). *N. Engl. J. Med.* **350:** 2247) suggesting no benefit of albumin over saline in critically ill patients (but this study included a hugely variable patient group, and not liver patients); only transient improvement in plasma oncotic pressure with HAS; and argue that adequate volume expansion, rather than HAS *per se*, is the key.
- End of the day, money will talk. With increased costs of blood products (500 ml 4.5% HAS x10 more expensive than 4% Gelofusin® solution), newer colloid starches with longer plasma half-life likely to be the future.

Alcohol dependency

Epidemiology

Alcohol is the third leading cause of preventable death in USA (behind smoking and obesity). Life-time prevalence of dependency approximately 10% in men, 4% in women in USA/Europe.

Clinical features

As well as <u>alcohol-related liver disease</u>, most other systems damaged: gastrointestinal (<u>oesophagitis</u>, <u>gastritis</u>, <u>acute</u> and <u>chronic pancreatitis</u>); neurological (cortical atrophy/dementia, <u>Wernicke's encephalopathy</u>, peripheral neuropathy); endocrine (pseudo-Cushing's, diabetes mellitus, hypoglycaemia, alcoholic ketoacidosis, hypoandrogenization); cardiovascular (dilated cardiomyopathy, conduction defects). Important cause of malnutrition, and increased risk of range of malignancies (e.g. <u>pancreatic/oesophageal</u>/<u>gastric cancer</u>, <u>hepatocellular</u>, bladder carcinoma).

Assessment

- Dependency is not defined by a given quantity of alcohol consumed.
- On examination, features of chronic liver disease may be present (see <u>Approach to gastrointestinal examination</u>).
- Although blood tests may suggest alcohol excess (↑AST> ALT, ↑ GGT, ↑ MCV, ↓ platelets), at least 3 of the 8 DSM-IV criteria for alcohol dependency should be met (see box).

Management

Many physicians have a nihilistic view towards the patient with alcohol dependency but a number of interventions are of benefit. Aim of treatment is to stop alcohol, or reduce to manageable levels (complete cessation is usually the most effective option in the patient with dependency).

- Psychological assessment and support is the cornerstone of treating dependency. First step involves an unequivocal clarification of the problems being caused by alcohol, and an assessment of the patient's 'readiness for change'.
- Specialist alcohol support agencies are available (e.g. Alcoholics Anonymous (AA)), and the patient should be given clear details of how to access services.
- Range of medications have been used to maintain abstinence in conjunction with psychological input, including disulfuram (which causes nausea and vomiting with coincident alcohol), and acamprosate (stimulates GABA transmission, and maintains abstinence in 12–18% of patients, compared with 5–7% on placebo).
- In the patient with severe physical dependency (e.g. marked withdrawal symptoms), who is committed to stopping, admission to hospital for acute detoxification may be indicated, and <u>alcohol withdrawal</u> pre-empted and treated prophylactically.

Criteria for alcohol dependency
- Continued drinking despite physical or psychological consequences caused or excacerbated by alcohol
- Neglect of other activities
- Inordinate time spent drinking or recovering
- Drinking more or over a longer period than intended
- Inability to control drinking
- Tolerance (defined as increased amounts needed for effect)
- Withdrawal symptoms on cessation of alcohol
- Drinking to relieve or avoid withdrawal symptoms

CAGE questionnaire is also a useful screening tool for problem drinking
1. Have you ever felt the need to **C**ut down on your drinking?
2. Have people **A**nnoyed you by criticizing your drinking?
3. Have you ever felt bad or **G**uilty about your drinking?
4. Have you ever had a drink first thing in the morning to steady your nerves or hangover (**E**ye-opener)?

Alcoholic liver disease

Epidemiology and pathogenesis

- Alcohol accounts for 40–80% of cases of cirrhosis in the developed world, and 1:6 of all casualty admissions in the UK. Consumption usually reported as units (1 unit = 1 glass of wine, 1/2 pint/270 ml of 4% beer, or small measure of 40% spirit), with safe limit debated, but currently set in UK at 21 units/week for women, 28 units for men. In individuals drinking > 40 units/week, 6–8% will develop cirrhosis within 12 years, with 20–30% of long-term heavy drinkers developing significant liver disease.
- Alcohol excess very strongly linked to anti-social behavior and domestic violence, and risks of binge drinking amongst young people are increasingly recognized. See also <u>alcohol dependency</u>.
- Number of clinical patterns of disease may occur.

Alcohol-induced fatty liver

Results from heavy alcohol intake over months. Usually asymptomatic, but associated with hepatomegaly, mildly elevated transaminases, and increased liver echogenicity on <u>ultrasound</u>. History should allow differentiation from <u>non-alcoholic fatty liver disease (NAFLD)</u>. Although usually resolves after several weeks of abstinence, progression to cirrhosis in 20% who continue to drink, and very rarely may present with <u>acute liver failure</u>.

Alcoholic hepatitis

Usually develops in those drinking very large amounts over a long period. An undefined trigger (usually develops in absence of recent increased intake) initiates severe proinflammatory response, associated with oxidant injury and neutrophilic liver infiltration. In those who recover from alcoholic hepatitis, cirrhosis develops in >10% per year.

Clinical features: Acute onset of malaise, jaundice, anorexia, diarrhoea, and nausea. Tender hepatomegaly and signs of decompensated liver disease (e.g. ascites, <u>hepatic encephalopathy</u>), which may worsen after hospital admission, despite stopping alcohol. Malnutrition is common, correlates with poor prognosis, and > 50% of total energy intake in these patients comes from alcohol. Mortality 60% in alcoholic hepatitis relates to the sequelae of liver failure—sepsis, renal failure, and variceal bleeding.

Investigations

- FBC may show ↑WCC (50% cases), ↓platelets (direct toxic alcohol effect, or due to hypersplensim), ↑MCV.
- U&Es may show ↓Na$^+$, K$^+$, Ca^{2+}, Mg^{2+}. Renal failure may be due to sepsis, dehydration, or <u>hepatorenal syndrome</u>.
- <u>Liver function tests</u>: AST/ALT characteristically < x3 ULN, with AST > ALT in > 70%. ↑ bilirubin and PT incorporated into discriminant function (DF) test (see box) predicts mortality (DF > 31 correlates with >35% 4 week mortality), but does not differentiate alcoholic hepatitis from end-stage liver failure/cirrhosis.

- ↑ Acute phase markers (CRP, ferritin).
- <u>Liver biopsy</u> establishes diagnosis (and excludes/identifies underlying cirrhosis), with features of hepatocyte ballooning and necrosis, Mallory bodies, and neutrophil infiltrate.

Management

- General supportive measures are paramount, with diligent care of IV lines and prevention of sepsis. No role for antibiotic prophylaxis (fever and ↑ WCC, ↑ CRP may be feature of alcoholic hepatitis *per se*), but culture of blood, urine, ascites, and use of broad spectrum antibiotics essential in setting of clinical sepsis (e.g. 3rd generation <u>CEPHALOSPORIN + METRONIDAZOLE, PIPERACILLIN/TAZOBACTAM</u>), ideally guided by culture results. If sepsis continues, consider systemic antifungal treatment (e.g. fluconazole, amphotericin). See <u>ANTIBIOTICS</u> and <u>ANTIFUNGALS</u>.
- Insert urinary catheter and monitor output if impaired renal function/poor urine output.
- Insert CVP line if patient shocked, bleeding, or in renal failure.
- Vitamin K 10 mg IV for 3 days.
- Thiamine 100 mg od (prophylaxis against <u>Wernicke's encephalopathy</u>)
- Protein supplements (>1.2 g/kg/day) speed nutritional recovery and liver function tests, and do not appear to precipitate or worsen encephalopathy. Parenteral feeding should be avoided if at all possible, because of risks (sepsis, bleeding). Nasogastric feeding can be safely given (and probably reduces bacterial translocation).
- Role of <u>CORTICOSTEROIDS</u> remains controversial, but consensus for use (e.g. commencing prednisolone 40 mg od) in severe disease (DF > 31) with encephalopathy. Variceal bleeding and sepsis are contraindications.
- Specific management of complications may be necessary—see:
  - Approach to ascites.
  - <u>Hepatorenal syndrome.</u>
  - Variceal bleeding—See <u>Acute upper GI bleeding.</u>
  - <u>Hepatic encephalopathy.</u>
  - <u>Alcohol withdrawal syndrome.</u>
- *N*–<u>ACETYLCYSTEINE</u>, pentoxifylline 400 mg tds PO (non-selective phosphodiesterase inhibitor), and <u>liver support devices</u> have shown some promise, but their exact role is still to be defined.

Discriminant function (DF) in alcoholic hepatitis

DF = 4.6 (prolongation of PT in sec) + (bilirubin in μmol/l/17.1)

Consider corticosteroids if DF > 31 (see text)

Alcoholic cirrhosis

Clinical features of cirrhosis due to alcohol are similar to those of other causes, ranging from entirely asymptomatic disease to severely decompensated liver failure (see Approaches: well patients with abnormal liver tests; recent-onset jaundice; cirrhosis and chronic liver disease). Histology may show micronodular cirrhosis. In alcoholic cirrhotics with ascites, 5 year survival is 16–25%. Mortality at 5 years is reduced by 50% through abstinence, irrespective of degree of liver dysfunction. Death occurs due to complications of cirrhosis, including hepatocellular carcinoma.

Management includes patient education as to the effect of abstinence on prognosis, and management of complications of cirrhosis—see:

- Portal hypertension.
- Emergencies—Acute upper GI bleeding.
- Hepatic encephalopathy.
- Hepatorenal syndrome.
- Approach to ascites.
- Approach to cirrhosis and chronic liver disease.

Most centres require patients to be abstinent for at least 6 months prior to liver transplantation, although 5 year survival post-transplatation is equivalent between those with alcoholic and non-alcoholic indications.

'Long quaffing maketh a short lyfe' John Lyly (1554–1606)

'Alcohol is the cause and the solution to many of life's problems'. Homer Simpson (1956–)

Alcohol withdrawal and delirium tremens (DT)

Abrupt cessation of alcohol in patient with history of chronic excess (see alcohol dependency, alcoholic liver disease) may lead to clinical features that, in their severest form (DT occurs in 5% with alcohol withdrawal), may carry mortality of 5–35%. On stopping alcohol, a decrease in the inhibitory neurotransmitter GABA results in unopposed increase in sympathetic activity.

Clinical features

- Alcohol withdrawal symptoms may develop < 8 hours since last drink (usually peaking at 48–72 hours)—confusion, hallucinations (auditory, visual, or olfactory), agitation, insomnia, nausea, vomiting. Generalized epileptic fits may occur. Signs of sympathetic drive: ↑HR, ↑BP (systolic > 160mmHg, diastolic > 100 mmHg), sweating, tremor, dilated pupils, fever.
- Delirium tremens signs and symptoms include all of the above, but to a greater severity. Neuropsychiatric manifestations prominent. > 20% mortality if untreated; 5% with treatment. Death is often due to complications of hyperthermia, electrolyte imbalance, volume depletion, infection, hypertensive crisis, or cardiovascular collapse.

Diagnosis

Largely clinical diagnoses. Always consider in any recently admitted agitated, confused inpatient (see Approach to agitation and confusion in the GI patient). Important differential diagnoses include drug intoxication (alcohol or other drugs), Wernicke-Korsakoff's syndrome, hepatic encephalopathy, or intracranial haematoma.

Investigation

- Bloods:
  - FBC: ↑WCC, ↑MCV, ↓platelets may be seen.
  - Clotting: ↑PT/APPT suggests significantly impaired liver function.
  - U&E, LFTs: dehydration common; abnormal liver function tests not a prerequisite for alcohol withdrawal; Mg^{2+} levels often ↓.
  - Glucose: seizures may occur secondary to hypoglycaemia.
  - Detectable alcohol during 'withdrawal' suggests an other diagnosis.
  - Measure serum anticonvulsant levels if patient taking these (often the case in alcoholics).
- ECG: excludes other causes of tachycardia (e.g. AF common).
- CT brain: in any patients with history of head injury, atypical presentation, focal neurology, or prolonged post-ictal phase.
- CXR, and cultures (e.g. blood, urine, sputum) if any sign of sepsis.

Management

- Manage patient in calm, safe environment. Monitor vital signs (HR, BP, temperature).
- Peripheral IV cannula. Give fluids (e.g. 5% dextrose 1 l over 8 hours).
- Thiamine 100 mg IV/PO/IM initially, then 100 mg PO daily. Magnesium sulphate 1 g IM/IV (note IM injection is painful) 6 hourly for 24 hours if required.
- Benzodiazepines of proven benefit (e.g. lorazepam 1 mg = diazepam 5 mg = chlordiazepoxide 25 mg), but no universally agreed protocol. Shorter acting lorazepam favoured in liver disease, and midazolam increasingly used.
- Mild–moderate alcohol withdrawal:
  - 'Symptom triggered' regimens (e.g. Chlordiazepoxide 50–100 mg PO every 2 hours until symptoms controlled, then prn) give better control and shorter treatment duration than 'fixed-schedules'.
  - 'Fixed-schedule' regimen shown in table.
- Severe withdrawal/DTs:
  - Lorazepam 1–4 mg IV every 1–3 hours (interval dosing). Onset of action occurs 2–5 minutes after IV injection, but peak plasma levels 1–6 hours. Close monitoring for respiratory depression essential. Adjust dosage and frequency to patient response (aim for calm, but awake). Dosage not to exceed 240 mg/24 hours.
  - Haloperidol given in addition if severely agitated. 3 mg IV, with doubling of successive doses every 30 minutes until calm.
- Other drugs for withdrawal (e.g. barbiturates, propofol, carbamazepine, clonidine) should not be used as first-line therapy.

'Fixed schedule' chlordiazepoxide oral regimen for alcohol withdrawal

	Dose	Frequency
Day 1	50 mg	4 hourly
Day 2	50 mg	6 hourly
Day 3	25 mg	4 hourly
Day 4	25 mg	6 hourly

Alpha-1-antitrypsin deficiency

Epidemiology + pathology. Autosomal recessive condition, commonest in Caucasians (1:1800 homozygous deficient (PiZZ)). Impaired cellular transport of α_1-antitrypsin with intrahepatic accumulation appears to underlie liver injury, but mechanism unclear.

Clinical features. Neonatal cholestasis and jaundice develop in 10% of homozygotes, with subsequent hepatomegaly and portal hypertension. Liver function tests show raised cholestatic enzymes and transaminases. Presentation in adulthood occurs in 10% of homozygotes, with cirrhosis or emphysema (rarely both in the same patient). High rates of portal hypertension and hepatocellular carcinoma reported.

Investigations. Diagnosis made by finding: serum α_1-antitrypsin level < 75% of lower limit of normal (80 mg/dl); ↓ α_1-globulin level on protein electrophoresis; genetic phenotyping by immunofixation; periodic-acid Schiff +ve globules in periportal hepatocytes on histology.

Management. Prevention of hepatic insults (e.g. alcohol), adequate nutrition, avoidance of smoking (with respect to chest). **Ursodeoxycholic acid** may help with neonatal cholestasis. Liver transplantation remains only treatment for advanced disease, with 80% 5 year survival in children. Inhaled α_1-antitrypsin has been used to treat pulmonary disease.

Alpha chain disease

Also known as immunoproliferative small intestinal disease (IPSID). A disorder of B lymphocytes involving proliferation of lamina propria plasma cells in the upper small intestine and associate mesenteric lymph nodes. Seen in Mediterranean countries, South America, Far East. Usually affects lower socioeconomic groups in areas with poor hygiene and a high incidence of bacterial and parasitic GI infection. Plasma cells produce truncated monoclonal heavy chains that lack associated light chains. Presentation is with malabsorption and diffuse lymphoid infiltration of the small bowel. Diagnosis made by detecting alpha chains in serum. Initial response to antibiotics (tetracyclines), but late stage disease is characterized by lymphoma.

Alpha-fetoprotein (AFP)

Protein normally produced by the liver and fetal yolk. Serum levels elevated (> 10 ng/ml) in a range of cancers, including hepatocellular carcinoma (HCC), germline tumours (e.g. testicular seminoma, teratoma, ovarian tumours), and metastasic liver deposits, but also in active liver disease, and in mothers pregnant with babies carrying neural tube defects or Down's syndrome.

AFP and liver disease. Although level of AFP may correlate with size of HCC, it is not elevated in 30% of HCCs. It is therefore not of use alone as a screening or surveillance test. It may also be elevated in 5% of patients with chronic liver disease (particularly during flare of disease, as indicated by raised ALT/AST). However, AFP > 100 ng/ml always necessitates the exclusion of HCC, by means of U/S, contrast-enhanced CT scan, and occasionally angiography.

Aminosalicylates

See: 5-AMINOSALICYLATES (5-ASA) preparations.

Amoebiasis

Epidemiology + pathology. *Entamoeba histolytica* is pathogenic in man and causes amoebic colitis and <u>liver abscess</u>. Cysts can live outside the hosts or be carried asymptomatically in the stool, while trophozoites, passed by people with invasive disease, cannot survive outside the host. The presence in stool of trophozoites with intracytoplasmic red blood cells is pathognomonic for infection by *E. histolytica*.

Clinical features. Varies from asymptomatic to a life-threatening fulminant colitis. Misdiagnosis as <u>ulcerative colitis</u> and treatment with <u>CORTICOSTEROIDS</u> may predispose to perforation and systemic sepsis.

- Colonoscopic appearance of shallow ulcers, commonest on right side of colon. Ulcers may erode into blood vessels or cause intestinal perforation and peritonitis.
- Systemic dissemination may involve brain, lungs, pericardium, liver.
- <u>Liver abscess</u> in approximately 4% of patients, with male predominance (despite equal sex distribution for colitis). Clinical features of abdominal pain, fever, and constitutional symptoms, but jaundice in < 15%.
- Colonic narrowing may be due to amoeboma (this should be managed medically because surgical resection has high complication rate).

Investigation. Diagnosis involves careful stool microscopy to look for cysts or trophozoites. Usually few leucocytes in the stool. Sigmoidoscopy can help but rectal involvement is less frequent than caecal involvement; colonoscopy is therefore investigation of choice. Liver abscess identified on <u>ultrasound</u> or <u>CT scan</u>, and enzyme immunoassay (EIA) serological test has sensitivity of 99% and specificity > 90% in patients with amoebic liver abscess, and is more reliable than stool microscopy.

Management is with <u>METRONIDAZOLE</u>: cure in 90%; treatment usually given for 10 days for intestinal disease. Diloxanide is recommended to eradicate cysts. Therapeutic needle aspiration/catheter drainage of liver abscess only considered if:

- Abscess > 5 cm, therefore at risk of rupture.
- Left lobe liver abscess, which carries increased risk of intraperitoneal/pericardial rupture.
- Failure to gain a clinical response to therapy within 1 week.

Ampullary cancer

- Rare cancer (< 0.5% of GI cancers) that may present with painless obstructive jaundice. May develop in villous adenoma, in association with <u>familial adenomatous polyposis</u> (FAP), or occur spontaneously.
- Abnormal, ulcerated ampulla at ERCP. Dilated pancreatic and common bile ducts ('<u>double duct sign</u>') may mimic <u>pancreatic cancer</u>. <u>CT scan</u> ± <u>endoscopic ultrasound</u> to define local invasion.
- Approximately 50% of ampullary cancers are resectable, with > 80% 5 year survival following <u>Whipple's resection</u> in those without local invasion (i.e. much better than for <u>pancreatic cancer</u>). Non-operative cases treated with endoscopic biliary stenting. Palliative chemotherapy has poor efficacy.

Amylase

- Pancreas produces 40% of serum amylase; salivary glands the rest. Total serum amylase (pancreatic isoenzymes are highly sensitive and specific, but rarely needed clinically) increases 6–12 hours after onset of <u>acute pancreatitis</u> (AP), and levels > 1000 U/l are strongly indicative of this diagnosis in the correct clinical setting. Amylase may be elevated, but usually < 1000 U/l, due to a wide range of abdominal causes, including acute <u>appendicitis</u>, <u>cholecystitis</u>, <u>choledocholithiasis</u>, viscus perforation, and salpingitis. Disease of the salivary glands (e.g. mumps), lung and ovarian tumours, head injury, and diabetic ketoacidosis can all cause elevation. Chronic elevation of serum amylase occurs in macroamylasaemia. Condition is of no clinical relevance (beyond confusing the diagnosis of AP), and can be differentiated from pancreatic amylase by the absence of amylase in urine.
- Diagnosis of AP should not rely solely on the level of amylase, which may not be significantly elevated due to underlying <u>pancreatic insufficiency</u> (i.e. with acinar cell loss, therefore unable to make amylase), or if AP due to hypertriglyceridaemia (an amylase inhibitor may be present). Level of amylase in AP does not predict prognosis. Serum lipase sensitive and specific for AP, and raised levels persist for longer, but less readily available than amylase.
- High levels of amylase within <u>pancreatic pseudocysts</u> help to differentiate them from <u>pancreatic cystic tumours</u>, and high amylase levels in ascitic fluid are diagnostic of pancreatic ascites, related to pseudocyst or pancreatic duct rupture.

Amyloidosis

Group of diseases characterized by extracellular deposition of abnormal fibrillar proteins. Classification is by capital A for amyloid followed by an abbreviation for a fibril protein.

- **Light chain (AL) amyloidosis** involves clonal excess of immunoglobulin light chains and can manifest as multiple myeloma. GI manifestations include macroglossia, GI bleeding, and motility problems. Management is with haematological chemotherapy.
- In **reactive systemic (AA) amyloid** the precursor protein is the acute phase reactant serum amyloid A. It occurs in less than 2% of patients with Crohn's and is very rare in UC. Presentation is usually with nephrotic syndrome but the liver and spleen may also be affected.
- Familial Mediterranean fever also involves AA protein; in this disease colchicine has been shown to prevent renal failure from amyloid deposition.
- Gastroenterolgists are sometimes called to help make the diagnosis of amyloid: rectal and duodenal biopsies are positive in over 80% of cases if submucosa is present in the biopsy.

Anal cancer

Rare (incidence 1 per 100 000 per year comprises 1–2% of colonic cancers). Risk factors include genital warts and history of receptive anal sex; human papilloma virus type 16 for squamous tumours.

- Mean age at presentation 60 years, with bleeding, pain, and pruritus, but 25% of patients are asymptomatic. Adenocarcinomas of the anal canal behave like adenocarcinomas of the rectum and are treated in a similar way with abdomino-perineal resection and pre- or post-operative chemoradiation for large or invasive tumours.
- 80% of cancers are squamous cell cancers and for this group treatment with chemoradiotherapy has replaced aggressive surgery and results in improved 5 year survival rate of 70%.
- Non-epidermal tumours are very rare, and include melanomas, intraepithelial neoplasia (also known as Bowen's disease), and Paget's disease, which is an intraepithelial mucinous adenocarcinoma arising from dermal apocrine sweat glands.

Anal fissure

Epidemiology + pathology

Painful linear ulcers in the anal canal. Young and middle-aged adults most commonly affected (M = F). 90% of primary fissures are in the posterior midline. Fissures can also be secondary to Crohn's disease, anal cancer, and infection (e.g. syphilis, TB)—in which case they are usually more lateral.

The elliptical arrangement of the fibres of the anal sphincter is supposed to offer less muscular support to the mucosa posteriorly, predisposing to traumatic tears after passage of a large hard stool. Repeated trauma can lead to chronic fissures—in these patients, resting anal tone is high (though whether this is cause or effect is unclear) and this may produce a degree of ischaemia that can lead to fibrosis.

Clinical features

The hallmark is severe sharp pain during and after defecation with scanty bright red bleeding. Digital examination or proctoscopy is usually too painful without topical anaesthesia. Simple inspection may reveal the diagnosis. A sentinel pile (fibrotic nubbin of skin at the anal verge) is common.

Treatment

Stools must be made soft and easy to pass (ensure high fluids: use nonstimulant osmotic <u>LAXATIVE</u>). Topical anaesthetics and frequent baths can reduce sphincter spasm. Medical treatment with topical nitrates or diltiazem is effective at increasing fissure healing. Surgical therapy includes sphincterotomy, which lowers sphincter tone: lateral sphincterotomy has better results than midline sphincterotomy with fissurectomy. The procedure of manual dilatation under anaesthetic produces very uncontrolled results, frequent complications, and is now discredited.

Anaphylaxis

May occur due to IgE-mediated hypersensitivity to foods. Localized to oropharynx (oral allergy syndrome), with pruritus, angio-oedema of the tongue, lips, palate, and throat, or generalized gastrointestinal anaphylaxis associated with allergic reactions in other organs (e.g. skin, airway). Symptoms develop minutes to 2 h after eating food, with nausea, vomiting, abdominal pain, diarrhoea. Diagnosis established by history and food-specific IgE antibodies: oral food challenge should be performed with caution but can occasionally be useful in confirming a diagnosis. Strict elimination of the offending allergen with scrutiny of food labels is the only proven therapy: histamine antagonists and steroids are of minimal overall efficacy. See Ramrakha PS and Moore KPK (2004) *Oxford Handbook of Acute Medicine* 2nd edn (Oxford, Oxford University Press) for management.

Angiodysplasia (see Colour Plate 3)

Gastrointestinal mucosal vascular ectasia not associated with cutaneous lesions, systemic vascular disease, or a familial syndrome (see also <u>gastric antral vascular ectasia</u> and <u>hereditary haemorrhagic telangiectasia</u>).

Most commonly found in patients > 60 years, and in 1–2% undergoing upper GI endoscopy for any indication, 4% if being endoscoped for bleeding (and more if being investigated for anaemia), and 3–6% in those undergoing colonoscopy.

Aetiology may be degenerative, relating to chronic low grade obstruction of mucosal veins, or alternatively result from mucosal ischaemia. Much quoted (and debated) association of angiodysplasia with aortic valve disease may be linked to an acquired form of von Willebrand disease.

Clinical features. Always through bleeding, which can range from haematemesis to PR bleeding to occult anaemia. In majority bleeding not life-threatening, but 15% patients with colonic angiodysplasia have acute massive haemorrhage.

Investigation. Diagnosis usually endoscopic (see Colour Plate 3). Although lesions may be indistinguishable from those of <u>hereditary haemorrhagic telangiectasia</u> (Osler–Weber–Rendu syndrome), Turner's syndrome, and the CREST syndrome, the other extra-intestinal signs of these various disorders are not seen. Small intestinal angiodysplasia can be diagnosed by push enteroscopy or wireless capsule endoscopy (see <u>enteroscopy</u>). Colonic lesions can be diagnosed at colonoscopy or at angiography.

Specialized diagnostic tests include radionuclide scanning with labelled red cells, but the intermittent nature of bleeding from angiodysplasia limits utility of this test. Historically intraoperative enteroscopy has been helpful in the diagnosis of distal small bowel lesions, although this will be partially replaced by the advent of wireless capsule endoscopy.

Management most often with endoscopic obliteration procedures (see <u>endoscopic haemostasis</u>), although the rebleeding rate is substantial. In patients unfit for surgery, transcatheter <u>embolization</u> using coils or gelfoam has been successful in stopping acute bleeding. Surgery may be definitive treatment if the bleeding source has been clearly defined. Medical treatment with oestrogen-progestogen therapy (0.05 mg ethinyloestradiol and 1 mg norethisterone given daily) has been tried, in the hope of optimizing coagulation, microvascular circulation, or endothelial integrity. Efficacy has not been fully established.

Angio-oedema

Hereditary angio-oedema is an autosomal dominant disorder caused by a deficiency of C1 esterase inhibitor, a regulator of the activated first component of complement. Pathogenesis not fully understood, but kinin release may mediate increased vascular permeability.

Clinical features include recurrent oedema of skin and mucous membranes. Although there can be tingling or burning at the onset, the lesions are painless and, unlike urticaria, pruritus is absent. Onset is usually in childhood and a family history is usually present. Attacks may be precipitated by local trauma, dental extractions, or surgery. Laryngeal oedema can cause airway obstruction. Gastrointestinal involvement includes colicky pain, diarrhoea, and vomiting. Fluid loss can lead to hypotension and shock: fever and leucocytosis are absent, bowel sounds may be increased, and there is no peritonism.

Diagnosis involves finding reduced C4 levels and a reduction in C1 esterase inhibitor.

Treatment. Anabolic steroids such as danazol and stanozolol can prevent attacks, but may have other actions than simply raising levels of C1 esterase inhibitor since patients often respond to low doses that are insufficient to raise complement levels. Doses are tailored to clinical rather than biological response. In known cases, premedication with C1 esterase inhibitor concentrates should be considered before interventional procedures such as upper GI endoscopy.

Anorectal abscesses

Usually result from infection of the anal glands along the dentate line. Acute infection may cause an abscess and lead to a chronic anorectal fistula. Abscesses are classified according to where they extend to and may be perianal, ischiorectal, intersphincteric, or supralevator (see Fig. 2.2). Commonest type is perianal (40–50%) and least common type is supralevator (5–10%).

Diagnosis can be difficult because there may be no external signs and rectal examination may be painful. Examination under anaesthetic, MRI scanning or intra-anal ultrasound can all be very helpful in establishing a diagnosis.

Treatment requires incision and drainage. Culture of pus is not usually necessary. Antibiotics alone are inadequate, although METRONIDAZOLE and CIPROFLOXACIN have an important adjunctive role: in particular, intravenous antibiotics may be needed if the patient is immunocompromised diabetic or shows sign of systemic sepsis.

Anorectal fistulae

A complication of a perianal abscess, resulting in a connection between the anorectum and the skin at the anal verge or elsewhere in the perineum. Any discharging area or area of granulation around the anus should be assumed to connect with the anorectum unless proved otherwise. Most surgeons will use operative exploration and their first diagnostic test for a fistula, but MRI is very useful in defining complex cases. The external and internal openings must be defined and the presence of any extensions established. An underlying disease process such as Crohn's disease, ongoing infection of the presence of a foreign body must not be missed. Biopsy is often needed.

Classification (Parkes, AG et al. (1976) Br. J. Surg. **63**: 1–12) is by their relation to the internal and external sphincters. There are 4 major categories: intersphincteric, trans-sphincteric, extrasphincteric, and suprasphincteric.

Preoperative assessment of sphincter function by anorectal manometry and an anorectal ultrasound is wise when any degree of sphincter damage is anicipated. Only those tracks passing through distal parts of the sphincter can be laid open without fear of incontinence. For fistulae not amenable to fistulotomy, rather than cutting and repairing the sphincter which often does not heal well, the insertion of a *seton suture* is a safer option. Complex or high fistulae require complex surgery.

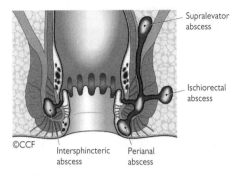

©CCF

Supralevator
abscess

Ischiorectal
abscess

Intersphincteric   Perianal
abscess   abscess

Fig. 2.2 Classification of anorectal abscesses. Reproduced from Feldman M,, Friedman LS, and Sleisenger MH (2003). *Sleisenger and Fordtran's Gastrointestinal and Liver Diease*, p2286, with permission from Elsevier

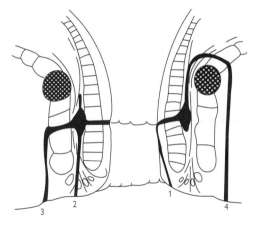

Fig. 2.3 Classification of anorectal fistulae. 1) Superficial; 2) Inter-sphinctreric; 3) Trans-sphincteric; 4) Supra-sphincteric

Anorectal manometry

An important technique in the evaluation of problems with defecation. Perfused probes or pressure sensitive transducers are introduced into rectum to record anal sphincter pressures, sensitivity to rectal distension, and the presence of the recto-anal inhibitory reflex.

Clinical assessment of anal sphincter tone by digital examination is very inaccurate so manometry is indicated in patients complaining of constipation or faecal incontinence, where clinical assessment of sphincter function is important. Resting anal pressures and maximal voluntary squeeze pressures can be measured: if there is a high resting pressure, the normal reflex relaxation response to rectal distension is assessed: this is absent in Hirschsprung's disease. High threshold for initiation of reflex anal relaxation may indicate a problem with rectal compliance (e.g. Hirschsprung's megarectum) or afferent sensory pathways (e.g. spinal cord injuries). Defects in voluntary squeeze suggest abnormal innervation of the external sphincter. A normal voluntary squeeze but low resting pressure suggests a problem in the internal sphincter, which can occur after haemorrhoid surgery or in conditions such as diabetes and systemic sclerosis. In constipated patients with normal resting pressure and normal recto-anal inhibitory reflex, anatomical abnormalities such as accentuated puborectalis angulation or internal rectal prolapse should be considered.

Anorexia nervosa

An eating disorder characterized by a distorted body image, an inability to interpret hunger and satiety, and a paralysing sense of ineffectiveness (also see bulimia).

Aetiology and pathogenesis. Not a true loss of appetite, rather a preoccupation with food and eating. Recently reported incidence of 30–150 per 100 000 in 16–25 year old women, making it the third commonest illness in the age group after obesity and asthma. Role of psychosocial factors is much studied and outside our scope here.

Clinical features include hypothermia, bradycardia, hypotension, acrocyanosis, carotinaemia giving a yellow appearance to face and hair, thin hair (lanugo) over face, arms, and back, and amenorrhoea.

Investigation may reveal hypokalaemia, hyponatraemia, and 'sick euthyroid' indices (low free thyroxine with a normal TSH).

Complications Arrhythmias, effects on bone mineralization/osteoporosis, and depressed menstruation and reproductive function. Gastrointestinal complications include constipation, pancreatitis, oesophagitis, peptic ulceration, abnormal liver function tests (and biochemical hepatitis), malabsorption, and reduced taste.

Treatment is difficult and centres on an interlocking approach to the psychological, nutritional, and medical problems. Sadly, while early mortality remains around 5%, late mortality can be as high as 20%, with suicide, arrhythmias, and infections the leading causes of death.

Antibiotic-associated diarrhoea (AAD)

Common—occurs after 5 to 25% antibiotic courses.
   Two main forms:

- Idiopathic, with no known pathogen (90% cases). Characteristic features are onset during antibiotic exposure, dose-related frequency, resolution when the antibiotic is discontinued, absence of inflammation on colonic biopsy or stool examination for leucocytes, and a benign course.
- Diarrhoea associated with *Clostridium difficile* (about 10% of all cases of AAD), which may present with pseudomembranous colitis. See clostridial infections of GI tract.

Mechanisms

- Direct effects of antibiotics on intestinal mucosa.
   - E.g. neomycin and clofazimine.
   - Erythromycin is prokinetic because of motilin receptor stimulation.
- Possible effects on gut ecology.
   - Altered bile acid metabolism.
   - Altered carbohydrate fermentation.
   - Overgrowth of pathogens.

Management

- Meta-analyses show a benefit of probiotic administration with lactobacillus or saccharomyces in AAD.
- AAD due to direct antibiotic effect may respond rapidly to cessation of antibiotic.
- Also see clostridial infections of GI tract and Approach to acute diarrhoea.

Antibiotic prophylaxis in endoscopy

Incidence of endocarditis due to endoscopy very low and evidence that antibiotic administration alters this is scanty (Vander Meer, JTM *et al.* (1992) *Lancet* **339**: 135). Conditions associated with an increased risk of endocarditis are shown in the first box. Antibiotic prophylaxis currently recommended for higher risk conditions but not moderate or low risk conditions.
   Risk probably relates to the incidence of bacteraemia, (although asymptomatic bacteraemia is common after tooth brushing): this is highest for endoscopic dilatation, variceal sclerotherapy (less for band ligation), laser therapy, and colonoscopy.
   Current antibiotic regimens are shown in the second box.
   Indications for antibiotic prophylaxis prior to endoscopy in those with biliary tract disease are debated, but recommendations for use include:

- Biliary obstruction (especially where high risk of incomplete drainage at ERCP (e.g. primary sclerosing cholangitis)).
- Pancreatic pseudocyst puncture.

- <u>Endoscopic ultrasound</u>-guided aspiration of suspected <u>pancreatic cystic tumour</u>.
- Prophylaxis needs to cover predominantly Gram-negative rods (e.g. <u>CIPROFLOXACIN</u> 500 mg PO 1 hour before, and 12 and 24 hours after procedure).

Sepsis after PEG placement. There is good evidence that a single dose of cefuroxime 750 mg IV reduces the incidence of peristomal wound infection after PEG placement.

Conditions associated with risk of endocarditis

Higher risk: prosthetic heart valve, previous endocarditis, synthetic vascular graft, severe neutropenia
Moderate or theoretical risk: mitral prolapse with heart failure, rheumatic valve disease, HOCM, heart transplant
No increased risk: pacemaker, coronary artery grafts, isolated mitral valve prolapse, uncomplicated ASD.

Suggested antibiotic regimens for endocarditis prophlaxis in GI endoscopy (BSG guidelines (1991): BNF (2004))
1. No allergy to penicillin, and no more than 1 course of penicillin in the previous month
   Adults amoxicillin 1 g IV plus gentamicin 120 mg IV, plus amoxicillin 500 mg PO 6 h after procedure. Child under 5, quarter adult dose amoxicillin, gentamicin 2 mg/kg; child 5–10, half adult dose amoxicillin, gentamicin 2 mg/kg
2. Penicillin-allergic or more than 1 course in the previous month
   Adults 1 g vancomycin by slow (over at least 100 mins) IV infusion plus gentamicin 120 mg IV. Children under 10: vancomycin IV 20 mg/kg, gentamicin 2 mg/kg.

Anti-reflux procedures

In those patients with persistent problems related to gastro-oesophageal reflux, despite maximal medical therapy (see <u>Approach to dyspepsia and gastro-oesophageal reflux</u>), a range of mechanical interventions are available. These aim to reverse mechanical and physiological abnormalities of gastro-oesophageal reflux disease (which should be proven by <u>oesophageal manometry</u>). Endoscopic and surgical options are available.

Endoscopic approach

- **Endoscopic gastroplication** was developed in the 1990s by Swain; currently there is only one commercial application (Endocinch, BARD), although other suturing devices are under development.

- **Radiofrequency-induced collagen remodelling** has been commercialized in the Stretta procedure. Using a dedicated catheter a balloon is inflated up to 3 cm and four needle electrodes are deployed into the muscular layer of the oesophagus. Each needle produces a lesion through a controlled rise in temperature up to 85°C. By rotating the catheter, a total of 50–60 lesions can be created in the area around the gastro-oesophageal junction.
- **Endoscopic submucosal injection** into the cardia is best developed in the Enteryx procedure, using a non-biodegradable polymer which is injected into the muscle of the cardia. This transforms on contact with water into a foamy particle: repeated injections result in circumferentially distributed patches of injected material. A similar principle is followed by the Gatekeeper system developed by Medtronic.

Surgical approach

Procedure performed laparoscopically or as open operation, and involves mobilization of lower oesophagus, reduction of hiatus hernia, and wrapping of gastric fundus around lower oesophagus, either totally (e.g. Nissan 360° fundoplication—see opposite) or partially (e.g. Toupet 270° fundoplication). Re-establishes competence of anti-reflux barrier and increases resting lower oesophageal sphincter pressure.

Patient selection difficult, as no direct comparisons of medical therapy versus anti-reflux surgery, but indications may include:
- Failed medical therapy, with persistent symptomatic <u>oesophagitis</u>.
- Young healthy patient who responds to medical therapy, but unable/unwilling to take long-term medication.
- Recurrent reflux complications (e.g. laryngitis, asthma, pneumonia).

Complications include dysphagia and air trapping, which may require reoperation, and have been reported in >10% following laparoscopic fundoplication. Mortality rate of 0.2%, is of significance in a condition that runs a benign course in the great majority. No good evidence that surgical fundoplication reduces risk of <u>oesophageal tumours</u>.

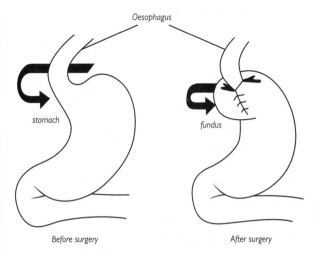

Oesophagus

stomach

fundus

Before surgery

After surgery

Fig. 2.4 Nissan fundoplication

Outcome of anti-reflux procedures

Clinical outcome after endoscopic procedures is currently (2004) dependent on open label studies, except for 1 sham controlled randomized trial for the Stretta procedure. Available outcome data suggest a significant reduction in both symptoms and oesophageal acid exposure for the Endocinch, Enteryx, and Stretta procedures but controlled data is needed. Incidence of adverse events is falling with increasing operator experience: the current serious complication rate is estimated at 0.25%.

Long-term outcome data are awaited: the role of endoscopic anti-reflux procedures relative to maintenance medical therapy and surgical anti-reflux approaches remains to be defined.

Aorto-enteric fistulae

Nearly always occur after reconstructive aorto-iliac surgery: frequency is about 1 in 200 patients at an average 3–5 years after operation. Usually affects third part of duodenum, so out of reach of standard upper GI endoscopy. Diagnosis requires enteroscopy or CT. **Always suspect the diagnosis if there is any hint of upper GI bleed** in a patient with appropriate surgical history: there is classically a self-limiting 'herald bleed' which may be the only chance to save the patients life, since this is often followed by a second massive life-threatening bleed.

Pathogenesis is usually subtle infection with *Staph. aureus* or *E. coli*, so beware of low grade fever, unexplained fatigue, raised inflammatory markers, or leucocytosis in the right clinical setting.

Aphthous ulcers

See: mouth ulcers.

Appendix and appendicitis

Acute appendicitis remains the commonest surgical emergency and may involve gangrene or perforation into the abdominal cavity. Although its function remains unknown, the high concentration of lymphoid tissue has always suggested an immune regulatory function. Recent epidemiological data shows that appendicectomy has a protective effect in ulcerative colitis and Crohn's disease, and the course of ulcerative colitis seems milder following a history of appendicectomy (Sacher, DB (2002). *Gut* **51**: 764). At present it is not clear if it is the appendicectomy itself or the prior appendicitis that is protective.

Argon plasma coagulation ('APC', 'argon beamer')

A relatively new approach for the endoscopic treatment of bleeding and superficial mucosal lesions. Allows controlled non-contact electrocoagulation by means of high frequency energy delivered to tissue through ionized gas. Application and control is easier than for free beam lasers, but depth of tissue injury is more superficial and not sufficient to effect relief of dysphagia associated with oesophageal carcinoma. Particular use for angiodysplasia, gastric antral vascular ectasia, and bleeding related to radiation damage.

Ascites

See: Approach to ascites.

Atrophic gastritis

A histological diagnosis, requiring endoscopic biopsy (2 biopsies from body, 2 from antrum, 1 from incisura). Findings include chronic gastric inflammation with loss of gastric glands and replacement by intestinal-type epithelium and fibrous tissue.

Two main causes:

- **Type A or auto-immune atrophic gastritis**. This is mainly restricted to the gastric corpus with sparing of the gastric antrum. It is characterized by auto-antibodies against gastric parietal cells and intrinsic factor, and often leads to <u>pernicious anaemia</u>.
- **Environmental factors** usually produce multifocal gastritis, involving antrum and corpus. Examples include dietary factors (e.g. nitroso compounds produced by bacterial metabolism of dietary nitrates) and <u>*Helicobacter pylori*</u>. *Helicobacter*-associated gastritis results from release of bacterial and inflammatory toxic products, and can result in either antral-predominant gastritis or multifocal gastritis affecting corpus, fundus, and antrum, with partial replacement of gastric type epithelium by intestinal epithelium. Mucosal inflammation, and therefore atrophic gastritis, is more marked with cagA positive strains of HP. Antral predominant gastritis is commonly found in infected patients with peptic ulcers, while mutifocal gastritis and autoimmune gastritis are associated with the development of gastric carcinoma.

Autoimmune hepatitis (AIH)

Aetiology + epidemiology

Necroinflammatory liver disease of unknown aetiology. Estimated prevalence of 50–100 cases per million population (F:M ratio 4:1). Strongly associated with HLA alleles DR3 (often younger at onset, more severe course) and DR4 (older, more benign course).

Clinical features

- Bimodal age distribution at disease onset—10–30 years and > 40 years. Young women commonly affected, but found in all other groups.
- Presentation with acute hepatitis in up to 40%, but <u>acute liver failure</u> very rare. Many present with gradual onset of jaundice, fatigue, abdominal pain, and fever, and 30–80% have cirrhosis at presentation.
- Associated with other autoimmune diseases in 48% of cases—thyroid disease, arthritis, vitiligo, <u>ulcerative colitis</u>, diabetes mellitus, lichen planus, alopecia, mixed connective tissue disease.
- Prior to immunosuppression, 50% 3–5 year mortality reported. When disease remission induced, 90% 10 year survival, even with <u>cirrhosis</u> at outset.
- Overlap syndromes may occur. In the presence of clinical features of AIH, anti-mitochondrial Abs (AMA) and <u>cholangitis</u> are seen in 8%, suggesting overlap with <u>primary biliary cirhosis</u> (PBC), and biliary disease suggestive of <u>primary sclerosing cholangitis</u> (PSC) occurs in 6%. Anti-LKM1 Abs shown in 2–5% of patients with HCV infection.

Investigations

Definitive diagnosis requires: circulating autoantibodies > 1:80 titre; IgG > x 1 ULN; all other causes of chronic liver disease excluded.

Incorporation of clinical, laboratory, and histological parameters into standardized scoring systems may aid diagnosis where classical features are absent (Johnson, PJ and McFarlane, IG. *Hepatology* 1993; **18**: 998).

Characteristic elevation of transaminases (ALT/AST) by > 1.5 x ULN for > 6 months. ALT > 1000 U/l rarely seen (note: ALT > 1000 U/l usually due to drugs, viral hepatitis, or ischaemia).

3 subtypes of AIH categorized, according to serological results:

- **Type 1.** 80% of cases of AIH, 70% female < 40 years. Antinuclear Ab (ANA) ± smooth muscle Ab (ASM) +ve. Elevated IgG in 97% of cases. Good response to immunosuppression in 80% of patients, but 25% have cirrhosis at presentation.
- **Type 2.** Very rare in USA; may account for 20% of AIH cases in Europe. Usually diagnosed in children. Associated with anti-liver–kidney microsomal Abs (anti-LKM1) and anti-LC-1 Abs, but ANA/ASM usually negative. Rapidly progressive, and poor response to immunosuppression.
- **Type 3.** Similar clinical pattern and treatment response to type 1 AIH, but ANA/ASM/anti-LKM1 negative. Anti-soluble liver antigen (anti-SLA) associated.

Liver biopsy. Periportal/lobular hepatitis characteristic, but no pathognomonic features in AIH. Histological grade (inflammation) and stage (fibrosis) predict prognosis (bridging necrosis/multilobular necrosis/cirrhosis probably predicts worse outcome). Repeat biopsy on treatment predicts likelihood of maintained remission off treatment.

Management

Treatment indicated when ALT/AST > 1.5 x ULN, IgG > 2 x ULN, and moderate–severe periportal hepatitis on biopsy. Absolute indication if ALT/AST > 10 x ULN, severe hepatitis and necrosis, or disease progression.

- <u>CORTICOSTEROIDS</u>. Mainstay of treatment, with 80% biochemical and histological remission within 2–4 years. Initiated alone or with <u>AZATHIOPRINE</u>. Usual starting dose prednisolone 30–50 mg od PO for 2/52, with aim of reduction of 5 mg every 10 days, to maintenance at 5–15 mg/day or less. Drug withdrawal should not be attempted <2 years after starting treatment, and then should be guided by histology (100% relapse if on-treatment progression to cirrhosis, 20% if histological resolution). Disease flares may occur whatever the response. Progression in 10% despite steroids.
- <u>AZATHIOPRINE</u>. No role as monotherapy for inducing remission. Very useful in combination with steroids, allowing steroid reduction, and as maintenance therapy after steroid withdrawal (maintains remission in > 80% over 1–10 year follow-up). Usual dose 1–1.5 mg/kg/day in combination, increasing to 2–2.5 mg/kg/day as monotherapy after remission achieved. Important side-effects (see drug section), and checking <u>TPMT</u> levels prior to commencing treatment is essential.

- New immunosuppressants. Effectiveness of tacrolimus, cyclosporin, mycophenolate, and others reported, and may be considered for treatment failures, but no established role yet.
- <u>Liver transplantation</u>. Consider in patients with progressive disease, especially if no response after 4 years of treatment, or early hepatic decompensation. Five and 10 year survival post transplant of 90% and 75% respectively. AIH may recur in graft, but rarely leads to graft loss.

Autoimmune pancreatitis

- Rare condition, mainly reported from Japan. May clinically mimic pancreatic cancer, and is a cause of chronic pancreatitis and pancreatic insufficiency. Also associated with intrahepatic biliary strictures similar to primary sclerosing cholangitis.
- Characterized by:
  - Diffuse pancreatic enlargement ('sausage pancreas').
  - Pancreatic duct abnormality.
  - Low common bile duct stricture.
  - Lymphoplasmacytic infiltrate on biopsy.
  - Raised serum IgG4 levels.
  - Associated autoimmune disease (e.g. Sjögren's, Crohn's disease).

Response to CORTICOSTEROIDS.

Autonomic neuropathy

Aetiology. Autonomic neuropathy affecting the gastrointestinal tract occurs as a complication of diabetes mellitus and Parkinsons's disease. Less common causes include rare types of amyloid, Fabry's disease, and porphyria.

Clinical features. Symptoms relate to postural hypotension and genitourinary involvement (impotence, loss of morning erections, urinary urgency). Gut stasis can give rise to bacterial overgrowth, which can produce diarrhoea and malabsorption. Nausea, vomiting, abdominal pain, and distension can all occur as a presenting problem.

Examination. In the gastrointestinal system, test for a succussion splash suggestive of gastroparesis, and look for faecal impaction.

Investigations. Autonomic function tests may help. Endoscopy is a poor test for motility: better to get a video swallow, barium meal, or gastric emptying study. Colonic motility can be assessed using a shapes test where clearance of differently shaped radio-opaque markers is assessed on sequential plain abdominal X-rays.

Treatment. Small frequent meals and avoiding anticholinergics, narcotics, and sympathomimetics.

B

Bacterial overgrowth

Refers to an increase in the normally low bacterial colonization of the GI tract upstream of the distal ileum. Produces symptoms of vitamin malabsorption, malnutrition, and weight loss.

Aetiology and pathophysiology

Contributing factors are shown opposite.
- Fat, protein, carbohydrate, and vitamin malabsorption result from poor enterocyte function and bacterial transformation of nutrients into nonabsorbable and toxic metabolites.
- Anaerobes deconjugate bile acids, preventing bile acid function and enterohepatic circulation. Deconjugated bile acids induce watery diarrhoea.
- Carbohydrate intolerance results from reduction of brush border disaccharidases: increased amounts of osmotically active carbohydrate fragments contribute to the diarrhoea associated with bacterial overgrowth.
- Anaerobes compete with the host for vitamin B12 which results in B12 deficiency and macrocytic anaemia.

Clinical features. Diarrhoea, weight loss, possibly neurological features associated with <u>vitamin B12</u> deficiency, abdominal pain, and symptoms of impaired absorption of fat-soluble <u>vitamins A, D, E, K</u>.

Investigation

Microbiological culture is the most direct method (> 10^5 colonies/ml after duodenal aspiration and culture). <u>Breath tests</u> are less invasive. The SeHCAT test is useful in testing for <u>bile acid malabsorption</u>. Also see <u>Approach to malabsorption and steatorrhoea</u>.

Treatment

If surgical correction of the underlying abnormality leading to stasis is not possible, antibiotics and treatment of dysmotility are the mainstays of treatment. Antibiotic regimens are usually empirical and involve drugs with activity against aerobic and anaerobic bacteria. Tetracycline 250 mg qds is a traditional choice, with augmentin, trimethoprim sulphamethoxazole (Septrin), and ciprofloxacin as alternatives. Often a single 7–10 day course can relieve symptoms for months, but sometimes continuous rotating antibiotics are necessary. So far, trials of probiotic therapy have given negative or inconclusive results.

Balloon dilatation

See: <u>endoscopic dilatation</u>.

Causes of bacterial overgrowth

Reduced host defences
- Hypogammaglobulinaemia
- Immunodeficiency (e.g. <u>HIV</u>)
- Old age
- <u>Chronic pancreatitis</u>

Excess bacterial entry to small bowel
- Atrophic gastritis/gastric acid suppression (e.g. proton pump inhibitors)
- Gastrojejunostomy/<u>Roux-en-Y anastomosis</u>
- <u>Gastrectomy</u>
- Enteral fistulae

Delayed small bowel clearance
- Small bowel/<u>jejunal diverticula</u> (e.g. <u>scleroderma</u>)
- Strictures (e.g. <u>Crohn's disease</u>, post-surgical)
- <u>Pseudo-obstruction</u>
- <u>Amyloidosis</u>
- <u>Autonomic neuropathy</u> (e.g. <u>diabetes</u>, post-vagotomy)

Barium contrast studies

Contrast studies of the GI tract can be performed using single- or double-contrast techniques. Barium is the agent of choice unless there are worries about bowel viability or perforation, in which case barium is avoided because free barium in the peritoneal cavity causes an inflammatory reaction. Single contrast uses low density barium to look for filling defects or contour abnormalities. Double contrast uses smaller amounts of high contrast barium with gas and gives much better resolution of fine mucosal detail.

Barium swallow and contrast examination of the upper GI tract

Traditionally a barium swallow was the initial investigation of dysphagia but with the use of endoscopic intubation under direct vision most clinicians now use endoscopy as first choice of investigation. However, video fluoroscopy with water soluble contrast is the preferred method of assessing swallowing dysfunction.

Contrast studies can be useful in demonstrating a sliding hiatus hernia or gastro-oesophageal reflux, and in giving information about structures that may be impassable endoscopically, e.g. in the oesophagus or duodenum.

Small bowel studies

The traditional techniques of small bowel meal and small bowel enteroclysis remain very useful in evaluating a variety of small bowel disease including tumours, inflammatory pathology such as Crohn's disease, and Meckel's diverticulum. Contrast studies can be useful in diagnosing the level of small bowel obstruction, although in this situation water soluble contrast should be used. The diagnostic yield of small bowel contrast studies in obscure GI bleeding is poor and techniques of <u>enteroscopy</u> are preferred.

Barium studies of the colon

This technique is becoming less common because of the availability of colonoscopy and the development of CT colonography, but the barium enema remains a commonly used technique for evaluating the colon. Contraindications include toxic megacolon, ischaemic colitis, or other diseases where the bowel wall is friable and more likely to perforate.

Barrett's oesophagus

After Norman Barrett, British surgeon (died 1979) although the condition was first described by PR Allison in 1948.

Definition. Presence of columnar epithelium lining the lower oesophagus (see Colour Plate 4). Because of imprecision in defining endoscopic landmarks (see practice point box), definition of classical Barrett's is usually restricted to columnar mucosa extending 3 or more cm into the tubular oesophagus. Less than this is 'short segment Barrett's'. Importance/relevance of short segment Barrett's is endlessly debated at meetings, with no clear message at the time of writing (2004).

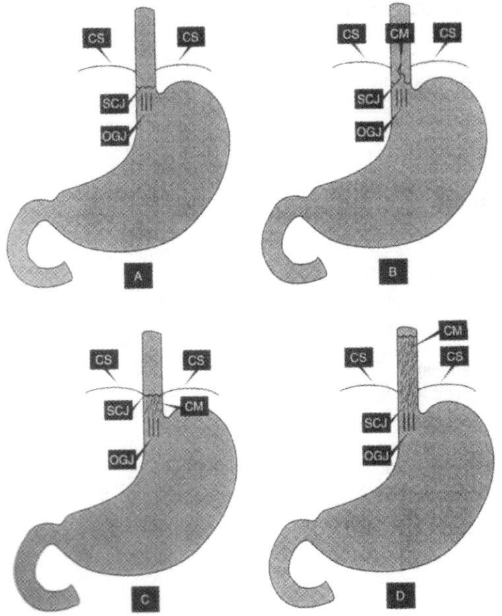

Fig. 2.5 Barrett's oesophagus. The relation of the oesophagogastric junction (OGJ: upper limit of gastric rugal folds), the squamocolumnar junction (SCJ), and the diaphragmatic crural sling (CS). A, normal situation. B, a tongue of columnar mucosa (CM), confluent but not circumferential. C, Short segment Barrett's: the columnar mucosa is confluent and circumferential but less than 3 cm long. D, segment Barrett's: circumferential columnarization longer than 3 cm. Reprinted with permission From Bloom S (2001). *Practical gastroenterology: A Comprehensive Guide.* Taylor & Francis Group Ltd.

Practice point: diagnosis of Barrett's oesophagus

Correct endoscopic identification of anatomical landmarks is vital (also affects interpretation of histology). Diagnosis of Barrett's oesophagus is often imprecise because of a failure to document (see Fig. 2.5).

• Level of diaphragmatic crus (usually 40 cm in males, 38 cm in females)
• Gastro-oesophageal junction (where the gastric rugal folds peter out into the tubular oesophagus)
• Squamo-columnar junction

All endoscopy reports should include these values if there is any question of Barrett's oesophagus. Failure to do this in so many studies has generated more heat than light over this controversial topic.

Pathogenesis + epidemiology. Usually arises as an adaptive change to reflux oesophagitis. Columnar mucosa is more resistant to acid than squamous epithelium, but the price for protection may be high, as epithelium can become metaplasic and premalignant. The incidence of developing adenocarcinoma (see <u>oesophageal tumours</u>) is approximately 1 in 100 patient years, representing approximately a 30-fold increase in risk. Frequency studies suggest it is more common than originally thought and moreover may be increasing.

Clinical features. May be entirely asymptomatic, or associated with symptoms of <u>oesophagitis</u>.

Diagnosis requires oesophageal biopsies showing columnar epithelium. Endoscopy alone is not sufficient.

In general the risk of malignancy seems associated with the presence of intestinal metaplasia on biopsy.

Note. Do not confuse Barrett's with an inlet patch of columnar mucosa in the upper oesophagus. This is usually congenital and is not exposed to enough acid to produce significant inflammation. It is not premalignant.

Treatment. No convincing data that either medical or surgical intervention results in clinically meaningful regression of Barrett's epithelium or reduces the risk of it undergoing malignant transformation. Because of the high mortality of surgery (about 7%), some centres are using lasers with or without photosensitizing agents, to ablate dysplastic Barrett's (see <u>photodynamic therapy</u>). This can lead to regrowth with squamous epithelium but long-term follow up data are awaited. Issue of <u>Barrett's surveillance</u> is controversial.

Barrett's surveillance

Most patients with Barrett's have normal lifespan and die of unrelated disease (Cameron, A J et al. (1985) *N. Engl. J. Med* **313**: 857). Endoscopic surveillance is frequently recommended **if the length of columnar epithelium is 3 cm or more and if there is intestinal metaplasia on biopsy.** Surveillance is recommended to detect <u>dysplasia</u> and asymptomatic adenocarcinoma. Cancers in Barrett's evolve slowly and there is some evidence that early resection carries a better prognosis than the 5 year survival of 17% reported for symptomatic adenocarcinomas (see <u>oesophageal tumours</u>).

Recommendations

- **No dysplasia.** Survey every 2 years by taking 4 quadrant biopsies using jumbo forceps every 2 cm throughout the length of Barrett's.
- **Low grade dysplasia.** First get a second pathology opinion for confirmation. Give a high dose PPI to minimize inflammation that makes pathological interpretation more difficult; then take repeat biopsies. In established low grade dysplasia, take biopsies every 6 months for 1 year, then yearly if no high grade dysplasia is seen.
- **High grade dysplasia** (which should be verified by 2 experienced pathologists) has long been regarded as an indication for oesophagectomy because cancer is found in 30–50% of specimens resected for such lesions. But the mortality is 5–10% and because of this **endoscopic ablative therapy** has been proposed as an alternative.

Non-endoscopic balloon cytology of Barrett's has been suggested as useful in surveillance—a small study suggested 85% sensitivity for HGD or carcinoma but only 25% for LGD. It is much cheaper than endoscopic surveillance and further studies seem warranted.

Behçet's syndrome

After H. Behçet, Turkish dermatologist, died 1948.

- Vasculitis affecting several organ systems. Said to occur along the old silk road from the Middle East to Japan: Incidence is highest in Turkey (370 cases per 100 000), Iran (16–100 per 100 000), Saudi Arabia and Japan (13 per 1 000 000). Onset typically in 3rd and 4th decades, more common in males in Middle East but females in Far East.
- Pathophysiology unknown, the basic lesion is a vasculitis. Neutrophil function is abnormal (enhanced neutrophil–endothelial cell adhesion, positive pathergy test).
- Diagnostic criteria include: oral aphthous ulcers (which are recurrent, painful, and non-scarring) plus 2 of: genital ulcers, uveitis (anterior or posterior), pustular vasculitis, synovitis, menigoencephalitis, and exclusion of patients with IBD, SLE, Reiter's, and herpes. Aphthoid ulcers may occur anywhere in the GI tract, most commonly in the ileo-caecal region, but also right colon and oesophagus.
- GI lesions are usually treated with steroids, 5-ASA, or thalidomide: colchicine and azathioprine are used for systemic manifestations.

Beriberi

Clinical manifestation of <u>vitamin B1</u> (thiamine) deficiency. Cause is inadequate intake (including diets high in polished rice which contains thiaminase: also alcoholics). Affects cardiovascular system (wet beriberi: sodium retention oedema, high output left ventricular failure) and nervous system (dry beriberi: motor and sensory neuropathy and Wernicke–Korsakoff psychosis). Associated with reduced red cell cell transketolase which requires thiamine as a cofactor. Those with <u>alcoholic liver disease</u> have reduced capacity to absorb thiamine so always give thiamine supplements.

Bezoars

From a Persian word for counterpoison, because they were originally thought to be antidotes for snake bites and insect stings.

Defined as persistent concretions of foreign matter found in the GI tract: nearly always in the stomach. Usually composed of plant and vegetable fibres, hair, or medications (aluminium antacids, enteric-coated tablets, bismuth). They are not common but occur when material that enters the stomach cannot exit because of size, indigestibility, obstruction, or poor motility. Symptoms depend on the size and location. Endoscopy is the most sensitive test. While surgical removal is sometimes needed, non-operative strategies include enzymatic digestion, mechanical disruption using endoscopic forceps and snares, and even laser treatment.

Bile acid malabsorption

Background

- Enterohepatic circulation of bile acids involves excretion from liver into bile of water soluble conjugated bile acids (cholic and chenoxydeoxychoilc acid). Deconjugation by intraluminal gut flora to insoluble dihydroxy bile acids (deoxycholic acid and lithocholic acid) allows 95% reabsorption of bile acids from terminal ileum and, via portal venous system, circulation back to liver. This process conserves bile acids, providing adequate intraluminal bile acids to allow micelle solubilization, and absorption of lipids and fat soluble vitamins (<u>vitamins</u> A, D, E, K).
- Bile acid malabsorption is usually secondary to other causes, including ileal resection/<u>Crohn's disease</u>, ileal radiation enteritis, <u>cholecystec-tomy</u> ('post-cholecystectomy diarrhoea'), <u>chronic pancreatitis</u>, <u>coeliac disease</u>, <u>cystic fibrosis</u>. Rare primary disease due to congenital defi-ciency in sodium–bile acid co-transporter.

Clinical features

- Bloating, abdominal discomfort.
- Steatorrhea: due to fat <u>malabsorption</u> secondary to reduced bile acids in small bowel.
- Diarrhoea. Increased concentrations of deconjugated bile acids in colon inhibit carbohydrate transporters, reduce intraluminal pH, and directly damage enterocyte.
- <u>Gallstones</u>: due to ↓bile acid pool and production of lithogenic bile.
- <u>Oxalate stones</u>.

Investigation

- High level of clinical suspicion often raised by associated clinical problems (e.g. terminal ileal <u>Crohn's disease</u>).
- Range of tests available, many of which are cumbersome and impractical (e.g. 72 hour stool collection for bile acid absorption test).
- Other approaches include:
  - Trial of bile acid sequesters. Failure to improve diarrhoea within 3 days of starting <u>CHOLESTYRAMINE </u>makes bile acid malabsorp-tion an unlikely cause of diarrhoea. However, cholestyramine may occasionally worsen symptoms if malabsorption severe.
  - Selenium-75 labelled homotaurocholic acid test (SeHCaT). Radio-active taurocholic acid given orally, and serial whole body scintigraphy over 4–7 days used to demonstrate abnormal absorption. Test is time-consuming and difficult to standardize.

Management

- Treatment of underlying cause.
- Use of bile acid sequesters (See above, and index of drugs).
- Maintain adequate fluid intake to reduce risk of <u>oxalate stones</u>.
- Replacement of fat soluble <u>vitamins A</u>, <u>D</u>, <u>E</u>, <u>K</u> may be necessary.

Biliary atresia

Congenital anomaly affecting 1:14000 live births, with fibrosis and destruction of biliary tree at different sites.
● Type 1 – common bile duct.
● Type II – common hepatic duct.
● Type III – liver hilum (85% of cases).
  Presents with progressive jaundice and hepatomegaly by week 2 post-partum, with other defects (e.g. dextrocardia) in 25%. Diagnosis suggested by abdominal U/S or hepatobiliary scintiscan in neonate with persistent jaundice, and made by cholangiography, either via ERCP, transhepatic puncture, or more usually intraoperatively. Liver biopsy may be charac-teristic (portal tract expansion, bile plugging of ducts).
Treatment is surgical, usually through Roux-en-Y anastomosis, with loop of small bowel anastomosed to hepatic ducts at hilum (Kasai porto-enterostomy). This is effective in > 50%, but only 35% 10 year survival due to complications, including secondary biliary cirrhosis. Liver transplantation may be required.

Biliary bypass procedures

Resection of extrahepatic bile duct, or biliary diversion, may be indicated for a range of biliary problems, including:
● Iatrogenic/traumatic bile duct injury (e.g. post-cholecystectomy), which is not amenable to endoscopic stent insertion.
● Biliary stone disease (e.g. Mirrizzi's syndrome).
● Persistent biliary stricture (e.g. secondary to pancreatic cancer or chronic pancreatitis).
● Choledochal cyst.

Operative approaches include:
● Whipple's procedure (distal common bile duct (CBD), duodenum, and pancreatic head resection).
● Hepatico-jejunostomy: Roux-en-Y anastomosis, with jejunal loop on to common hepatic duct.
● Choledochoduodenostomy: usually side-to-side anastomosis of lower CBD on to duodenal bulb. Used for very distal strictures.
● Cholecyst–enterostomy: anastomosis of gallbladder on to small bowel—rarely performed.
Practical point. In patient with hepaticojejunostomy, subsequent ERCP to access biliary tree is usually impossible, due to Roux-en-Y anastomosis and long jejunal loop.

Biliary reflux

- Refers to the reflux into the stomach and oesophagus of biliary fluid from the duodenum. Alkaline bile is an irritant to oesophageal squamous mucosa. Factors associated with biliary reflux include duodenal pathology (e.g. distal duodenal stricture), hiatus hernia, and surgery (e.g. Billroth II partial <u>gastrectomy</u>, with reflux of bile from afferent loop into stomach). Symptoms are similar to those of gastro-oesophageal reflux, but pH oesophageal monitoring (also see <u>oeso-phageal manometry</u>) demonstrates increased pH in association with reflux symptoms, and acid suppression provides no benefit.
- Treatment includes prokinetic agents (metaclopramide, domperidone (see <u>DOPAMINE RECEPTOR ANTAGONISTS</u>)) and mucosal protection (<u>sucralfate</u> 2 g bd PO). Surgery is sometimes necessary—a <u>Roux-en-Y anastomosis</u> allows diversion of bile flow further down jejunum.

Biliary strictures

May develop at any point within biliary tree, but site may give some clue to aetiology (see table): e.g. low common bile duct (CBD) stricture more likely due to <u>pancreatic cancer</u>, chronic <u>pancreatitis</u>; mid-CBD due to <u>Mirrizzi's syndrome</u>, <u>gallbladder cancer</u>; and hilar structuring may be due to <u>primary sclerosing cholangitis</u>, <u>cholangiocarcinoma</u>.

Clinical features. Jaundice (see <u>Approach to recent-onset jaundice</u>), right upper quadrant pain, <u>cholangitis</u> (fever, rigors), abnormal <u>liver func-tion tests</u>, or rarely the complications of secondary biliary cirrhosis.

Investigations
- Bloods may show ↑ Bn, cholestatic LFTs (↑ALP, GGT).
- U/S accurately demonstrate biliary dilatation, presence of gallbladder stones, and possible mass lesions.
- <u>CT scan</u> and <u>MRI/MRCP</u> are non-invasive tests of choice to define exact site of stricture, aetiology, and surrounding structures.
- <u>ERCP</u> allows delineation of stricture/biliary tree, cytological brushings, endobiliary biopsies, and therapy (e.g. stone extraction, biliary stenting).
- <u>Endoscopic ultrasound</u>, including intraductal miniprobe ultrasound, may be available in specialist units, and may delineate nature of stricture further (e.g. <u>cholangiocarcinoma</u>).

Management depends on defining the cause of the stricture (see relevant A–Z sections). Simplistically, treatment involves endoscopic resolution of stricture (e.g. sphincterotomy for ampullary stenosis, balloon dilatation of benign stricture), endoscopic stenting, or surgery (which may include <u>cholecystectomy</u> for <u>Mirizzi's syndrome</u>, or <u>biliary bypass procedure</u>).

Causes of biliary strictures

Primary sclerosing cholangitis	HIV cholangiopathy (see HIV and the liver)
Cholangiocarcinoma	Autoimmune pancreatitis
Gallbladder cancer	Pancreatic cancer
Extrinsic compression by hilar nodes	Ampullary cancer/stenosis
Mirizzi's syndrome	Bile duct stone-related stricture
Cholecystectomy-related bile duct injury	Clonorchis infection
Ischaemic stricture	Bile duct (peri-dochal) varices/cavernoma
Acute/chronic pancreatitis	

Biliary tree variations

- Most variations in the anatomy of the biliary tree appear to result from alterations in the budding from the foregut of the embryonic liver and biliary tract. Minor anomalies usually cause no clinical problems, but may be of great relevance to the biliary surgeon.
- An accessory bile duct from right hepatic duct to cystic duct/gall bladder ('duct of Lushka') may result in biliary leak post-<u>cholecystectomy</u>. In 5% the right hepatic duct inserts low down in common hepatic duct, and may be mistaken for cystic duct. In 20% the cystic duct does not pass straight into the common hepatic duct, but runs parallel to it, down towards the papilla ('low inserting cystic duct'), with a risk of incorrect ductal ligation at surgery, and incorrect stent placement at ERCP.
- Gall bladders may be congenitally bilobed, double, intrahepatic, or absent. Other congenital abnormalities may cause symptoms through predisposing to bile stasis, stone formation, or malignancy (see <u>Caroli's disease</u>; <u>choledochal cysts</u>).

Bilharzia

See: <u>Schistosomiasis</u>.

Bilirubin metabolism

- Bilirubin is an end product of haem degradation, derived from red blood cells (70–80% of total) and extrahaematopoietic tissues (mainly liver). Approximately 4 mg/kg of bilirubin produced/day.
- Bilirubin produced by initial conversion of haem to biliverdin (via haem oxygenase), and then biliverdin to bilirubin (via bilverdin reductase).
- Unconjugated bilirubin circulates in plasma bound to albumin. After uptake into hepatocytes (? by organic anion transporting polypeptide (OATP)) it undergoes conjugation in endoplasmic reticulum by bilirubin glucuronyltransferase (UGT-1) (defective enzyme activity associated with <u>Gilbert's syndrome</u>). Conjugation converts hydrophobic bilirubin into water-soluble form (80% as bilirubin diglucuronides), which is excreted into bile via an ATP-dependent export pump (site of defect in <u>Dubin–Johnson syndrome</u>).
- Resorption of conjugated bilirubin from the gut is minimal, but it may be hydrolysed by bacterial β-glucuronidase interminal ileum/colon, with this unconjugated bilirubin subsequently converted to colourless urobilinogen. Approximately 20% of urobilinogen is resorbed, and excreted in the urine.

Billroth

See also <u>gastrectomy</u>. Christian Billroth (German–Austrian surgeon, 1829–1894).

Billroth pioneered many surgical operations including <u>gastrectomy</u>. Billroth 1 operation involves directly joining gastric remnant after partial gastrectomy onto the duodenum; Billroth II operation involves closing the duodenal stump and making a gastroenterostomy. Billroth I is preferred because of a lower incidence of <u>dumping</u> and weight loss. Billroth II is used if duodenal inflammation makes a Billroth I technically difficult.

Biofeedback

A process of behavioural retraining (usually applied in gastroenterology to toileting behaviour) using sensory training, electromyographic feedback, or manometric feedback. The sensory component teaches the patient to perceive smaller volumes of rectal distension, which are often insensible to constipated patients. The motor component is performed with a pressure probe in the anal canal, to monitor anal sphincter pressure. Patients become accustomed to visual feedback of sphincter activity on voluntary sphincter contraction. This can demonstrate failure of sphincter relaxation or failure of pelvic floor function and many patients can be taught to improve this. About two-thirds of patients with long-term intractable constipation report improvement with the technique (Bassotti, G et al. (2004) Br. Med. J. **328**: 393). Technique is less successful in patients with psychiatric comorbidity or poor compliance with home practice.

Blastocystis

Previously considered a yeast; recently reclassified as a protozoan. Associated with GI symptoms, but may simply be an indicator of exposure to faecal infection with 'true pathogens' such as E. histolytica. 60% of patients with Blastocystis hominis but no other stool pathogens have underlying disease associated with some immunosuppression, and most have symptoms lasting 3–10 days. Reasonable to treat symptomatic patients where no other stool pathogens have been identified and and who have moderate to heavy infection (more than 5 B. hominis per high power field on microscopy). Treatment is usually with <u>METRONIDAZOLE</u>; furazolidone and co-trimoxazole are inhibitory in vitro.

Blind loop

Surgical alterations of intestinal anatomy with creation of pouches or long segments of diverted intestine (entero-enteric anastomoses, Billroth II, jejuno-ileal bypass, Kock distal ileal pouch for continent ileostomy) interfere with peristalsis and can lead to <u>bacterial overgrowth</u>.

Body mass index (BMI)

Also known as the Quetelet index. Defined as body weight (kg) divided by height (m) squared (see BMI chart in Appendix 2). It correlates well with obesity but is not a direct measure of adiposity. The World Health Organization definitions of body weight categories are shown in the table opposite. See also Approach to obesity and obesity surgery.

Bone densitometry

See also osteoporosis. A method of measuring bone mineral density (BMD) to detect osteopenia or osteoporosis, which can be expressed as the number of standard deviations (SD) above or below the mean BMD for young adults (T score) or the mean BMD for age-matched controls (Z score). The risk of fracture increases 2–3 times for each SD decrease in BMD. WHO criteria for defining osteoporosis includes a T score in the hip and/or spine that is 2.5 or more SD below young adult mean value. Osteopenia is a T score of 1 to 2.5 SD below mean value. The best technique currently involves dual energy X-ray absorptiometry (DEXA). Note that lumbar spine measurements are unreliable in the elderly due to presence of osteophytes, extraskeletal calcification, and vertebral or spinal deformity.

Boerhaave syndrome

Herman Boerhaave (1668–1738), Dutch, one of the most revered teachers of his day. Best known for his description of oesophageal rupture in the grand admiral of the fleet van Wassanaer. Said to have written a book containing all the secrets of medicine: after he died it was opened and all the pages were blank except one on which was written 'keep the head cool, the feet warm and the bowels open'.

- Oesophageal rupture caused by vomiting against a closed glottis: common after excess alcohol intake. Rupture usually occurs at the weakest point (at the lower end on the left side), but may occur in the mid-oesophagus on the right. The lack of serosa in the oesophagus may make it more prone to rupture. Gastric contents spill into the thorax. Pain is severe, upper abdominal, and may radiate to the back. Examination may reveal dyspnoea, sepsis, hypovolaemic shock, and cyanosis. Surgical emphysema may be found in the neck.
- Early diagnosis reached by clinical suspicion and a gastrograffin swallow. CXR may show air in mediastinum.
- Initial management is to keep patient strictly nil by mouth and give IV antibiotics (e.g. 3rd generation CEPHALOSPORIN and METRONIDAZOLE), but most patients should be managed surgically. Early surgery (within 6h) may be life-saving. Primary closure may be possible if surgery is not delayed: in late cases alternatives are drainage with a cervical oesophagostomy and gastrostomy, or transhiatal oesophagectomy. Mortality for cases diagnosed and treated within 6–12h is 10–15%, rising to over 50% for those diagnosed after that time.

Body weight categories

Category	Body mass index (kg/m^2)
Underweight	< 19
Normal weight	19–24.9
Mild overweight	25–29.9
Moderate overweight	30–39.9
Severe overweight	> 40

Botulism

Rare food-borne illness usually due to neurotoxins produced by *Clostridium botulinum,* although there are recent cases due to contaminated drugs injected subcutaneously (also see <u>Clostridial infections in GI tract</u>). Toxin produces gastrointestinal symptoms within 18 to 36 h, followed by constipation with dry mouth, diplopia, blurred vision, dysarthria, dysphagia, and muscle weakness, with a classical symmetrical descending paralysis.

Therapy includes supportive ventilation and antitoxin if disease is diagnosed early.

Bougies

General term used for dilators of luminal strictures in the GI tract. Derived from the Algerian town of Bouginhay, medieval capital of the wax candle trade, because wax dilators were used in the middle ages for food impaction. A cork-tipped whalebone was used to dilate an achalasia patient in the 16th century. Bougies are widely used in <u>endoscopic dilatation</u>.

Bowel preparation

Bad bowel prep is the bane of colonoscopy. Some sort of bowel preparation is almost always needed. For examination of the left colon a phosphate enema should be given 15–60 minutes pre-procedure but, in patients with diverticular disease or strictures, full bowel prep may be needed. Frail, ill, and elderly may need inpatient preparation.
- **Modification to diet and medication.** Iron should be stopped 1 week prior to colonoscopy. Constipating agents should be avoided for 24 hours pre-procedure: some centres suggest stopping antiplatelet agents including aspirin for 7 days to reduce the risk of immediate or delayed bleeding after polypectomy, but this is not evidence based and not part of current guidelines. Colon cleansing is aided by a liquid diet for 24 hours prior to examination.
- **Purgative regimens** (author's note: remember the difference between regimen and regime, the latter a term reserved for authoritarian dictatorships—such as Chile under Pinochet (or the NHS target culture)): see opposite.

Breath tests

A wide variety of volatile compounds in expired air relate to aspects of digestive function. For urea breath tests, see *Helicobacter*.

Hydrogen breath tests. Sole source of hydrogen in mammals is bacterial fermentation. Increased breath hydrogen can be easily detected using a hand-held meter and does not involve radioactive substrates. A rise of breath hydrogen of > 20 parts per million (ppm) compared with baseline after oral ingestion of 50 g lactose identifies <u>lactose intolerance</u>.

Bowel cleansing regimens for colonoscopy

Preparation	Advantages	Disadvantages	Notes
Non-absorbable carbohydrate (mannitol, lactulose sorbital) act as osmotic laxatives)	Avoids cramping effects of purgatives	Sweet, unpalatable in large volume needed	Not recommended—hydrogen gas produced by fermentation gives risk of explosion during electrosurgical procedures
Polyethlylene glycol based solutions (e.g Kleenprep)	Safe, effective	Large volume (4L) often difficult for patients to manage	Widely used in UK
Magnesium salts—have strong purgative and osmotic effects	Magnesium citrate has a milder flavour than magnesium sulphate	Need to drink 2L of fluid	Widely used in UK. Effective when combined with oral senna
Low volume sodium phosphate	Well tolerated—2×45ml aliquots of sodium phosphate taken orally the evening before and 4 hours prior to colonoscopy produce a vigorous catharsis	Fluid balance shifts or hyperphosphataemia can be significant, especially in the presence of cardiac or renal disease	

General advice given to patients on preparing for colonoscopy
- Stop Iron tablets 7 days before the exam; continue all other medications and laxatives until the procedure.
- Taka a low residue diet for 1–2 days before the examination (no cereals, nuts or muesli).
- No solid food after lunch on the day preceding the colonoscopy, but take plenty of clear fluids to avoid dehydration.
- After the exam, it is better not to use public transport, but if essential the patient MUST be accompanied.
- No alcohol or operation of heavy machinery for 24 hours after procedure.
- No driving on day of procedure if sedation has been given or signing of legal documents.

An early rise in breath hydrogen is seen within 2 hours of glucose or lactulose ingestion in patients with small intestinal <u>bacterial overgrowth</u> (all people show a late rise due to colonic fermentation); conventional testing uses a rise of 20 ppm, which has good specificity but poor sensitivity especially if low doses (< 20 g) of test carbohydrate are used. Sensitivity can be improved by ensuring the dinner preceding the overnight fast contains readily absorbed carbohydrates to avoid a high basal level on the day of the test, measuring the increase at 6 hrs rather than 4 and having a cutoff of 10 ppm over baseline for diagnosing malabsorption. Despite these precautions and the attractions of ease of performance and avoidance of a radioactive tracer, many authorities regard hydrogen breath tests as insufficiently sensitive or specific.

Carbon breath tests. The ^{14}C-triolein breath test measures $^{14}CO_2$ in breath after ingestion of labelled trigyceride. The test utility is insufficient to justify the equipment expense and radiation exposure and the test is not widely used. The sugar xylose is catabolized by aerobic Gram-negative overgrowth flora; following a 1 g oral dose of ^{14}C-D-xylose, elevated $^{14}CO_2$ is found in 85% of people with small bowel <u>bacterial overgrowth</u>.

Brush border

The terminal products of luminal stomach digestion, as well as diasaccharides such as sucrose and lactose, cannot be absorbed intact and must be hydrolysed by brush border membrane hydrolases, maximally expressed in the villi of duodenum and jejunum. Impaired activity of these enzymes may occur if the brush border is damaged (by, for example, infective gastroenteritis, chemotherapy, <u>coeliac disease</u>, <u>HIV</u>)—although there are also rare congenital causes of carbohydrase deficiency. This results in non-absorbable carbohydrates passing into the colon where they are metabolized by bacterial flora, producing osmotically active short-chain fatty acids. This leads to gaseous distension and diarrhoea if the colonic capacity to absorb short chain fatty acids is overwhelmed.

Budd–Chiari syndrome (BCS)

Definition and pathogenesis. BCS refers to obstruction of main hepatic veins (HVs) by thrombus, and is viewed as separate from <u>veno-occlusive disease</u>, which involves hepatic venules. Causes of BCS include generalized thrombophilia in > 40% (e.g. myeloproliferative disorders, factor V Leiden deficiency), <u>hepatocellular carcinoma</u>, and anomalies of inferior vena cava. In clinical practice the diagnosis is rarely made unless it's considered.

Clinical features. Usual pattern involves abdominal pain, ascites, and hepatomegaly developing over several months, but <u>acute liver failure</u> may rarely occur. Jaundice is variable. Features of <u>portal hypertension</u>, including splenomegaly and bleeding varices, may develop. Clinical course varies considerably, but 3 year survival in chronic BCS of 50% has been reported.

Investigation. Diagnosis usually made with Doppler <u>ultrasound</u> or contrast <u>CT scan</u> (but alert radiologists to clinical possibility!) Venography and venous pressure measurement allow the site of obstruction to be defined. Caudate lobe hypertrophy (due to separate drainage into inferior vena cava) on imaging is a characteristic, but only seen in 50% of cases. Unlike in most cases of portal hypertension, the ascitic fluid in acute Budd–Chiari syndrome is often an exudate (i.e. SAAG < 11 g/dl. See <u>Approach to ascites</u>). Perform thrombophilia screen to identify underlying cause (see <u>portal vein thrombosis</u>).

Management. In acute BCS, thrombolysis and subsequent anticoagulation has been used, to attempt recannulation of HVs, and in the rare cases of <u>acute liver failure</u> (see emergencies) <u>liver transplantation</u> may be required. In chronic BCS anticoagulation should also be considered, but management of complications is central, including ascites and <u>portal hypertension.</u> Ascites is diuretic-resistant in 30% from presentation. <u>Liver transplantation</u> probably carries better prognosis than surgical portocaval shunting, but <u>TIPSS</u> has been used to good effect.

Bulimia

Initially used to describe a syndrome of gluttonous overeating and induced vomiting; more recently applied to the psychiatric diagnosis of **bulimia nervosa**, which centres on a maladaptive behaviour employed to control calorie consumption and promote weight loss. As with <u>anorexia nervosa</u>, incidence has increased in recent years: it is more common than anorexia and estimated to affect 2–5% of school and college aged females. Hallmark personality features are loss of control, low self-esteem, and guilt. Most bulimic individuals are of normal weight and perceive their eating behaviour as problematic, often seeking medical help (unlike the patient with <u>anorexia nervosa</u>). Important physical signs are salivary gland hypertrophy, dental enamel erosion, excoriations on knuckles (caused by digitally induced vomiting), and chronic sore throat. Medical complications can include electrolyte disturbances (hypokalaemia, hypomagnesaemia, hypoglycaemia, hyperprolactinaemia) as well as oesophagitis, pancreatitis, abdominal pain, constipation, and cathartic colon.

B vitamins

See: <u>vitamins</u> and <u>cobalamin</u>.

C

Campylobacter

Motile Gram-negative rods that have emerged since the 1970s as a major cause of acute dysentery, accounting for up to 20% of positive stool cultures in patients with acute infective bloody diarrhoea. Two main species are responsible, *C. jejuni* and *C. coli*: both affect the colon, producing an acute febrile syndrome in children and adults resembling <u>*Shigella*</u> infection.

Epidemiology. Similar to <u>*Salmonella*</u>. Person–person transmission is common: poultry and eggs the commonest source of infection.

Pathogenesis may involve epithelial invasion or toxin production.

Clinical features. Children and young adults are most susceptible. Incubation period 1–6 days. There is a prodrome of fatigue and myalgia for 24 hours; then nausea, abdominal cramps, tenderness, and bloody diarrhoea are typical. Disease spectrum ranges from asymptomatic carriage to life-threatening colitis with <u>toxic megacolon</u>. <u>Reiter's syndrome</u> and <u>haemolytic–uraemic syndrome</u> can all occur. About 30% of patients with Guillain–Barré syndrome have evidence of *Campylobacter* infection (either stool culture or antibodies to *C. jejuni*). Antibodies to *C. Jejuni* share epitopes with brain gangliosides suggesting that cross-reacting antibodies may contribute to the development of nerve damage following campylobacter enteritis.

Diagnosis. Made on stool cultures, which seldom remain positive for more than 2 weeks. 90% have negative stool cultures after 5 weeks.

Therapy. Mainstay is replacement of fluids and electrolytes. Recurrent or severe disease, or arguably disease that is diagnosed early, can be treated with antibiotics: erythromycin 250 mg Po qds for 5 days and <u>CIPROFLOXACIN</u> 500 mg Po bd are effective: ciprofloxacin has the advantage of being effective against <u>entero-toxigenic *E.coli*</u>, <u>*Shigella*,</u> and <u>*Salmonella*</u>. Quinolone resistance reaches 50% in some areas but most are sensitive to azithromycin. Also see <u>Approach to acute diarrhoea.</u>

Candida

Epidemiology. A frequent commensal of healthy people (found in 40–65% normal faecal flora), it is also the commonest fungal human pathogen. The clinical syndrome depends largely on the host immune status, although there are also fungal virulence factors.

Clinical features. Two main patterns:

• Mucocutaneous candidiasis rarely causes death, although in patients with refractory HIV infection can become resistant to antifungal therapy and lead to severe oropharyngeal/oesophageal involvement.

• Disseminated candidiaisis has a high mortality but is comparatively rare. In the GI tract the commonest lesions associated with *Candida* are single or multiple ulcerations: white plaque and thickened mucosal folds can be seen at endoscopy. Apart from oropharynx, oesophagus is the most commonly affected site within the GI tract, but gastric and small intestinal infection can also occur. The commonest symptom associated with intestinal candidiasis is diarrhoea: since the organism is so often present, a small bowel biopsy with histologic evidence of invasion is necessary for diagnosis.

Differential diagnosis includes other diseases affecting the GI tract in immunocompromised hosts: other mycoses, TB, ischaemic bowel, typhlitis, *Mycobacterium avium*.
Treatment. Fluconazole and nystatin commonly used for mucocutaneous disease including oropharyngeal candidiasis. For disseminated disease, amphotericin B is recommended with fluconazole as second-line therapy. See ANTI-FUNGALS.

Risk factors for *Candida*

- HIV (see HIV and the gut)
- Immunosuppression
- Parenteral feeding
- Urinary catheters
- Broad spectrum antibiotics
- CORTICOSTEROIDS
- Burns, trauma
- Recent surgery
- Haemodialysis

Capsule endoscopy

See <u>enteroscopy</u>.

Carcinoembryonic antigen (CEA)

A glycoprotein discovered in 1965 in association with <u>colorectal cancer</u> and embryonic and fetal gut tissues. Elevated in various malignant diseases (breast, lung, <u>gastric</u>, and <u>pancreatic cancers</u>) and also in nonmalignant conditions (heavy cigarette smoking, chronic bronchitis, and pancreatitis). Measuring CEA is not useful as a screening test, even when applied to patients with gastrointestinal signs or symptoms. CEA level is a poor measure of tumour bulk because the level is highest when the liver is involved, even to only a minor degree, and may be barely elevated in patients with a bulky intra-abdominal recurrence. With these caveats, there are some defined roles for CEA (see box opposite).

Carcinoid

Tumours arising from enterochromaffin cells (derived from neural crest cells: also called APUD cells (**A**mine **P**recursor **U**ptake and **D**ecarboxylation)) at the base of intestinal crypts. GI carcinoids account for 95% of all carcinoids and about 1.5% of all GI tumours. They secrete a range of hormones, including 5-HT (serotonin—metabolized in the liver by monoamine oxidase into 5-hydroxy-indole-acetic acid (5-HIAA) and excreted in the urine), ACTH, histamine, bradykinin, and kallikrein.

Clinical features. Most patients are asymptomatic but can present with pain, obstruction (20%), weight loss (15%), palpable mass (15%), or perforation of haemorrhage (rare).

Carcinoid syndrome arises when the hormonal load exceeds the capacity of the monoamine oxidase in the liver and lung to metabolize serotonin—most patients with carcinoid syndrome have liver metastases from a bowel carcinoid.

Clinical features of carcinoid syndrome include diarrhoea and abdominal cramps (70%), flushing of skin and telangiectasia, right-sided heart failure from right-sided endocardial fibrosis leading to tricuspid regurgitation, and pulmonary valve stenosis.

Carcinoids at different sites of the GI tract can behave rather differently:

- **Foregut carcinoids** are rare: tumours are usually slow growing and benign. Gastric carcinoids have been classified into type I (small benign tumours associated with chronic <u>atrophic gastritis</u> and hypergastrinaemia), type II (large, polypoid lesions, prone to metastases, and associated with <u>multiple endocrine neoplasia</u> type 1 (MEN-1) and Zollinger–Ellison syndrome (see <u>gastrinoma</u>), and type III (large, solitary, sporadic tumours not associated with raised gastrin levels).
- **Midgut carcinoid.** Most commonly occurring tumour of the small bowel. Ileum is commonest affected site (90%). Tumours may be multiple, and liver metastases occur in 25%.

Rules for measuring CEA

1. Preoperative CEA level is related to the stage of <u>colon cancer</u> and may serve as a predictor of surgical incurability: values greater than 5.0 ng/ml have been associated with a poor prognosis, independent of surgical stage
2. Postoperative CEA level may serve as a measure of the completeness of tumour resection. If a preoperatively elevated CEA value does not fall to normal levels within 4 weeks (a period that is twice the plasma half-life of CEA) after surgery, the resection was probably incomplete or occult metastases are present
3. The CEA level may serve as a useful monitor of tumour recurrence
4. The CEA assay may serve as a monitor of response to treatment of metastatic disease. Serial CEA values parallel either tumour regression or tumour progression. A rising CEA level is incompatible with tumour regression, whereas CEA values decrease in most patients who have responded to treatment.

- **Hindgut carcinoid.** Colonic carcinoids account for 0.3% of colon tumours. 75% occur in the ascending colon. A carcinoid may be an incidental finding on examination of a removed appendix, usually in patients aged 20–40 years. In patients with a tumour at the base of the appendix or if the tumour is larger than 2 cm, a right hemicolectomy is indicated. In patients with carcinoid at the <u>appendix</u> tip, appendicectomy alone is adequate.

Differential diagnoses include <u>pancreatic endocrine tumours</u>, or rare abdominal tumours such as desmoids.

Investigations. Elevated hormone output demonstrated with <u>gut hormone screen</u> (e.g. ↑ chromogranin A), and 24 hour urine collection for 5-HIAA (note: may be falsely ↑ by bananas, avocado, pineapple, walnuts, coffee, and chocolate). <u>Ultrasound</u> is not specific, but may lead to more appropriate investigation. <u>CT scanning</u> is better at providing anatomical information, and <u>endoscopic ultrasound</u> and angiography may be necessary. Barium studies are of low yield. The most promising techniques include octreotide and MIBG (metaiodobenzylguanidine) scanning. <u>PET scanning</u> increasingly used to identify metastatic lesions.

Management. Surgical cure may be possible for isolated lesions (or limited liver metastases). For those with carcinoid syndrome <u>OCTREOTIDE</u> (see index of drugs) may effectively control hormone release, but other symptomatic approaches may also be necessary (e.g. loperamide for diarrhoea). Palliative approaches to reduce tumour load include hepatic artery embolization for large hepatic metastases; <u>INTERFERON-ALPHA</u>; chemotherapy (e.g. streptozocin, 5-fluorouracil, and doxorubicin); radio-isotope iodine (I^{131}) MIBG or octreotide therapy. Carcinoid tumours are generally slowly progressive (> 80% 5 year survival in surgically treated patients, and even in those with metastatic disease median survival > 2 years). Also see <u>pancreatic endocrine tumours</u>.

Caroli's disease

Congenital segmental cystic dilatation of intrahepatic bile ducts, thought to relate to a ductal plate malformation, and associated with autosomal recessive polycystic kidney disease. Sometimes classified as type 5 <u>choledochal cyst</u>. Hepatic fibrosis may occur, but the extrahepatic tree is unaffected. Often presents in early 20s, and clinical features include jaundice, <u>cholangitis</u>, and intraductal stones. <u>Cholangiocarcinoma</u> (reported in 7%) and <u>portal hypertension</u> may develop. Diagnosis often made with non-invasive imaging (e.g. <u>U/S</u>, <u>CT</u>, <u>MRCP</u>). Endoscopic biliary drainage may be attempted, but is of limited use in draining intrahepatic ducts. Hepatectomy is effective if disease confined to one lobe, but <u>liver transplantation</u> may be indicated for recurrent cholangitis and extensive disease.

Caustic injury

80% of caustic ingestions occur accidentally in children: ingestion in adults usually indicates intent of suicide or self-harm. Most ingested corrosives are alkaline (bleach and other household cleaning agents) or acids (toilet cleaners, battery acids, swimming pool cleaners). Risks to the GI tract are of oesophageal necrosis and perforation and later sequelae such as oesophageal scarring and stricture formation. However, most deaths following acid ingestion relate to systemic effects (renal failure, liver failure, DIC).

Clinical features can be dramatic: mouth and chest pain, with painful swallowing (odynophagia), dysphagia, excess salivation, and epigastric pain.

Management

- Gastric lavage and induced emesis are contraindicated. Activated charcoal not recommended. Water of no proven use.
- Prophylactic antibiotics are often given parenterally.
- CXR may show free air in the mediastinum or under the diaphragm.
- Water soluble contrast agents such as gastrograffin conventionally recommended over barium, especially if perforation needs excluding, but in the author's opinion <u>CT scanning</u> can give the same information.

Endoscopy

- The oropharynx may need to be examined by laryngoscopy, since a supraglottic or epiglottic burn with erythema and oedema formation may be a harbinger of airway obstruction and should be seen as an indication for early endotracheal intubation or tracheostomy.
- Endoscopy serves a dual purpose:
  - Patients with no evidence of gastrointestinal injury can be discharged, provided there are no other complications. More than 50% of patients with history of caustic ingestion have no endoscopic evidence of injury.
  - Those with evidence of severe injury can be managed appropriately.
- Endoscopy should preferably be performed < 12 hours and generally not > 24 hours since ingestion (although some authors state that endoscopy can be safely performed up to 96 hours post-ingestion). Severity of mucosal damage on endoscopy within 24 hours predicts mortality (overall 2–14%, with increased rate after acid, due largely to systemic complications—renal/liver failure, haemolysis, DIC). Wound softening begins after 2 to 3 days and lasts up to 2 weeks making endoscopy risky during this period.

Contraindications to endoscopy

- Evidence of full thickness injury, with possible perforation, shock, or acidosis.
- Third-degree burn of the hypopharynx seen at laryngoscopy.
- Perforation complicating endoscopy is rare but attempts to continue past circumferential burns are associated with increased risk.

Complications of caustic ingestion

- Stricture formation in 15% of cases. Early use of IV <u>CORTICOSTEROIDS</u> may reduce risk of stricture formation but this is controversial. <u>Endoscopic dilatation</u> rarely provides long-term cure, necessitating surgery in most cases.

Role of surgery

- If there is perforation or gastric necrosis, surgery is mandatory: 50% of patients with oesophageal perforation die. Options include oesophagectomy and gastrostomy if the stomach is intact, or gastrectomy and jejunostomy if the stomach is necrotic.

Cestodes

See: tapeworms.

Chagas' disease

See: trypanosomiasis.

Child–Pugh score

Widely used grading system in patients with chronic liver disease, as it is easy to calculate and uses straightforward clinical parameters (see table opposite).

This grading system is of prognostic use, and is widely used as the basis for assessing patients with cirrhosis for liver transplantation (e.g. Child–Pugh score > 7 as indication for referral).

Cholangiocarcinoma

Definition and pathogenesis

- Primary malignancy arising from intrahepatic or extrahepatic biliary tree, which causes 1.5% of all cancers; the rate is increasing. An important cause of biliary strictures.
- Associations include primary sclerosing cholangitis (PSC) (> 20% of cases of longstanding PSC develop cholangiocarcinoma, but PSC associated with only 5% of cases), gallstones, choledochal cysts, Caroli's disease, and biliary infestation with oriental liver fluke *Clonorchis sinensis*.
- Approximately 20–25% of tumours intrahepatic, 50–60% perihilar ('Klatskin' tumours involve confluence of left and right hepatic ducts in 20%), and 20–25% distal bile duct.

Clinical features

Abdominal discomfort, weight loss, and obstructive jaundice are the commonest presenting symptoms, similar to those of pancreatic cancer.

Investigations

- See Approach to recent onset jaundice
- Site, size, and vascular involvement of tumour may be demonstrated with CT and MRCP. Biliary anatomy well shown with MRCP, but ERCP allows intraductal U/S and endoscopic stenting to be performed (see Bismuth classification in figure). PET scanning may find a role.
- Tissue diagnosis may be made by endoscopic biopsies or brushings, or percutaneous biopsy. Diagnosis particularly difficult to confirm in patient with PSC and intra/extrahepatic duct strictures.
- Tumour marker CA19-9 ↑ in 85% of cases, but diagnostic role limited as may be elevated in biliary obstruction *per se*. Staging by TNM (see tumour staging).

Child's grading (with Pugh's modifications)

Criteria	Points		
	1	2	3
Hepatic encephalopathy grade	None	1–2	3–4
Serum bilirubin (μmol/l)	<35	35–50	>50
(In primary biliary cirrhosis)	<70	70–170	>170
Serum albumin (g/l)	>35	35–28	<28
Prothrombin time prolongation (sec)	1–4	4–10	>10
Total score	5–6	7–9	10–15
Child's grade equivalent	A	B	C

Percentage survival in chronic liver disease			
Child's grade	1 year	5 years	10 years
A	84	44	27
B	62	20	10
C	42	21	0

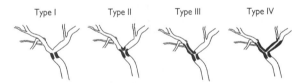

Fig. 2.6 Bismuth classification of cholangiocarcinoma. Type I, involvement of common hepatic duct, but below confluence of right and left ducts; type II, involvement of origin of left and right ducts at confluence; type III, involvement of secondary left or right intrahepatic ducts; type IV, involvement of secondary intrahepatic ducts bilaterally.

Management
- Surgical resection possible in only 10–15% of cases. 5 year survival post-surgery 9–18% for proximal tumours, 20–30% for distal bile duct lesions. <u>Liver transplantation</u> is rarely performed (because of very high rates of recurrence), but very highly selected patient groups may show up to 53% 5 year survival, with emerging data on aggressive neo-adjuvant therapy prior to transplantation showing some promise.
- Effective palliative endoscopic or percutaneous transhepatic stenting (plastic or self-expanding metal stents) is vital to preserve liver function and prevent cholangitis.
- Conventional chemotherapy (e.g. gemcytabine regimens) may provide partial response in 20–30% of cases. Palliative <u>photodynamic therapy</u> shows promise and may help to maintain duct patency.

Cholangitis

Infection of the biliary tree, usually arising from combination of biliary obstruction (e.g. <u>biliary stricture</u>) and presence of bacteria (usually Gram-negative gut flora).

Aetiology + pathogenesis. Causes of obstruction include stones (see <u>choledocholithiasis</u>), biliary strictures (e.g. <u>primary sclerosing cholangitis</u>, <u>pancreatic cancer</u>, <u>cholangiocarcinoma</u>), infestation (e.g. <u>Clonorchis</u>), and following instrumentation (particularly if incomplete drainage achieved at <u>ERCP</u>).

Clinical features

Classic Charcot triad includes fever (>90% of cases), jaundice (65%), and right upper quadrant pain (>40%). The presence of all three strongly favours the diagnosis, but this combination occurs in <20% of cases at presentation. Septic shock and confusion may occur.
- Secondary complications include acute renal failure, disseminated intravascular coagulation (DIC), and <u>liver abscess</u> formation.

Investigation
- FBC shows ↑WCC (↑ neutrophils).
- U&Es. Renal failure associated with septic shock.
- LFTs: ↑Bn, and predominantly cholestatic pattern (↑↑ALP/GGT), but ↑ALT, AST often present.
- Blood cultures positive in up to 50% of cases.
- Urgent <u>U/S</u> or <u>CT scan</u> showing biliary dilatation in correct clinical setting strongly supports diagnosis. Loss of aerobilia (air in biliary tree) in patient with biliary stent *in situ* suggests blocked stent.
- After demonstration of dilated bile ducts, <u>ERCP</u> allows confirmation of biliary obstruction and therapy.

Management
- Fluid resuscitation and management in high dependency area if hypotensive with signs of septic shock.
- Broad spectrum IV antibiotics (e.g. IV <u>CEPHALOSPORIN</u> + <u>METRONIDAZOLE</u>, or <u>PIPERACILLIN/TAZOBACTAM</u>), but note that antibiotics alone rarely resolve cholangitis in presence of ongoing biliary obstruction.
- ERCP with biliary decompression (e.g. biliary sphincterotomy and stone removal/stent insertion) essential. Percutaneous transhepatic drainage (PTC) only used if ERCP fails/technically impossible, as complications higher (and puncture often increases bacteraemia acutely).
- Mortality rate 7–40%, with poor outcome closely correlated with delays in definitive management.

Cholecystectomy

- 700 000 cholecystectomies a year performed in USA, mainly for gallstones.
- Laparoscopic cholecystectomy (LC) in > 80% of cases, but conversion to open cholecystectomy (OC) needed in 5–10%. In patients with bile duct stones (choledocholithiasis), duct clearance and sphincterotomy usually done by ERCP prior to surgery, but laparoscopic bile duct clearance increasingly performed at time of LC.
- Major complications include wound infection, bleeding, abscess formation, or bile leak (arising from cystic duct stump, damaged common bile duct, or aberrant bilary ducts (e.g. duct of Lushka)). See biliary tree variants. Bile duct injury occurs in 0.1–0.2% of OC, 0.5–1% of LC. Complications due to biliary strictures may develop immediately or up to 20 years later. Mortality for cholecystectomy 0.2% overall (0.03% in <65 year olds).

Cholecystitis

Defined as inflammation of the gallbladder, which results from obstruction of the cystic duct by gallstones in 90% of cases, and occurs in 30% of patients with gallstones. Acalculous cholecystitis is related to biliary stasis (e.g. major surgery/trauma, sepsis, parenteral nutrition, sickle cell disease, diabetes mellitus). Bacterial infection is thought to be secondary to obstruction.

Clinical features

Most patients have a prior history of biliary colic (see gallstones), but pain of acute cholecystitis is more constant and severe and lasts for > 6 hours. It settles in most cases after 1–4 days.
- Fever, nausea, and vomiting often present.
- Examination may reveal fever and tachycardia, with tenderness in the right upper quadrant (Murphy's sign), with guarding and rebound. Palpable gallbladder in 30% of cases.
- Jaundice suggests choledocholithiasis or Mirizzi's syndrome.
- Gallbladder perforation occurs in 10–15% of cases, and gallbladder empyema may occur.

Investigation

- ↑ WCC (neutrophilia) is common.
- ↑ ALP in 25% of cases, but deranged liver function tests usually suggest associated biliary obstruction (CBD stones in 10% of patients with calculous cholecystitis).
- Transabdominal ultrasound is >90–95% sensitive, 80% specific for cholecystitis. Diagnosis suggested by pericholecystic fluid, gallbladder wall thickening >4 mm, and presence of gallstones. Wall thickness unreliable in patients with ascites and hypoalbuminaemia.
- CT scan 95% sensitive and specific for cholecystitis. Although less effective than U/S in detecting gallstones, it is more accurate in identifying complications (e.g. gallbladder perforation, empyema).
- Hepatobiliary scintigraphy (HIDA scan) may show impaired gallbladder emptying in an acalculous cholecystitis.

Management. Cholecystectomy.

Choledochal cyst

Cystic dilatation of the intra/extrahepatic bile ducts. Particularly reported in the Far East. Classified into several types: see Fig. 2.7.

Clinical features. Majority of patients present at <30 years, with pain and jaundice. Complications include rupture, <u>cholangitis</u>, cirrhosis, <u>acute pancreatitis</u>, <u>portal hypertension</u>, and <u>cholangiocarcinoma</u> (up to 50% of untreated patients by age 50).

Investigation. Diagnosis usually made by <u>CT scanning</u>, <u>MRCP</u>, or <u>ERCP</u>.

Management. Complete cyst excision is essential (in part to reduce risk of cholangiocarcinoma), with <u>Roux-en-Y</u> hepaticojejunostomy (see <u>biliary bypass procedures</u>). Recurrent symptoms are common, and secondary biliary cirrhosis may require <u>liver transplantation</u>.

Choledocholithiasis

Aetiology + pathogenesis. In 85% of cases common bile duct (CBD) stones have been formed in the gall bladder and passed into the CBD via the cystic duct (secondary stones). Primary stones within the bile duct may occur in association with biliary inflammation and/or bile stasis (e.g. <u>primary sclerosing cholangitis</u>, <u>choledochal cyst</u>, <u>biliary strictures</u>, *Clonorchis* infection).

Clinical features

- Asymptomatic CBD stones found in 7% of patients undergoing <u>cholecystectomy</u>, but symptoms develop in up to 50% if stones left in CBD.
- Obstructive jaundice, often associated with colicky right upper quadrant pain, is common. Pain, nausea, and vomiting often precede jaundice, which is associated with dark urine and pale-coloured stools. Examination reveals jaundice, right upper quadrant tenderness. Palpable gallbladder unusual, and suggests cause of CBD obstruction other than stones (see Courvoisier's law in <u>pancreatic cancer</u>).
- <u>Acute pancreatitis</u> (AP). Passage of stones is the cause of 50% of cases of AP, and this complication occurs in 4–8% of patients with gallstones.
- <u>Cholangitis</u>. Suggested by jaundice and fever. Unusual in patients with choledocholithiasis *per se*, but more common in association with biliary intervention (e.g. post-<u>ERCP</u>).

Investigation

- See also acute <u>pancreatitis</u>, <u>cholangitis</u>, <u>Approach to recent-onset jaundice</u>.
- In patients with obstructive jaundice <u>LFTs</u> show ↑ Bn, and predominant cholestatic derangement (↑↑ALP, GGT) (although ↑ALT, AST often also present).
- Abdominal <u>U/S</u> is first-line test, but only 50% sensitive in detecting CBD stones, but much more accurate at detecting CBD dilatation.

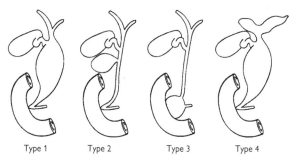

Type 1   Type 2   Type 3   Type 4

Fig. 2.7 Choledochal cysts.

Classification of choledochal cysts

Type 1: diffuse or fusiform dilatation of extrahepatic bile ducts (93% of cases)

Type 2: diverticulum arising from bile duct

Type 3: cystic dilatation of distal bile duct, within the duodenum

Type 4: type I and an intrahepatic cyst

(Type 5: <u>Caroli's disease</u>)

- ERCP > 95% sensitive and specific for CBD stones. Indicated in patients with high probability of bile duct stones (e.g. dilated CBD on U/S, jaundice, gallbladder stones) as allows therapeutic intervention.
- MRCP is risk free (in contrast to ERCP), with 60–90% sensitivity for bile duct stones. May fail to detect stones <5 mm, but increased role in patients with low–intermediate chance of CBD stones.

Endoscopic ultrasound may be used when low–intermediate chance of CBD stones, with sensitivity/specificity comparable to ERCP. CT scan has a sensitivity of 75–90% in the detection of CBD stones.

Management

ERCP allows performance of biliary sphincterotomy and stone clearance in 85–90% of cases. Reasons for failure to clear stones include altered duodenal anatomy (e.g. Billroth II gastrectomy), or large (>1.5 cm) impacted bile duct stones. Bile duct stenting performed if stone cannot be removed at ERCP.

- Cholecystectomy should be considered in all patients with secondary CBD stones, usually after ERCP and stone clearance. In expert hands laparoscopic cholecystectomy and bile duct stone clearance have a high rate of success, but are not widely available. It avoids the added risks of ERCP.
- In patients unfit for surgery, ERCP and biliary sphincterotomy may be performed without cholecystectomy, but >30% develop further episodes related to stones over 5 year period.
- URSODEOXYCHOLIC ACID (UDCA) may be used to prevent recurrence of primary CBD stones (e.g. in primary sclerosing cholangitis/benign biliary strictures), but >6/12 treatment needed for dissolution of even small stones (<5 mm). Occasionally used in conjunction with biliary stenting and extracorporeal shock wave lithotripsy (ESWL) for management of impacted CBD stones when surgery not an option.

Cholera

Kills 100 000 per year in Asia, Africa, and Latin America. Children aged 2–9 and women of child-bearing age are most at risk; mortality in children is 3–5% but in adults effective fluid replacement has reduced mortality to less than 1%.

Pathogenesis. There are about 10 species of *Vibrio* pathogenic to humans: *V. cholerae* and *V. parahaemolyticus* are the most important. Serotyping of *V. Cholerae* is according to O antigen of cell surface lipopolysaccharide: cholera is caused by group O1. Contaminated water is the main route of transmission: person to person transmission is rare.

Diagnosis is usually made presumptively or by laboratory identification of toxigenic vibrios.

Clinical features. Ingested cholera produces a toxin that switches on adenyl cyclase: the resulting increase in cAMP stimulates chloride secretion and reduces sodium reabsorption, producing large volume watery diarrhoea. The risks are those of metabolic acidosis, hyponatraemia, hypokalaemia, hypoglycaemia, and fits. Fever and abdominal pain are rare.

Outcome. Hypoglycaemia and altered conscious level are risk factors for death. Full recovery without antibiotics can be expected in 1–6 days with adequate fluid replacement.

Therapy. Oral rehydration (WHO) solution is effective in 95% cases.

Vaccination. Thrrere is an oral vaccine available for travellers to endemic or epidemic areas. The injectable vaccine uses a killed whole cell vaccine, gives only 50% protection for 3–6 months, and does not prevent the transmission of disease: it is no longer available in the UK.

Chromoendoscopy

First described in Japan in 1976, endoscopic spraying of the gastrointestinal tract with contrast dyes can highlight subtle irregularities in mucosa, improving sensitivity of endoscopic examination, particularly to identify preneoplastic and neoplastic lesions. Common dyes include indigo carmine as a contrast stain (0.1–0.4%) and methylene blue (0.1%) as an absorptive stain.

Recent developments in high-resolution and magnifying endoscopy appear to enhance the diagnostic usefulness of chromoendoscopy. Different staining patterns of colon polyps have been categorized (e.g. the 5 pit patterns described by Kudo), and appear to allow improved endoscopic prediction of histology. However, current systems are too cumbersome for routine use. Most promising techniques are the detection of squamous cell cancer of the oesophagus (see oesophageal tumours) with Lugol's solution, staining of Barrett's oesophagus by methylene blue, including potential to identify neoplasia, and demarcation of neoplasia with indigo carmine in stomach and colon for local endoscopic resection. Indigo carmine (0.1%) sprayed on to the colonic mucosa increases the yield of endoscopic detection of neoplastic lesions in ulcerative colitis and enables targeted biopsy of suspicious lesions (Rutter, MD *et al.* (2004) *Gut* **53** (2): 256).

Chronic granulomatous disease (CGD)

Rare genetic immune deficiency in which phagocytes are unable to kill bacteria and fungi as a result of defects in the electron transport chain underlying the respiratory burst. It is classified according to mode of inheritance and component of reduced NADPH oxidase affected. 65% are X-linked, the remainder are autosomal recessive.

GI involvement is common (30% of all cases; more common in X-linked patients) and involves an abnormal inflammatory response with persistent tissue granuloma formation (presumed due to inadequate clearance of bacterial or fungal antigens).

Clinical features. In most patients, GI involvement is granulomatous or ulcerative involving the colon. Symptoms include abdominal pain, diarrhoea (which may be bloody), and nausea and vomiting. In many cases the phenotype is clinically and radiologically indistinguishable from inflammatory bowel disease; the patchy distribution and presence of granulomas are more suggestive of <u>Crohn's disease</u> than <u>ulcerative colitis</u>. There is a high frequency of pyloric obstruction. Clinical similarity offers a tantalizing clue as to possible pathogenic mechanisms in inflammatory bowel disease. Recently reported association in <u>Crohn's disease</u> of mutations in NOD-2, which is involved in recognition of the bacterial product MDP, suggests that failure to deal adequately with bacterial infection could be common to CGD and <u>Crohn's disease</u>.

Management. Treatment of GI involvement in CGD is not well defined and usually involves <u>CORTICOSTEROIDS</u>. Treatment with gamma-interferon reduces serious infections but does not seem to aggravate GI inflammation in CGD.

The prognosis is poor: mean age of death in patients with GI involvement is 14 years.

Chronic pancreatitis

Definition and aetiology

Benign disease characterized by permanent alteration of anatomy and function due to chronic inflammation. Causes include <u>alcohol</u> (> 70% of cases); tropical pancreatitis (onset < 40 years in equatorial regions, and may be linked to protein–energy malnutrition); pancreatic duct obstruction (e.g. tumours, intraductal stones, traumatic strictures); <u>hereditary pancreatitis</u>; idiopathic chronic pancreatitis (20% of cases); intraductal papillary mucinous tumour (IPMT—see <u>pancreatic cystic tumours</u>); <u>cystic fibrosis</u>; and <u>autoimmune pancreatitis</u>. Episodes of <u>acute pancreatitis</u> may occur during course of chronic disease.

Clinical features

- Epigastric pain, often radiating to back, and associated with anorexia and weight loss. Pain resolves in 80% within 10 years of onset, often in parallel with development of endocrine and exocrine <u>pancreatic insufficiency</u>.
- Insulin-dependent diabetes develops in 40–70% of patients.
- Steatorrhoea (pale, loose, foul smelling stools that are difficult to flush).

Complications

- <u>Portal vein thrombosis</u> and <u>portal hypertension</u> in 1%.
- Jaundice due to low <u>biliary stricture</u>.
- <u>Pancreatic pseudocyst</u> formation.
- <u>Pancreatic cancer</u> develops in approximately 3% of patients (8-fold risk over general population).
- Life expectancy in patients with chronic pancreatitis is shortened by 10–20 years.

Investigation. Diagnosis made by assessing pancreatic structure and function.

Structure

- AXR may show pancreatic calcification (25–60% of cases).
- <u>CT, MRCP, ERCP</u>, and <u>endoscopic ultrasound</u> are complementary, and may show anatomical features of chronic pancreatitis: irregular main pancreatic duct, with dilatation and/or strictures; side branch irregularity; pancreatic parenchymal heterogeneity, enlargement, or atrophy.

Function

- Functional abnormalities in chronic pancreatitis include a decrease in stimulated secretory capacity, exocrine insufficiency (maldigestion and steatorrhoea), and endocrine insufficiency (diabetes mellitus).
- MRCP with secretin. Reduced secretin output, or obstruction of flow due to pancreatic stricture may be seen.
- Fasting glucose/glucose tolerance test. Serum <u>vitamins A,D,E,K</u>.
- Faecal elastase 1 produced by pancreas, and passed in stool largely unaltered (and unaffected by coadministration of <u>PANCREATIC ENZYME SUPPLEMENTS</u>). Highly sensitive and specific for exocrine function (except for falsely low levels with significant diarrhoea), and much easier to perform than urine pancreolauryl test or 3 day faecal fat (also see <u>pancreatic function tests</u>).

Management

- Remove precipitant (e.g. alcohol).
- <u>Pain control</u>. Start with simple non-opiates (e.g. paracetamol, NSAIDs), cautiously increasing to mild <u>OPIATES</u> (e.g. coproxamol, tramadol) and then stronger opiates (e.g. Fentanyl patches). Endoscopic removal of stones from pancreatic duct in head of pancreas may occasionally help. Coeliac plexus block (percutaneously or via <u>endoscopic ultrasound</u>) may be effective, but occasionally surgical drainage procedures or total pancreatectomy used.
- Treat diabetes (most patients require insulin, although doses may be low, due to associated loss of glucagon-producing α cells).
- In patients with exocrine insufficiency, oral <u>PANCREATIC SUPPLEMENTS</u> (see index of drugs) with meals (e.g. creon, nutrizym) may help reduce weight loss, malabsorption, and steatorrhoea (give with proton pump inhibitor to reduce inactivation of enzymes in stomach).
- Endoscopic stenting of <u>biliary strictures</u> may be required, but if no improvement in 12–18 months, consider surgery (see <u>biliary bypass procedures</u>).
- Nutritional support (± fat soluble vitamins).
- Surgery, including pancreatic resection (e.g. <u>Whipple's procedure</u>) or drainage procedure (e.g. Frey, Puestow) occasionally indicated.

Cirrhosis

See: Approach to cirrhosis and chronic liver disease.

Clonorchis infection

Chinese live fluke (*Clonorchis sinensis*) infects 30 million people worldwide, mainly in SE Asia. Life cycle involves passage of eggs in human faeces, ingestion by snail, subsequent ingestion of cercariae by fish, and consumption of fish and encysted larvae by man. 10–25 mm adult worms induce inflammatory response in biliary tree where they may persist for 30 years, leading to biliary strictures and obstruction, recurrent cholangitis, choledocholithiasis, secondary biliary cirrhosis, and cholangiocarcinoma. Diagnosis suspected in patient from high risk area with unexplained biliary stricturing/cholangitis, and confirmed on isolation of eggs in stool or duodenal aspirate. Treatment with praziquantel or albendazole, but biliary lesions may persist.

Clostridial infections of the GI tract

For *C. botulinum* see botulism.

Pseudomembranous colitis (PMC): synonymous with *Clostridium difficile* colitis

- *C. difficile* was discovered in 1935 but only associated with antibiotic-associated diarrhoea in 1978. It is a Gram-positive obligate anaerobe that can form spores, which facilitates antibiotic resistance. Can be found in the stools of healthy newborns, but seldom part of the normal commensal flora. Colonization normally follows antibiotic ingestion, cancer chemotherapy, or infection by other pathogens (*Salmonella, Shigella*).
- GI damage depends on two exotoxins, A and B. They are cytotoxic, destroying actin filaments making up the cell skeleton. Serum antibodies to toxins are common in the general population, although it is not clear if they confer protective immunity.
- Asymptomatic carriage is rare in healthy adults but not in hospital patients (7% positive on admission to hospital, rising during stay, but only 30% of these develop diarrhoea).

Risk factors

- Antibiotics. First seen with clindamycin, but amoxycillin and the cephalosporins are now most frequently implicated.
- Other risk factors are extremes of age, recent GI surgery, malignancy, and prolonged hospital stay.

Clinical features

- Diarrhoea and abdominal cramps usually occur within the first week but can be delayed up to 6 weeks.
- Nausea, fever, and dehydration can accompany severe colitis.
- Abdominal examination may reveal distension and tenderness.

- Sigmoidoscopy (not simple proctoscopy; the rectum is spared of pseudomembranes in 30%) reveals characteristic yellow-white raised plaques, 2–5 mm diameter. Biopsy reveals a characteristic 'summit lesion', an outpouring of pus from a microulceration of the surface epithelium (see Colour Plate 5).
- Fulminant *C. difficile* colitis can present acutely in the previously well, or develop during the course of milder infection. Look for fever, tachycardia, tenderness, guarding, and reduced bowel sounds. Plain radiograph may show <u>toxic megacolon</u>; the bowel wall may appear very thick on CT scanning.
- *C. difficile* infection can complicate <u>ulcerative colitis</u>: a 5 to 25% incidence of toxin positive stools has been reported, not always after antibiotic exposure. Always get a stool for *C. difficile* toxin in patients with relapses of IBD.

Diagnosis
- Stool culture is sensitive but needs anaerobic culture facilities, takes 2–5 days, and reveals toxigenic and non-toxigenic strains.
- Same day enzyme immunoassays are available for toxins A and B.

Management
- Oral <u>METRONIDAZOLE</u> 400 mg tds is recommended as first-line therapy but some clinicians feel this is less effective than vancomycin 125 mg qds, and this author recommends oral vancomycin as first-line treatment for severe or fulminant PMC.
- Relapse occurs in 20% of successfully treated patients. Options include withholding further antibiotics to allow normal flora to re-establish, giving probiotics (*Saccharomyces boulardi* reduces *C. difficile* recurrence rate) or a 14 day course of vancomycin followed by a course of anion-binding resin such as cholestyramine.
- There is no proven benefit in treating asymptomatic carriers.

Necrotizing enterocolitis
A severe and fulminating colitis classically occurring in neonates (although the association here with *Clostridium* is not proven) but in adults associated with gas gangrene of the bowel wall.

Clostridium perfringens
- A food-borne pathogen usually producing diarrhoea and vomiting due to enterotoxin prodiced by *C. perfringens* type A. 90% of cases caused by meat or poultry cooked adequately but then left to stand for 4–24 hours and then served cold or poorly rewarmed. Symptoms include cramps and diarrhoea and are usually short-lived (less than 24 h): vomiting and fever are unusual. Fatalities are very rare.
- In sporadic outbreaks especially in Papua New Guinea, the disease is called pig bel, resulting from feasting on poorly cooked pork contaminated with *C. perfringens* type C. A vaccine can prevent disease. Treatment includes high dose benzylpenicillin.

CLO (*Campylobacter*-like organism) testing

Endoscopic mucosal biopsies from gastric antrum can be inoculated into a medium containing urea and phenol red, a dye that turns pink in a pH of 6.0 or greater. The pH will rise above 6.0 when _Helicobacter pylori_ metabolizes urea to ammonia by way of its urease activity. This test is commercially available at low cost and provides 98% sensitivity and 100% specificity. However it depends on the patient being off antisecretory therapy (PPIs for 4 weeks, H2 receptor antagonists for 72 hours) and also takes 24 hours to read at room temperature (4 hours at 37°C). Sensitivity is maximal with 2 regular (or 1 jumbo) biopsies. Newer tests are becoming commercially available with reaction times of only a few minutes.

Cobalamin (vitamin B12)

Found in animal sources: vegetarians/vegans may have inadequate intake. Deficiency can be caused by disease at a number of sites: see box opposite.
Investigation. If not vegan, do parietal cell antibodies and intrinsic factor antibodies to exclude _pernicious anaemia_. Remember that severe vitamin B12 malabsorption can damage mucosa and affect absorptive capacity, so either wait 2 months before doing _Schilling test_ or repeat after treatment.
Treatment is usually by IM hydroxycobalamin (1 mg x 3/week for 2 weeks, then 1 mg every 3 months), although high dose oral cobalamin (1–2 mg/day) may be effective.

Coccidia

Intracellular protozoan pathogens. Genera *Cryptosporidium*, *Cyclospora*, *Isospora* can cause acute self-limiting diarrhoeal illness in immunocompetent hosts and severe chronic diarrhoea in the immunosuppressed. They all replicate in the enterocyte and can also shed cysts or spores that are excreted in the stool.

Cryptosporidium parvum

- Responsible for several large water-borne outbreaks of diarrhoeal disease. 15% to 30% people are seropositive in developed countries (higher in developing countries). Common cause of diarrhoea in AIDS and other immunosuppressed states.
- Mean incubation period 9 days; mean duration of disease 12 days. Watery but not bloody diarrhoea, abdominal cramps, mucus PR. Extraintestinal manifestations rare in the immunocompetent, but _cholecystitis_ in 10% AIDS patients, and has been implicated as cause of HIV cholangiopathy (see _HIV and the liver_). Diagnosed by finding oocytes in stool samples.

Causes of cobalamin (vitamin B12) deficiency
- Inadequate dietary intake
  - Vegans
  - Alcoholics
- Inadequate release of food bound cobalamin
  - Achlorhydria
  - <u>PROTON PUMP INHIBITORS</u>
- Loss of active intrinsic factor (IF)
  - <u>Pernicious anaemia</u>
  - <u>Gastrectomy</u>
  - Congenital lack/abnormality of IF
- Proximal small bowel disease and pancreatic disease
  - <u>Pancreatic insufficiency</u>
  - <u>Gastrinoma</u>
  - <u>Tropical sprue</u>
  - Small bowel <u>bacterial overgrowth</u>
  - Fish tapeworm *diphyllobothrium latum* (rare)
- Ileal disorders
  - Mainly loss of absorptive mucosa through surgery or mucosal disease
  - <u>Crohn's disease</u>
  - TB (see <u>TB and the GI tract</u>)
  - Lymphoma
  - Dysfunctionnal uptake and use of cobalamin by cells: R binder deficiency, transcobalamin II deficiency, some drugs (colchicine)
- Miscellaneous (rarely lead to clinical anaemia)
  - Pregnancy
  - Thyrotoxicosis
  - Erythroid hyperplasia
- Drugs
  - PAS
  - Colchicine
  - Neomycin
  - Metformin

- Treatment. Antibiotics not effective. Supportive treatment with fluid replacement is the main therapy. May resolve with immune reconstitution associated with HAART for HIV.

Cyclospora cayetanensis

- Discovered in the 1990s, Cyclospora appears a relatively common cause of diarrhoea in patients with AIDS in developing countries but is rare in
- Developed countries although sporadic outbreaks have been reported. The disease is self-limiting in immunocompetent hosts. Diagnosis is by stool microscopy, which reveals 8–10 μm spheres. Treatment with co-trimoxazole is effective.

Isospora belli

- Responsible for 15% cases of diarrhoea in AIDS patients in developing countries. Rare in immunocompetent people. Can cause eosinophilia. Sensitive to co-trimoxazole.

Coeliac disease

A disease involving abnormal small intestinal mucosa that reverts to normal when patients are treated with a gluten-free diet and that relapses when gluten is re-introduced.

Epidemiology and pathogenesis

- Prevalence through Europe is about 1:300, and is more common in Celtic populations. It also occurs in non-Caucasians but is very rare in Black populations. Females are slightly more commonly affected than men. Mortality is reduced by a therapeutic gluten-free diet, but remains higher than for a matched control population.
- The disease phenotype is produced in a susceptible host by intestinal atrophy and inflammation due to a T-cell mediated hypersensitivity reaction to a component of gluten.
- The precise structure of the protein antigen remains unknown, but recent studies suggest that enterotoxicity is produced by a peptide corresponding to amino acids 31–49 of A-gliaden. 10–15% of first-degree relatives are affected. Concordance rates for identical twins are 70–100%. There is a strong association with the histocompatability antigen HLA-DQ2, but other genes are also though to be involved in mediating genetic susceptibility. Genome-wide screening to identify susceptibility alleles is being undertaken in a number of centres.

Clinical features

- Coeliac disease can present at any age.
- In children, it classically occurs after weaning; there is failure to thrive with pallor, apathy, anorexia, abdominal distension.
- In adults the commonest age of presentation is 20s and 30s. Diarrhoea is usually present, as are constitutional symptoms of lassitude, weight loss, glossitis, angular stomatitis, and symptoms relating to anaemia. Vitamin D deficiency or osteoporosis may be the presenting problem in adults.

- Other presentations in adults include depression and a Korsakoff-like syndrome. 30% of women of child-bearing age are amenorrhoeic. Men with untreated coeliac disease have low sperm counts and reduced plasma testosterone levels.
- Although a bowel habit of 3–4 loose, pale, often offensive stools is a typical finding, normally formed and coloured stools do not preclude the diagnosis, and bowel habit depends on gluten intake. Severe pain is not a typical feature. Symptoms are often mild and non-specific. Given the recently recognized high prevalence, a high index of suspicion is appropriate, especially in patients with unexplained mild macrocytic anaemia with low serum <u>folic acid</u>.

Disease associations

- Link with organ-specific autoimmune diseases.
- Associated skin conditions include <u>dermatitis herpetiformis</u>, psoriasis, eczema, cutaneous vasculitis, epidermal necrolysis, mycosis fungoides.
- 10–15% of coeliacs have abnormal liver blood tests and there is a higher than expected incidence of <u>autoimmune hepatitis</u> and <u>primary biliary cirrhosis</u>.
- There is also an association with <u>inflammatory bowel disease</u>, especially ulcerative proctitis.
- Ulcerative jejunitis can be associated with coeliac disease and may be a variant of a T-cell proliferative condition that can result in a T-cell lymphoma.

Investigations

Blood tests may show anaemia, classically with iron or folate deficiency. The peripheral blood may show target cells, Howell–Jolly bodies, acanthocytes, and thrombocytosis. Biochemistry may show low calcium, vitamin D, zinc, and albumin. Useful **serological tests** include IgG and IgA gliadin, IgA reticulin, IgA anti-endomysial and tissue transglutaminase antibodies. Anti-endomysial antibodies are 90% sensitive and almost 100% specific. The antigen recognized is tissue tranglutaminase: specific transglutaminase antibodies may be even more sensitive.

2% of the general population are IgA deficient, so it is important to exclude IgA deficiency as a cause of false negative serological testing.

Small bowel biopsy remains essential. 4 biopsies from the second part of duodenum using standard or jumbo-sized forceps are recommended (difficulty in interpretation sometimes occurs because of normal villous mucosa overlying Brunner's glands). In severe cases loss of the normal circular fold pattern of the duodenum can be seen macroscopically, but this is not a reliable method of diagnosis.

Radiology. The barium follow through can be abnormal, with loss of fine feathery mucosal pattern. Radiology is important in the presence of abdominal pain to exclude a complicating jejunal stricture, lymphoma, or carcinoma. Abdominal CT may show splenic atrophy and an associated low grade lymphadenopathy.

Treatment

- Diet. A **gluten-free diet** should avoid wheat, rye, barley, and oats (although there is controversy about the toxicity of oats). Supplementation with fibre may be needed. Repeat biopsy at 6 months is necessary to assess response to diet. Further endoscopy after gluten challenge is not indicated if the patient has responded well to the diet with a corresponding histological response. Failure of response to the diet is usually (but not invariably) due to poor dietary compliance or inadvertent ingestion of gluten. Rarely, failure to respond is due to a small intestinal lymphoma or the presence of another disorder such as chronic pancreatitis.
- CORTICOSTEROIDS reduce the diarrhoea and facilitate weight gain and reduction in steatorrhoea, but the effects do not persist after stopping the drugs. Steroids may be useful in 10% and in these patients second line steroid-sparing agents such as AZATHIOPRINE can also be useful.

Complications. Most patients are lactose intolerant at the time of diagnosis, but this rarely persists after treatment. There are reported but poorly understood neurological complications including demyelination of the posterior and lateral spinal cord columns and cerebellar degeneration that may respond, at least partly, to supplementation with vitamins A, E, B, or calcium.

Collagenous colitis

See: microscopic colitis.

Colonic cancer

Epidemiology and pathogenesis. As with other malignancies, colonic cancer is an acquired genetic disease produced by exposure to environmental carcinogens; the damage caused by these accrues over many years. No single gene is so crucial that a mutation results in cancer.

In the UK there are approximately 30 000 new cases of colon cancer and 16 000 deaths from colon cancer per year (for the USA, figures are 135 000 and 60 000). Attack rates are lower in Japan and most developing countries. Rectal cancer is different in epidemiology, pathogenesis, and treatment.

Risk factors include:

- Cancer family syndromes: familial adenomatous polyposis (FAP) or Gardner's syndrome, HNPCC.
- Prior polyps (main determinants of risk are polyp size >1 cm and tubulovillous or severely dysplastic histology) and cancers (metachronous cancers in 5%).
- Inflammatory bowel disease: main determinants are duration of disease and extensive disease (approximately 10% after 30 years in patients with pancolitis).
- Diet: risk is modest at most. High fat and low fibre are the most common associations. Current advice is to reduce caloric intake, reduce dietary fat

to less than 25% of total calorie intake, enrich diet with 5 portions of fruit and vegetables per day, and include 25 g fibre in the diet per day.

Clinical features

Change of bowel habit in people >40 years is the classic symptom. Tumours often grow slowly and produce 4 main symptom patterns:

- Obstruction. Distension, pain, nausea, and vomiting. Obstruction is more common in the (narrower) sigmoid, descending and transverse colon than the caecum or ascending colon.
- Bleeding: usually occult but if visible, blood tends to be mixed in with the stool.
- Local invasion: often produces pain but can lead to e.g. ureteric obstruction, bladder invasion, or malignant fistulation.
- Wasting syndrome. Loss of appetite, weight, and strength. Can occur with any GI tract (and many other) malignancy: particularly involves loss of subcutaneous fat.

Investigations

- Colonoscopy is the most accurate and sensitive diagnostic modality: even if distal colonic tumours are found, full colonoscopic evaluation is required to detect synchronous lesions (5%).
- Barium enemas are still frequently used, but biopsy is not possible, patients find them unpleasant, and the diagnostic sensitivity is less (approximately 85%).
- CT pneumocolon (CT with air distension of the bowel) is increasingly used and some centres are combining CT scanning with positron emission tomography (PET): labelling of intestinal contents with oral contrast media and removal of these from CT scans by digital image manipulation should allow accurate radiological imaging of the bowel without the need for bowel cleansing in the near future.

Management. Central aim is to detect tumours early in their natural history and to intervene with appropriate surgery.

Preoperative workup includes

- CT scan of chest, abdomen, and pelvis to exclude metastases.
- Full colonoscopy to exclude a synchronous colonic tumour.
- Other tests include routine haematology (?iron deficient anaemia) and biochemistry and (arguably), testing for CEA.

Management depends on staging (see Dukes staging and tumour staging), and evidence of local or metastatic disease.

Local disease

Surgery. Curative treatment is surgical: local resection of tumour and regional nodes with clearance margins of 5 cm is the aim. Tumours proximal to the splenic flexure are removed by right hemicolectomy: tumour of the left colon are removed by left hemicolectomy. Sigmoid cancers are treated with low anterior resections but very low tumours may require a colostomy. The overall operative mortality for colorectal cancer is about 5%. Treatment of rectal cancer is covered elsewhere.

Adjuvant chemotherapy after 'curative' surgery. There is benefit in treating patients with Dukes stage C disease with 5FU and levamisole. No evidence of survival benefit is found in stage B disease. Newer regimens including oxaloplatin and irenotecan are being evaluated and may alter recommendations. Adjuvant radiotherapy for colon cancer outside rectum has no benefit.

Follow up. 30% of patients undergoing 'curative' surgery develop metastases. Colonoscopy should be carried out 3–6 months post-operatively and again at 12 months. A rise in CEA may indicate metastatic disease. Intensive follow up with either ultrasound or CT scanning has a minor impact, at considerable expense, on patient outcome.

Metastatic disease

Surgery. A single or small number of hepatic metastases should be considered for surgical resection because some patients will go on to experience a prolonged disease-free interval. A solitary lung metastasis less than 3 cm can also be considered for surgery but the impact on survival and cure rates is less clear.

Chemotherapy or non-surgical ablation techniques. Intra-arterial infusion of chemotherapeutic agents is reported to ablate or shrink a small number of tumours with less systemic drug toxicity. Radiofrequency ablation using transcutaneously positioned needles may also be effective.

Immunostimulant therapy is an attractive but unproven treatment option.

Prognosis

The pathological stage (see Dukes staging) is the best predictor of outcome. Crude 5 year survival rates (i.e. not adjusted for age-related mortality) are 85, 65, 40, and <5% for stages A, B, C, and D, respectively.

Metastatic disease occurs in 25% and carries an adverse prognosis: the mean survival period for patients with hepatic metastases (the commonest site) at diagnosis is 4.5 months. Other metastatic sites include regional lymph nodes, lung, peritoneum, and adrenals. There is a suggestion that with improving chemotherapy the natural history is changing so that metastatic disease to the lungs and brain, previously rarely seen, is becoming more common. CT is the most sensitive test for detecting occult metastases, but addition of PET scanning may further enhance early detection.

Prevention of colonic cancer

Diet. There is no clear association with high fat or low fibre intake that can be separated from overall calorie intake.

Micronutrients. There are theoretical benefits to calcium and selenium supplementation, not supported by clinical trials. Anti-oxidants including vitamins A, E, and beta-carotene have not been proven beneficial or to reduce the rate of polyp recurrence.

Aspirin and NSAIDs. Aspirin takers get fewer colon cancers and NSAIDs inhibit tumour development *in vitro*. The non-steroidal drug SULINDAC reduces polyp formation in familial adenomatous polyposis, but has shown conflicting results for sporadic colonic polyps.

There is early data suggesting that statins have a protective effect on cancer development: more data are awaited.

Colonic inertia

Defined as a delayed transit of radio-opaque markers through the proximal colon (see box on opposite page). Classically found in about 70% of patients (most often young to middle-aged women) consulting for infrequent defecation who are non-responsive to therapeutic intervention (see <u>LAXATIVES</u> in index of drugs, and <u>biofeedback</u>). Unlike patients with normal colonic transit, they show no sign of psychological distress and may have a physiological basis to their symptoms. Although resting motility appears normal, there seems to be a failure to increase motility after meals. This suggests an abnormality of the enteric plexus. Patients with severe colonic inertia may have reduced oesophageal motility, delayed transit through the small intestine, and a high incidence of bladder dysfunction.

Colonic polyps

There are four common types (only adenomas are neoplastic).
- Adenomas.
- Benign hyperplastic polyps.
- Hamartomatous polyps.
- Inflammatory polyps.

Adenomas

Can be pedunculated or sessile but are very common (up to 50% in autopsy studies, frequency increasing with age). Importance lies in the risk of malignant transformation, which relates to size (adenoma >2 cm has significant risk of containing cancer) and histology (can be tubular, villous (often sessile, more likely to contain focus of cancer), or tubulo-villous).

Aetiology. There is disordered and persistent cell replication coupled with retarded cell maturation.

Genetic factors include aneuploidy, tetraploidy, DNA hypomethylation. Altered expression of oncogenes *fos, myc, ras* occurs. Mutations in APC, DCC, p53 have been reported. See <u>adenoma–carcinoma sequence</u>.

Environmental factors may include diet (some but not conclusive evidence for the role of fat, fibre, bile acids, faecal bacteria). Nonsteroidal anti-inflammatory drugs may retard polyps in familial syndromes (familial <u>adenomatous polyposis (FAP)</u>, <u>hereditary non-polyposis colon cancer</u> (HNPCC), but seem ineffectual in sporadic adenomas.

Clinical features. Usually asymptomatic. Symptoms of rectal bleeding, prolapse, abdominal pain, or change in bowel habit usually occur with large polyps. There is no correlation with histology or location. Only polyps over 1.5 cm are associated with positive faecal occult blood tests. Large villous adenomas can produce watery diarrhoea and hypokalaemia.

Diagnosis. Barium radiology, endoscopy (sigmoidoscopy/colonoscopy), and more recently CT colonography can produce a diagnosis: endoscopy is currently the most sensitive and only endoscopy allows biopsy and therapeutic excision.

Colonic transit studies

Technique used to study patients with severe constipation and otherwise normal GI investigations. Patient takes a high fibre diet and avoids laxatives, enemas, or any medications that may affect bowel function.

Results can only be interpreted if procedure is strictly adhered to:

- **Day 1:** Patient takes 1 capsule (containing 20 radio-opaque markers) in water at 0900 h
- **Day 5:** 0900 h. Supine abdominal X-ray. If no markers seen, discontinue study (as no evidence of slow transit)
- **Day 7:** 0900 h. Supine abdominal X-ray. Slow transit constipation diagnosed if >80% of markers retained (i.e. at 1200).

When is a colonic polyp not a polyp?

Polyp means any tissue protrusion above the mucosal surface into the lumen.

Neoplastic polyps

(Adenomas and cancers): see text

Non-neoplastic polyps

Hyperplastic, inflammatory, hamartomatous

Other lesions

- Lipomas, fibromas, leiomyomas, and Kaposi's sarcoma are usually submucosal and less often diagnosed by biopsy
- Pneumatosis can also appear polypoid
- Angiomas can sometimes be sampled by hot biopsy but there is a risk of bleeding
- Benign lymphoid nodules can be mistaken for neoplasms or polyps, especially in the terminal ileum
- Occasionally metastatic tumours may be seen on colonoscopy
- <u>Carcinoids</u>

Natural history. Adenoma–carcinoma progression probably takes 5–10 years, possibly less in the case of HNPCC/microsatellite instability. Although polyps grow slowly and only perhaps 5% is destined for malignancy, the necessity of excision for histology underlies current advice that all colonic polyps should be removed if possible.

Therapy. See polypectomy.

Benign hyperplastic polyps

Usually <5 mm, often multiple, commonest in recto-sigmoid. About 50% of all polyps <5 mm are hyperplastic. Arise because of an increased number of epithelial cells per unit length, which causes buckling and a serrated surface. Traditionally thought not to be premalignant, but some genetic changes occur that overlap with adenoma–cancer sequence.

Hamartomatous polyps

An abnormal mixture of benign cells. See juvenile polyps, Peutz–Jeghers, and Cowden's disease.

Inflammatory polyps

Also called pseudopolyps. Common in ulcerative or Crohn's colitis but also seen after infective or ischaemic colitis. They represent islands of residual mucosa in a sea of previously sloughed healed mucosa.

Colonic transit studies

See: colonic inertia.

Colonoscopy

First used in the early 1960s, now a standard technique for assessing and treating colonic disease, because most colonic disease starts on the inner mucosal aspect. Caecal intubation is possible in 98% of colonoscopies in expert hands. Current areas of discussion include the following.

Making colonoscopy easier

Because of the tortuosity and lack of landmarks this remains an issue. Most significant recent developments are the introduction of the variable stiffness colonoscope and magnetic endoscope imaging. The variable stiffness instruments can help negotiate difficult sigmoid loops and splenic flexures, and magnetic endoscope imaging has been shown to facilitate negotiation of loops, improve success rates, and shorten procedure times.

See: bowel preparation.

Sedation

The need for and practice of sedation varies widely and depends on patient expectation as well as local practice. Some countries use general anaesthesia. Although some stretching of peritoneal attachments is almost inevitable, with a resulting visceral discomfort, total colonoscopy in unsedated patients is possible with expert endoscopists and motivated patients. In the UK routine practice involves intravenous administration of a benzodiazepine to provide anxiolysis and anterograde amnesia together with an opiate for analgesia. If this combination if used, the opiate should be given first and doses kept to a minimum. A common protocol is to use pethidine 25 mg and midazolam 2.5 mg.

Monitoring
Current guidelines include routine use of pulse oximetry and supplemental oxygen (2 l/min via nasal cannulae) given to all sedated patients.
Contraindications. See box below.
Risks. See <u>endoscopic complications</u>.

Comparison with barium enema and virtual colonoscopy
Miss rate of colonoscopy for lesions <1 cm can be substantial (up to 25%). Barium imaging using double contrast barium enemas can provide high quality imaging of the colon but operator skill is an important variable and poor prep, air bubbles, muscle spasm, diverticular disease, or convoluted loops may impair the view. Colons difficult to examine by colonoscopy are also those difficult to examine by barium. Colonoscopy is impossible in the presence of barium, so it is logical to attempt colonoscopy first. Barium enema or CT pneumocolon are effective in assessing colon morphology when there are strictures or fistulae that may be impassable to the endoscopist.

Contraindications to colonoscopy
- Avoid if possible for 4–6 weeks after proven myocardial infarction
- Because of the risk of perforation, colonoscopy is contraindicated in acute or abscess-associated diverticulitis
- Crohn's, ischaemic, or ulcerative colitis mandate particular care but colonoscopy can provide valuable information in these situations and benefit may outweigh risk.

Colorectal cancer screening and surveillance

- **Screening.** Testing of apparently healthy people who may be at average or increased risk of disease.
- **Surveillance.** Periodic testing of people at high risk for the disease who have previously tested negative.

Colorectal cancer (CRC) screening (see algorithm Fig. 2.8)

Average risk
(i.e. background population risk in people with no risk factors)
- Two screening modalities reduce mortality from colon cancer.
  - <u>Faecal occult blood test</u> (FOBT) provides up to 30% reduction in mortality if done annually with rigorous follow up of positives with endoscopy.
  - Endoscopic examination of the colon. Endoscopy reduces mortality from colon cancer: while this would seem to be confined to area of bowel visualized at endoscopy, controversy exists as to the incidence of proximal tumours out of reach of the flexible sigmoidoscope. One study reports less than 2% of people with a normal sigmoidoscopy have proximal tumours (Imperiale, TF et al. (2000) N. Engl. J. Med. **343:** 169).
- Other methods such as <u>CT pneumocolon</u> ('virtual colonoscopy') are still being evaluated.
- The best screening method for colon cancer has not been determined.
- Criteria include sensitivity, specificity, patient acceptability, and affordability.
- Recommendations published by the American Gastroenterology Association (AGA) are shown in the algorithm. In the UK, screening of average risk people for colon cancer using FOBT will begin in 2006.

Increased risk

Family history (excluding cancer family syndromes)
Familial clustering of colorectal cancer is common. Risk is increased depending on the number of affected relatives, their age of diagnosis, and the presence of adenomatous polyps in a first-degree relative under the age of 60 (see table).

How this affects screening is controversial and depends on the cutoff of acceptable risk. A family history of colon cancer should lead to screening with regular FOBT and 5-yearly sigmoidoscopy. Patients with multiple affected family members or an affected first-degree relative <55 years should have colonoscopy 5 years earlier than the earliest cancer in the family.

Cancer family syndromes
Genetic screening is valuable for syndromes relating to <u>familial adenomatous polyposis</u> (FAP); referral to a geneticist should be considered for confusing histories.

Familial colon cancer: relative risk

Relatives affected	Risk
None-1	in 35
One first-degree	1 in 17
One first-degree and one second-degree	1 in 12
One first-degree under 45	1 in 10
Both parents	1 in 8.5
Two first-degree	1 in 6
Three first-degree	1 in 2

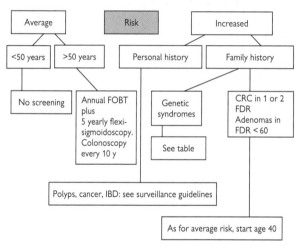

Fig. 2.8 Algorithm for colorectal cancer screening based on American Gastroenterology Association guidelines. CRC, colorectal cancer; FOBT, faecal occult blood testing; FDR, first-degree relatives; IBD, inflammating bowel disease.

Colorectal cancer surveillance (see table opposite)

High risk

- **Highly penetrant autosomal dominant syndromes.**
  - <u>Familial adenomatous polyposis.</u>
  - <u>Hereditary non-polyposis colorectal cancer</u>.
- Hamartomatous polyposis syndromes (<u>Peutz–Jeghers syndrome</u>, juvenile polyposis, <u>Cowden's disease</u>).
- Longstanding history of <u>inflammatory bowel disease</u> of the colon.
- Patients with <u>acromegaly</u>. Current recommendations are for 3 yearly colonoscopy from age 40.

Moderate risk

Prior history of adenomatous <u>colonic polyps</u>

- Solitary adenomas <1 cm diameter do not predict recurrent neoplasia and these lesions, especially in the elderly, do not need follow up.
- Surveillance colonoscopy is indicated for:
  - Adenomas >1 cm.
  - Villous or tubulo-villous histology.
  - Multiple adenomas.
  - Advanced dysplasia.
- 3-year interval is adequate for follow up colonoscopy if the colon has been cleared of polyps, with subsequent intervals of 5 years.

Prior history of colon cancer

- The anastomosis site should be examined at 3–6 months and perhaps again at 1 year (little evidence for this recommendation).
- After this examination is recommended every 3–5 years as for patients with advanced adenomas.

Inflammatory bowel disease. See box opposite.

Condition	Recommendation
<u>Familial adenomatous polyposis</u>	Genetic testing for APC mutations age 12. Yearly flexible sigmoidoscopy starting at age 12 in people with a family history of FAP. If polyps found, full colonoscopy with a view to prophylactic colectomy and surveillance of remaining rectum. In addition, upper endoscopic surveillance of stomach, duodenum, and periampullary region. Consider AFP for hepatoblastoma
<u>Hereditary non-polyposis colorectal cancer</u>	Individuals identified by family history (see Amsterdam criteria in <u>hereditary non-polyposis colorectal cancer</u>). Start colonoscopic surveillance (**not** flexible sigmoidoscopy because many tumours are right-sided) at 20–25 years at intervals of 1–2 years. Offer genetic testing to first-degree relatives of patients with known inherited mismatch repair defect
<u>Peutz–Jegher's syndrome</u>	2 yearly upper and lower GI endoscopy, barium follow through (?video <u>capsule endoscopy</u>). Polypectomy for large polyps to avoid intussusception. Surveillance for gonadal, breast, cervical cancer
<u>Juvenile polyposis</u>	Rare. No firm guidelines

Colorectal cancer surveillance in patients with IBD

This is a controversial area. Extensive <u>ulcerative colitis</u> or <u>Crohn's</u> colitis of long duration (>10 years for patients with disease proximal to splenic flexure, >15 years in patients with left-sided disease above the sigmoid: no increased risk in patients with proctitis alone) have an increased risk of colon cancer.

The magnitude of increased risk varies in different studies, partly due to referral bias reflecting hospital rather than community prevalence studies. Commonly quoted figures are an incidence of colon cancer of 7–15 % at 20 years after diagnosis of UC with an increasing incidence of about 1% per year after this. Long term treatment with 5-ASA may decrease the risk of colon cancer associated with IBD.

Risk is further increased in patients with
- <u>Primary sclerosing cholangitis</u>
- A family history of <u>colon cancer</u>
- (Possibly) young onset of disease
- Colonic stricturing

There is no evidence that endoscopic surveillance improves mortality from colon cancer in IBD. Areas of dysplasia are difficult to see macroscopically, so standard guidelines recommend surveillance with colonoscopic biopsies taken from 4 quadrants every 10 cm.

<u>Dysplasia</u> is a recognized predictor of malignancy, but there is inter-observer variability in interpretation. Alternative markers of pre-cancer include detection of aneuploidy, abnormal mucins, genetic markers, and optical reflectance characteristics ('optical biopsy').

CT (computed tomography) scanning

Collimated X-rays through the patient produce a series of attenuation profiles that are computed into cross-sectional images (usually 3–8 mm cuts dependant on machine/clinical indication). More recently continuous motion (helical or spiral CT) has replaced sequential acquisition. Tissue contrast achieved by the fact that tissues attenuate X-ray to differing degrees. Whole abdomen may be scanned within one breath hold. Adiposity improves definition on CT (in contrast to <u>ultrasound</u>). Sequentially timed imaging after injection of iodine-based IV contrast may produce characteristic appearances of lesions/disease in arterial, venous, or portal venous phases. Specific acquisition protocols used dependent on organ/clinical question.

Indications for CT in GI disease wide-ranging, including investigation of <u>acute abdominal pain</u>, cancer diagnosis and staging (e.g. <u>pancreatic</u> and <u>oesophageal cancer</u>), assessment of pancreatic, biliary, and liver disease, and investigation of intra-abdominal collections. <u>CT pneumocolon</u> is discussed separately. Targeted biopsy of lesions may be performed by CT or U/S, dependent on anatomical site/local expertise.

Contraindications are few, but include iodine allergy (discuss with radiologists if any useful information to be gained from unenhanced CT).

Radiation dose during abdominal CT is large (equivalent to 500 chest X-rays, or 3.3 years background radiation), so careful consideration of alternatives in young and in those needing repeated imaging. Avoid in pregnancy, especially first trimester.

Constipation

See: <u>Approach to constipation</u>.

Cowden's disease

Autosomal dominant condition relating to <u>juvenile polyposis</u>. Associated with a mutation of the PTEN gene on chromosome 10, resulting in multiple hamartomas of skin and mucous membranes. The hallmark is multiple trichilemmomas around the eyes, nose, and mouth. About 1/3 affected people have hamartomas scattered through upper and lower GI tract. They can be 1 mm to several cm diameter and include lipomas, juvenile polyps, inflammatory polyps, ganglioneuromas, and lymphoid hyperplasia. Glycogenic acanthosis can be seen in oesophageal lesions.

There is no increased risk of GI cancer but a 10% risk of thyroid cancer and a 50% risk of breast cancer.

COX-1 and COX-2

See: <u>Non-steriodal anti-flammatory drugs (NSAIDS) and the GI tract</u>.

Crohn's disease

After Burrill B. Crohn, a New York physician who published in 1932 on 'regional ileitis' with Ginsberg and Oppenheimer. Many believe Dalziel described the disease in 1912.

Definition. A chronic inflammatory condition that can affect any part of the gut from mouth to anus but most frequently the distal small intestine and proximal colon.

Epidemiology

- Accurate figures are difficult because of lack of gold standard for diagnostic criteria and global variations in case ascertainment.
- Found worldwide but incidence varies. In high incidence areas (UK, USA, northern Europe) the incidence is about 4–8/100 000. In Australasia and in white South Africans it is about 2/100 000. Low incidence areas include Asia, Japan, and South America, with estimates of 0.05 to 0.8/100 000 per year. In careful studies of stable populations in high incidence areas (USA and Denmark) the incidence increased 6-fold from 1950s to 1980s and appears to have stabilized since.
- Slightly more common in women, with peak incidence age 20–40 and a second smaller peak in older adults.

Aetiology and pathogenesis

- Almost 100 years after initial description, whether Crohn's disease represents an appropriate response to an unrecognized pathogen or an inappropriate response to an innocuous stimulus is not resolved.
- Resemblance of Crohn's disease to some animal diseases with known bacterial causes (John's disease in goats) and the proven role of gut pathogens in inducing inflammation in genetically susceptible animal models of inflammatory bowel disease strongly suggest a central role for bacterial antigens as triggering factors.
- A huge amount of experimental work has helped to define cellular and humoral immune events underlying mucosal inflammation. Evidence points to over-responsiveness of T cells to enteric flora in IBD, with T cells producing a Th1 cytokine response profile in Crohn's disease.
- Genetic diseases involving defects in bacterial killing and degradation (e.g. chronic granulomatous disease) produce a phenotype very like inflammatory bowel disease and this supports experimental evidence that the interaction between T cells and macrophages also appears central to the pathogenesis of Crohn's disease.
- The recent rise in incidence supports the importance of environmental factors.
- Diet and smoking are particularly important: some evidence suggests Crohn's patients have a problem handling saturated fatty acids, while smoking worsens disease possible due to its effect on microvasculature.

Genetics versus environment

- Strong genetic component in predisposing to Crohn's disease, with a high concordance rate among identical twins and higher incidence among Ashkenazi Jews. Techniques of genome-wide screening for linkage and association studies of candidate genes have revealed association with a locus on chromosome 16 as being due to gene CARD-15 (NOD-2),

which codes for receptor for muramyl dipeptide (MDP) a component of bacterial cell walls.
- The recent rise in incidence supports the importance of environmental factors.
- Diet and smoking are particularly important: some evidence suggests Crohn's patients have a problem handling saturated fatty acids, while smoking worsens disease possible due to its effect on microvasculature.

Pathology

The hallmark is focal intestinal inflammation: disease is classically discontinuous giving rise to 'skip lesions' unlike ulcerative colitis (UC), which is continuous. Early lesions include aphthous ulcers overlying lymphoid aggregates and support a role of luminal antigens initiating immune activation. Noncaseating granulomas, although characteristic of Crohn's disease, are neither unique to the disease nor universally found (occur in up to 70% of surgical resection specimens).

TNF is involved in granuloma formation: this is how anti-TNF strategies were developed for Crohn's.

Inflammation is transmural, and accounts for late development of large ulcers, sinus tracks, anal fissures, and anorectal fistulae. Concomitant attempts at healing lead to extensive fibrosis as major component of Crohn's disease. TGF beta is a key cytokine involved in this process.

Clinical features

Disease distribution. 40% have disease confined to terminal ileum and proximal colon, 30% have disease confined to the small bowel, and 20% have disease confined to the colon. The remaining 10% have disease elsewhere in the GI tract, particularly perianal disease although the mouth, oesophagus, and stomach can also be affected.

Symptoms. Classical symptoms are **abdominal pain and diarrhoea**. Weight loss, anorexia, and fever may be seen, and growth retardation is common and important in children. Gross rectal bleeding and acute haemorrhage are uncommon.
- **Anaemia** occurs in 30%, mainly as a result of iron deficiency but sometimes as a result of vitamin B12 deficiency in ileal disease or folate deficiency in proximal small bowel disease.
- Patients can present with small bowel **obstruction** or symptoms relating to small bowel **stricturing**. Colonic Crohn's disease may present with bloody diarrhoea but tenesmus is less common than in ulcerative colitis because the rectum is less commonly affected (although about 30% of patients with ileal disease have some degree of proctitis).
- Gastroduodenal Crohn's disease can present as *Helicobacter*-negative peptic ulcer disease.

Extraintestinal manifestations

Pauciarticular **arthropathy** affects 6% of patients with Crohn's, usually accompanying active intestinal disease and may include sacroilitis. There is an association with ankylosing spondylitis and Crohn's are HLA B27 positive. Polyarticular arthropathy affects about 4% of Crohn's patients.
- **Metabolic bone disease** is common, with osteopenia (T score on DEXA scanning of −1 to −2.49) found in up to 50% of patients; steroid usage is the main risk factor, but loss of bone density is an independent feature of disease.

- There is an association with venous and arterial **thrombo-embolic disease**. Hospitalization, immobility, and malnutrition contribute, but in addition platelets can be high and many clotting factors are increased. There is no independent association with factor V Leiden. Treatment with prophylactic anticoagulants is safe and effective.
- Mucocutaneous manifestations include aphthous ulceration, pyoderma gangrenosum, and erythema nodosum.
- Ocular manifestations (scleritis, episcleritis, and uveitis) occur in about 5% of Crohn's patients.
- Gallstones are twice as common in Crohn's as a control population, There is an association with fatty liver and autoimmune hepatitis as well as with primary sclerosing cholangitis.
- Terminal ileal disease is associated with renal oxalate stones.

Behaviour of disease

Disease can be stricturing, penetrating, or neither. This has been incorporated into recent classifications of Crohn's such as the Vienna classification (see box; Gasche, C. *et al.* (2000) *Inflamm. Bowel Dis.* **6**: 8).

Fistulae reflect the transmural character of Crohn's. Perianal fistulaes may occur in 15–30%, and enteroenteric, entero-vaginal, and entero-cutaneous fistulas can occur.

Establishing the diagnosis and evaluating the disease

History and examination. Focus on recent travel, antibiotic use, diet, family history, sexual activity, and ask about smoking. Examine carefully for signs of obstruction, tenderness, or a mass. Always examine the perianal region.

Laboratory tests. **Stool culture** is important, including examination for parasites and *Clostridium difficile* toxin. Check **full blood count** (look for anaemia, raised platelets as a surrogate sign of inflammation, leucocytosis) **haematinics** including iron and TIBC, B12 and folate levels, **LFT** (best test of liver function are albumin and INR: liver often switches out of synthesizing albumin and switches into making inflammatory mediators like CRP). Also remember to look for **vitamin and micronutrient** deficiency: calcium and magnesium levels can be low: zinc may be low in extensive small bowel disease and is a critical factor in tissue healing.

Special investigations

- Ultrasound, endoscopy, radiological (CT and barium) studies, and histopathology are all used to make the diagnosis.
- Endoscopy is probably the gold standard for diagnosing colonic and terminal ileal disease; it is the only diagnostic modality that readily permits mucosal biopsy and also allows for balloon dilatation of any strictures.
- Barium follow through is still a standard method for evaluating the small bowel, although capsule enteroscopy may have an important role if stricturing can be excluded.
- CT does not show mucosal detail but is very helpful in discerning extraluminal features. There is interest in using CT or MRI to assess regional blood flow in attempting to distinguish fibrostenotic Crohn's from inflammatory disease causing stricturing as the treatment implications are very different. MRI is the modality of choice for imaging perianal or pelvic fistulating disease.

Vienna classification of Crohn's disease		
Age at diagnosis	1 = <40 years 1 > 40 years	Time of histological, surgical, radiological, or endoscopical diagnosis; no retrospective time of diagnosis
Location	1 = Terminal ileum 2 = Colon 3 = Ileocolon 4 = Upper GI-tract	Maximum extent of the lesions at any time before resection Aphthous lesions or ulcerations of any size (mucosal erythema is not enough)
Behaviour	1 = Non-stricturing, non-penetrating 2 = Stricturing 3 = Penetrating	Inflammatory masses, abscesses, fistulae, perianal ulcers are defined as penetrating Strictures can be diagnosed radiologically, endoscopically, or surgically Postoperative complications are excluded

- Ultrasound is very useful in expert hands and is reported as having high sensitivity and specificity for detecting thickened bowel, abscesses, and fistulae.

Differentiating Crohn's from ulcerative colitis

This can be an issue when IBD is confined to the colon. Discriminating features include small bowel disease, mainly right-sided colonic disease, rectal sparing, fistulization, perianal disease, and granulomas, all of which favour Crohn's disease. Immunological markers may be of some help: pANCA is found in 70% of UC but only 15% of Crohn's and antibodies to *Saccharomyces cervisiae* are found in up to 50% of Crohn's but less often in UC. When done together specificity is further improved.

Assessing disease activity

It is usually sufficient to follow the patient's response to treatment, as well as simple markers of inflammatory activity such as the CRP. There are a number of scoring systems that are important research tools: see Crohn's disease activity indices.

Aims and principles of management

Since a cure is not available, goals of therapy are to induce and maintain remission. Medical therapies include AMINOSALICYLATES, ANTIBIOTICS, CORTICOSTEROIDS, and immunosuppressants including AZATHIOPRINE/ 6-MERCAPTOPURINE, and METHOTREXATE.

- AMINOSALICYLATES are superior to placebo in treating colonic disease and pentasa is effective for ileal disease in a dose of 4 g/day. The data as to the efficacy of 5-ASA in maintaining remission are contradictory: one meta-analysis has suggested some benefit in patients after ileal resection but a prospective randomized trial has not confirmed this result and the benefits seem marginal at best for this group of patients.
- ANTIBIOTICS have a role in treating infectious complications of Crohn's disease.
- METRONIDAZOLE is of proven efficacy in reducing post-surgical endoscopic recurrence after ileal resection and probably also has an effect

in healing perianal fistulae. The effect may not be totally due to its antibacterial properties since *in vitro* it inhibits neutrophil margination across endothelium. CIPROFLOXACIN is also used in treating complications of Crohn's with good effect.

- Claims have been made for multiple antibacterial therapy targeted against mycobacteria but the data to date are not compelling.
- Novel CORTICOSTEROIDS such as budesonide have been shown to be almost as effective as prednisolone with fewer side effects, but budesonide is not effective as maintenance therapy.
- CORTICOSTEROIDS still play a central role in many physician's management of Crohn's disease, although they do not heal the disease and the adverse side effects are well known. They are not effective as long term therapy, although many patients find difficulty in tapering the dose without recurrent symptoms.
- Convincing evidence of efficacy exists for azathioprine/6-mercaptopurine and METHOTREXATE. These drugs are widely and increasingly used in patients with active Crohn's who fail to respond to first-line therapies or who fail to taper steroids.
- Data on cyclosporin and mycophenolate do not indicate a major role for these drugs in the management of Crohn's.
- A number of newer 'biological' therapies have been introduced in recent years. INFLIXIMAB is a chimeric antibody to TNF alpha and has an evolving role in managing Crohn's disease. New agents being developed include anti-IL-12 antibodies, anti-adhesion molecule antibodies, growth factors, and inhibitors of NFκβ.

Nutritional therapy targets both repletion of specific nutrient deficits and also primary therapy of the disease. Elemental diets are as effective as corticosteroids in inducing remission, particularly in children.

Surgery

- 75% of Crohn's patients will have surgery within 20 years of diagnosis. Indications for surgery include complications such as intra-abdominal masses, medically intractable fistulae, fibrotic strictures with obstruction, toxic megacolon, haemorrhage, and cancer.
- Details of surgical procedures vary with site of disease and to some extent with country, but can be classified as:
  - Resections with or without anastomoses.
  - External or internal bypass surgery.
  - Surgical procedures to repair or resect fistulae.
- Recurrent disease is common after surgery and has been assessed endoscopically as approaching 80%. About 50% of patients undergoing surgery will need another operation within 10 years.

Crohn's disease in pregnancy

Active disease is probably associated with reduced fertility, which may relate to chronic inflammation, undernutrition, or reduced libido. Women with quiescent disease at conception have the same rate of recurrence as non-pregnant women. Among women with active disease at conception, one-third get better, one-third get worse, and one-third do not change during pregnancy. Most pregnancies carried by women with Crohn's are normal, and perianal complications develop infrequently in women who deliver vaginally with an episiotomy.

Course and prognosis

The rate of relapse in the first 1–2 years correlates with the risk of relapse in the ensuing 5 years. About 25% of patients will maintain long periods of remission, 25% experience chronically active symptoms, and 50% have a course that fluctuates between active and inactive disease.

Risk of cancer

When Crohn's affects the colon, the risk of <u>colon cancer</u> appears to be similar to that for cancer in <u>ulcerative colitis</u>. Surveillance colonoscopy is recommended from 10 years after diagnosis. Data from radiological studies in the 1970s suggests that stricturing disease of the colon has a higher risk of malignancy, of approximately 7%. There is an increased risk of small bowel adenocarcinoma in small bowel Crohn's disease, and probably a small increased risk of Hodgkins and non-Hodgkins lymphoma.

Crohn's disease activity indices

Symptoms and clinical signs of Crohn's disease do not always correlate with inflammatory severity; the cardinal features of abdominal pain and diarrhoea may be due to superimposed irritable bowel, previous surgical resection, or complications such as strictures or fistulae.

The most widely used activity index is the **Crohn's disease activity index (CDAI)** developed by Best (see box opposite; Best, WR *et al.* (1976) *Gastroenterology* **70**: 439). The main criticisms are the excessive weight put on the number of bowel actions per day, which can be influenced by many factors apart from disease activity, and the inclusion of haematocrit as a marker of activity. Many research studies use a fall in the CDAI as a primary endpoint of efficacy: traditionally a fall of 70 points has been required, but recently this has been revised so that a fall of 100 points is currently required for evidence of efficacy.

The **Harvey–Bradshaw index**, proposed in 1980, is a simplified form of the CDAI and also in widespread use in research studies of disease intervention.

Endoscopic activity scores such as the **Crohn's disease endoscopic inflammation score** (CDEIS) are also widely used, as for instance in work of Rutgeerts showing early endoscopic recurrence after resectional surgery for Crohn's disease that predates symptomatic recurrence.

Cronkite–Canada syndrome

Reported in 1955, it is a non-inherited syndrome occurring in middle-aged or older people. It consists of diffuse polyposis, dystrophic changes of fingernails, alopecia, cutaneous hyperpigmentation, and a malabsorption syndrome with diarrhoea, weight loss, and abdominal pain.

The malabsorption is progressive and the prognosis poor. Bacterial overgrowth can be a complicating factor.

Cryptosporidium

See: Coccidia.

Calculating the Crohn's disease activity index

$$CDAI = 2 \times 1 + 5 \times 2 + 7 \times 3 + 20 \times 4 + 30 \times 5 + 10 \times 6 +$$
$$6 \times 7 + (\text{weight factor})_8$$

where

1 = Number of liquid or very soft stools in one week
2 = Sum of seven daily abdominal pain ratings:
   (0 = none, 1 = mild, 2 = moderate, 3 = severe)
3 = Sum of seven daily ratings of general well-being:
   (0 = well, 1 = slightly below par, 2 = poor, 3 = very poor,
   4=terrible)
4 = Symptoms or findings presumed related to Crohn's disease
   (score 1 for each)
   • arthritis or arthralgia
   • iritis or uveitis
   • erythema nodosum, pyoderma gangrenosum, aphthous
     stomatitis
   • anal fissure, fistula, or perirectal abscess
   • other bowel-related fistula
   • febrile (fever) episode over 100 degrees during past week
5 = Taking lomotil or opiates for diarrhoea
6 = Abnormal mass
   0 = none; 0.4 = questionable; 1 = present
7 = Haematocrit [(Typical – Current) × 6]
   Normal average: for male = 47, for female = 42
8 = 100 × [(standard weight – actual body weight)/standard weight]

An on-line calculator for this index can be found at: http://www.
ibdjohn.com/cdai/

CT pneumocolon ('virtual colonoscopy')

Technique of imaging the colon using helical CT scanning. Colon is usually cleansed using the same <u>bowel preparation</u> as in conventional colonoscopy, although there is interest in 'tagging' intestinal contents with orally ingested contrast agents and then subtracting tagged material at the image processing stage to enable colonic imaging without bowel prep.

CT images can be reconstructed to give a 'virtual colonoscopy' that can include views behind folds that can be difficult with conventional colonoscopy. The role of CT pneumocolon is still being evaluated but it may have an important role in screening for colorectal disease, particularly in the setting of incomplete colonoscopy; in this area CT pneumocolon is often used as an alternative to barium enema. A recent review (Van Dam, J et al. (2004) *Gastroenterology* **127**: 970) highlights the wide variation in results of clinical trials investigating CT as a screening tool for <u>colon cancer</u>. At least one of these trials reports similar sensitivity of virtual and conventional colonoscopy in detecting colon polyps over 6 mm diameter. CT pneumocolon will have a significant effect on the practice of gastroenterology but the magnitude of this effect is unclear.

Cyclospora

See: <u>*Coccidia*</u>.

Cyclosporin (ciclosporin)

See: index of drugs.

Cystic fibrosis (CF) and the GI tract

Epidemiology + pathogenesis

Autosomal recessive condition, with disease prevalence of 1:3000 northern Europeans and gene carriage in 1:25. CF results from mutations in gene for the cystic fibrosis transmembrane conductance regulator (CFTR), a cAMP-activated chloride channel found in secretory epithelia. Major complications of pulmonary and GI system, due to production of dehydrated protein-rich secretions.

Clinical features

- GI tract complications increasingly common, due in part to improved management of pulmonary complications and longer life expectancy (median 30 years).
- CF is the commonest cause of exocrine <u>pancreatic insufficiency</u> in childhood (occurs in 90–95% of children with CF), and severity of pancreatic disease parallels lung involvement. Presents with failure to thrive, steatorrhoea, colicky abdominal pain. Predisposes to malabsorption of fat-soluble <u>vitamins</u> A, D, E, and K. Diabetes mellitus in 8–12% of patients >25 years.
- Bile duct plugging due to secretions may lead to indolent development of secondary biliary cirrhosis and <u>portal hypertension</u>. Hepatic congestion due to pulmonary hypertension/right heart failure. <u>Fatty liver</u> in 20%; <u>gallstones</u> in 15% of young adults with CF.
- CF may result in meconium ileus at birth (12% of neonates with CF) and in distal intestinal obstruction syndrome (DIOS) later. Intestinal obstruction, intussusception, rectal prolapse may occur. Excessive <u>PANCREATIC ENZYME SUPPLEMENTS</u> associated with colonic strictures (fibrosing colonopathy).

Investigations

- Diagnosis usually made in infancy, based on typical pulmonary ± GI tract manifestations, a family history, and positive results on sweat test. Confirmation by genetic testing in most cases.
- Investigation of GI complications dependent on specific presentation.
- Check vitamin A,E,D,K levels.

Management

- Multidisciplinary approach to care, with expert nutritional support.
- Replace <u>vitamin</u> deficiencies
- <u>PANCREATIC ENZYME SUPPLEMENTS</u> for exocrine insufficiency (see index of drugs).
- Lung and <u>liver transplantation</u> has been successful.
- Gene therapy remains the ultimate goal for treatment of CF.

CF mutations and pancreatitis

Recent observations suggest that heterozygosity for CFTR may be linked to recurrent <u>acute pancreatitis</u> and idiopathic <u>chronic pancreatitis</u>. Few of these patients have any evidence of pulmonary disease or abnormal sweat tests.

Pathogenic importance of these findings remain controversial.

Cytomegalovirus (CMV)

50–80% people are seropositive for CMV. Primary infection in immuno-competent hosts causes few or no symptoms.

Immunosuppression can lead to CMV retinitis, pneumonitis, colitis, and oesophagitis. CMV is third commonest pathogen in AIDS after pneumo-cystis and candida (see <u>HIV and the gut</u>).

CMV colitis (see Colour Plate 6)

Occurs in 2–15 % of patients with solid organ transplants (average time is 5–7 months after transplant) and 3–5% patients with HIV/AIDS. It is rare in immunocompetent hosts but can complicate ulcerative colitis, especially in patients receiving steroids. Patients with steroid-dependent colitis who present with refractory disease should be assessed for CMV infection.

Diagnosis. Sigmoidoscopy or colonoscopy allows mucosal visualization and biopsy. Histology may reveal inclusion bodies and immunohistochem-istry may show CMV antigen.

CMV oesophagitis (see Colour Plate 6)

Unknown in healthy hosts, Found in 10–25% patients with AIDS undergo-ing upper GI endoscopy. Symptoms include odynophagia, nausea, vomit-ing, fever, diarrhoea, weight loss, chest pain. Diagnosis usually involves upper GI endoscopy and biopsy: appearances are classically of large shallow ulcers.

Therapy. Intravenous <u>GANCICLOVIR</u> for 3 weeks.

D

Defecography studies

- A method of evaluating defecation in patients who complain of excessive straining, or who employ digital manipulation to facilitate evacuation. Barium, thickened to a consistency that approximates stool, is introduced into the rectum. Evacuation of the barium is monitored by fluoroscopy (see Fig. 2.9 on opposite page). This allows assessment of anorectal anatomy, and measurement of the anorectal angle (the angle made between the axis of the rectum and the axis of the anal canal: usually about 90 degrees) at rest and during defecation. Rectoceles and intussusceptions not seen at rest may be seen during evacuation. The degree of perineal descent can also be assessed, which gives information on the integrity of the puborectalis and other muscles of the pelvic floor.
- Magnetic resonance imaging (MRI) using an endoanal receiving coil can give good anorectal imaging and also dynamic information about rectal emptying.

Dentate line

This represents a border between the distal squamous mucosa and a transitional area of squamous/nonsquamous mucosa within the anal canal (see Fig. 2.10 opposite). It is usually located in the middle portion of the internal anal sphincter. Four to eight anal glands drain into the columns of Morgagni at the level of the dentate line, and most rectal abscesses and fistulae originate in these glands. The dentate line also delineates where sensory fibres end; proximal to this line the rectum is supplied by stretch nerve fibres but not pain nerve fibres (so allowing surgical procedures to be performed without anaesthesia above this point).

Dermatitis herpetiformis

An itchy, papular, vesicular eruption symmetrical on elbows, buttocks, knees, sacrum, face, neck, and trunk. Very closely associated with coeliac disease: nearly 100% have abnormal jejunal mucosa. Characterized by IgA at the dermo-epidermal junction away from sites of blistering. Pathogenesis unknown. Treatment involves dapsone 1–2 mg/kg. All patients should go on to gluten-free diet. See Colour Plate 7.

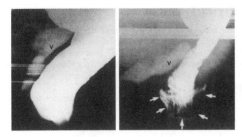

Fig. 2.9 Defecating proctogram showing rectal intussusception. Left, normal rectum prior to defecation. Right, attempted defecation leads to intussusception. Reproduced from Feldman M, Friedman LS, and Sleisenger MH (2003). *Sleisenger and Fordtran's Gastrointestinal and Liver Disease*, with permission from Elsevier

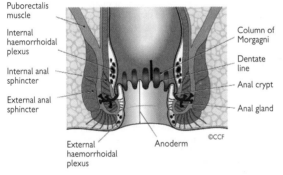

Puborectalis muscle

Internal haemorrhoidal plexus

Internal anal sphincter

External anal sphincter

Column of Morgagni

Dentate line

Anal crypt

Anal gland

External haemorrhoidal plexus

Anoderm

©CCF

Fig. 2.10 Anatomy of the anal canal. The heavy vertical line denotes the transition zone 1 to 1.5 cm proximal to the denate line.

Dermatomyositis

- Acquired muscle disease, with autoimmune basis, characterized by primary muscle weakness, endomysial inflammation, and ↑serum muscle enzyme levels (e.g. creatine kinase, AST, lactate dehydrogenase (LDH)). Other clinical features include heliotropic (purplish-blue) rash around eyes, proximal myopathy, Raynaud's phenomenon.
- GI involvement includes:
  - Dysphagia, due to striated muscle involvement in upper one-third of oesophagus (15–50% of cases).
  - GI tract ulcers and bleeding.
  - Vasculitis with abdominal pain, and bowel infarction.
  - Acute pancreatitis (rare).
  - Association with internal malignancy (e.g. with gastric cancer) in 10–20% of patients.
- Diagnosis made on basis of: clinical history; ↑serum muscle enzymes; antinuclear antibodies (present in 80%); needle EMG showing myopathic features with indications of muscle irritability; muscle biopsy findings of inflammation and perifascicular atrophy.
- Oesophageal involvement may be demonstrated by oesophageal manometry (see oesophageal motility studies).
- Management includes immunosuppression with steroids.

Diabetes and the GI tract

Altered gut motility due to autonomic neuropathy can result in:
- **Diabetic gastroparesis.** Delayed gastric emptying on scintigraphy is found in up to 50% of unselected patients. About 25% of insulin-dependent diabetics with peripheral neuropathy report nausea, vomiting, anorexia, and heartburn. Suspect the diagnosis in a patient with appropriate symptoms and a negative endoscopy or barium study. Pathophysiology is complex and may involve impaired visceral sensation, gastric smooth muscle degeneration, a local myopathic effect of hyperglycaemia, or altered secretion of gut hormones. Management centres on small frequent meals, tight control of blood sugar, and PROKINETICS such as domperidone or erythromycin. Jejunostomy feeding tubes occasionally needed. External electrical pacing has been suggested to improve gastric emptying but is not widely used.
- **Diabetic diarrhoea.** This occurs in association with long-standing insulin-dependent diabetes and is associated with autonomic neuropathy and occasionally faecal incontinence. It may also be associated with bacterial overgrowth. In some patients exocrine pancreatic insufficiency may contribute to the pathogenesis. Management is with anti-diarrhoeal agents such as loperamide or codeine. OCTREOTIDE has been useful in selected patients.

Fatty liver. Abdominal ultrasound will often include a report of 'fatty liver', reflecting the accumulation of lipid in hepatocytes. This occurs as part of a **metabolic syndrome** incorporating obesity, hypertension, and diabetes. A proportion of patients with non-alcoholic fatty liver disease (NAFLD) will have steatohepatitis, which may progress to fibrosis and cirrhosis and is not the benign process it was once considered to be.

Diaphragmatic herniae

Can occur through the oesophageal hiatus (see <u>hiatus hernia</u>), through other openings (foramina of **Bochdalek**, at the lumbocosatal margins of the diaphragm posterolaterally or **Morgagni**, at the sternocostal margins of the diaphragm anteriorly) or through post-traumatic defects.

Congenital hernias occur in 0.1 to 0.5 per 1000 live births. In neonates they are mostly Bochdalek hernias. Morgagni hernias occur mainly in adults and 80% are on the right side. They may contain omentum, stomach, colon, or liver. Repair is possible through open, thoracoscopic, or laparoscopic techniques.

Dieulafoy lesion

First described by Georges Dieulafoy, a French surgeon, in 1898, this lesion is a rare cause of <u>acute upper GI bleeding</u>. It consists of an arteriole that protrudes through a 2–5 mm mucosal defect, and is found in the stomach, within 6 cm of the gastro-oesophageal junction, in 75–95% of cases. Rarer sites include the distal oesophagus, small intestine, colon, and rectum. Diagnosis made on endoscopy, and endotherapy (e.g. electrocoagulation, adrenaline injection, haemoclipping). Results in permanent haemostasis in 85% of cases. See Colour Plate 8.

Disinfection of endoscopes

A range of infections has been transmitted during endoscopy, including bacteria (<u>Salmonella</u>, <u>Pseudomonas</u>), and viruses (<u>hepatitis B</u>, <u>hepatitis C</u>). The theoretical risk of prion disease (Creutzfeldt–Jakob disease (CJD)/variant-CJD) transmission necessitates careful consideration of merits of endoscopy in patients with any possibility of having these diseases, as conventional sterilization is ineffective, and long-term quarantine/destruction of endoscopes is required if used. A multistep process is involved in cleaning and sterilizing an endoscope after use.

- **Manual cleaning.** Blood/mucus/debris wiped off after use; suction and accessory channels washed through with dilute detergent, and brushed. It is likely that all endoscopy accessories wil become single use only in the near future.
- **Washer disinfection.** Cycles of disinfection, washing, and drying, usually performed over 30 minutes in automated washing system.
- **Sterilization.** Usually achieved by steam autoclaving.

Selection of disinfectant

The ideal agent must be effective against pathogens including spores, *Mycobacterium* TB, and blood borne viruses, be compatible with instruments and washers, non-irritant and affordable.

Glutaraldehyde is widely used but all aldehydes can be irritants and sensitizers and this may limit long-term utility. Peracetic acid and chlorine dioxide are both effective. Further information can be found in the report of a working party on cleaning and disinfection of endoscopes of the BSG Endoscopy Committee ((1998) *Gut* **42**: 585).

Diversion colitis

Development of inflammation in the distal bypassed colon after colostomy or ileostomy performed for cancer, diverticulitis, inflammatory bowel disease, or trauma. First reported by Morson in 1972.

Inflammation is seen endoscopically in 90% of patients: most (95%) are mild or moderate, with only 5% severe. However symptoms present in a minority—less than 10%. Symptoms are more common in patients operated on for IBD and develop within 1–9 months after faecal diversion.

Pathogenesis. Because inflammation resolves after restoration of the faecal stream, luminal nutrient deficiency is the favoured mechanism. Roediger showed that luminal short chain fatty acids (SCFA) are the main fuels for the distal colonocyte (butyrate provides 70% oxidative energy for epithelial cells: acetate, ketone bodies, and glutamine are alternatives). SCFA enemas can be therapeutic but do not always work. Other luminal factors (growth factors, dietary constituents, or bacterial products) may be involved in the pathogenesis. See short chain fatty acids.

Diagnosis and pathological findings. Where there was no preoperative inflammation, diagnosis is straightforward: flexible sigmoidoscopy with biopsy and culture of stools for ova cysts, parasites, and pathogens (including *C. difficile* toxin) will establish the severity of inflammation. Radiology does not help unless a fistula or abscess is suspected, in which case CT is indicated: remember to consider radiation or ischaemic colitis in the appropriate clinical context.

Differentiating recurrent Crohn's disease from diversion colitis. This can be difficult: endoscopic features favouring Crohn's disease are longitudinal ulcers and strictures: ulcers are usually small in diversion colitis. Absent preoperative rectal involvement can be helpful. Pathological features are compared in the table opposite.

Treatment. SCFA enemas may work (60 mM lactate, 30 mM proprionate, 40 mM butyrate) but they smell awful and this limits compliance. Steroid enemas do not work but 5-ASA enemas have been used successfully.

Diverticular disease (diverticulosis, diverticulitis, and diverticular bleeding)

A diverticulum (pleural: diverticula) is a sac-like protrusion of the intestinal wall. Most diverticula of clinical interest occur in the colon, but also see duodenal diverticulum, Meckel's diverticulum, jejunal diverticulum, and Zenker's diverticulum (see pharyngeal pouch).

Colonic diverticula do not contain all bowel wall layers because the mucosa and submucosa herniate through the muscle layers of the colon at the points where the vasa recta penetrate the circular muscle layer.

Diverticulosis. Prevalence increases with age (5% at age 40: 65% by age 85) and also seems to have increased markedly in the last century. In Western countries it is common and usually left-sided: in the Far East it is rarer, more commonly right-sided, and affects younger people. Pathogenesis is commonly held to relate to low dietary fibre.

Diversion colitis	Crohn's disease
Granulomas can occur but are usually mucinous. Transmural changes usually absent	Transmural inflammation, crypt architectural changes (suggests lonstanding inflammation) and epithelioid granulomas
Lymphoid hyperplasia with frequent germinal centres is very prominent	Lymphoid hyperplasia can occur
Very few macrophages and plasma cells	

Diverticulitis. Inflammation of the wall and surrounding tissues leads to a variable clinical picture ranging from subclinical inflammation to life-threatening peritonitis.

Simple diverticulitis is characterized by constant left lower quadrant pain, nausea, or vomiting in 20–60%, and change of bowel habit. Physical signs include lower abdominal tenderness and an abdominal mass (in about 20%). Low grade fever and leucocytosis are common but about 50% have a normal white cell count. Urinalysis may reveal sterile pyuria secondary to adjacent inflammation. **Complicated diverticulitis** may be accompanied by signs of peritonitis, abscess formation, or fistulation. Faecal discharge from the vagina is diagnostic of a colo-vaginal fistula.

Diagnosis. Plain abdominal films can help in excluding other causes of abdominal pain and in showing free intraperitoneal air. For further diagnostic information, contrast-enhanced CT scan is preferred. CT can identify complications: peritonitis, fistula formation, obstruction, and abscess formation. It can also function as an aid to therapeutic abscess drainage. In about 10%, CT is unable to distinguish acute diverticulitis from colon cancer as both produce focal bowel wall thickening.

Treatment

- Depends on the individual and severity of inflammation. Most patients with simple diverticulitis can be treated conservatively with broad spectrum ANTIBIOTICS with cover directed towards Gram-negative rods and anaerobes (e.g. CEFUROXIME or CIPROFLOXACIN plus METRONIDAZOLE).
- Patients with complicated diverticulitis (free intraperitoneal perforation, obstruction, abscess, or fistula formation) will often need surgery. In the emergency situation, a two-stage procedure is commonly employed, with resection of the diseased colon, oversewing of the rectum, and an end colostomy (a Hartmann procedure). The colostomy can be closed 3 months later.

Diverticular bleeding. Local trauma to the vasa recti within diverticula can lead to arterial bleeding. Diverticular bleeding is the commonest cause of acute massive colonic blood loss. Although bleeding may stop spontaneously, rebleeding is common and often comes from the right colon, even though most diverticula are left-sided.

Management of diverticular bleeding. After resuscitation, the principles are to diagnose and locate the source of bleeding, and to treat the cause (see also acute lower GI bleeding). Colonoscopy is reasonable in most patients because blood is cathartic and visualization of a bleeding source may allow endoscopic haemostasis to be achieved. Some clinicians employ bowel preparation: recommendations include the use of balanced electrolyte solutions, e.g. kleenprep given via NG tube. In patients where colonoscopy is unsuccessful, the bleeding is massive, or the patient remains haemodynamically unstable, options include angiography or surgery. Diagnostic angiography can be combined with a trial of octreotide infusion to stop the bleeding and allow bowel prep for future operative intervention, or selective embolization of a bleeding vessel or area of angiodysplasia. It is however important to exclude upper GI sources of bleeding. Surgical options usually involve segmental colectomy.

Double duct sign

Term used to describe appearance on ERCP, MRCP, or CT, of stricture (and upstream dilatation) of common bile duct and pancreatic duct, usually in patient with biliary obstruction. Often associated with pancreatic cancer (in head of pancreas, as shown on ERCP in Fig. 2.11 opposite), but rarer causes include focal pancreatitis or ampullary cancer/ stenosis.

Down syndrome and GI tract

Trisomy 21 affects 1:1000 babies in UK, and is characterized by a wide range of phenotypic abnormalities, including short stature, learning difficulties, wide epicanthic folds, and macroglossia. GI problems can be subdivided into the following.

Embryological. Imperforate anus; duodenal/jejunal atresia; Hirschsprung's disease (2% of cases).

Motility. Feeding problems; constipation, gastro-oesophageal reflux.

Immunological

- Coeliac disease: affects > 5% of people with DS (> 40-fold increase over non-DS population).
- Autoimmune hepatitis: probable increased frequency.
- Hepatitis B and associated autoimmune thyroiditis: increased rate of HBV infection may relate to history of institutional living, but high frequency of chronicity probably due to inherent immune defects in DS.

Drug-induced hepatotoxicity

Background. Accounts for < 5% of cases of jaundice, but 30–50% of cases of acute liver failure. Incidence approximately 1:10 000 to 1:100 000 persons exposed to drug. Risk factors for drug reaction include: female sex; old age (may relate to reduced hepatic blood flow and renal clearance); obesity (e.g. methotrexate-induced hepatic fibrosis); fasting (e.g. paracetamol/acetaminophen); multiple drug use (induction of cytochrome P450 may be important); alcohol (especially paracetamol, isoniazid, methotrexate); chronic liver disease (increased risk of anti-TB and HAART-related liver reactions in patients with chronic viral hepatitis).

The injury caused can be considered in terms of the mechanism of toxicity, and the site of injury within the liver.

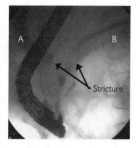

Fig. 2.11 ERCP showing 'double duct sign'. Stricture of (A) common bile duct and (B) pancreatic duct, in this case associated with pancreatic cancer (in head of pancreas).

Common causes of drug-induced liver injury

Injury	Common examples	Comments
Hepatocellular	Paracetamol	Hepatic necrosis
	Methotrexate, tetracycline, valproate, herbal remedies, HAART, amiodarone	Steatosis
	Isoniazid, sulfonamides, disulfuram, aspirin, ketoconazole, terbiafine, minocycline	Acute or chronic hepatitis
Cholestasis	Amoxicillin–clavulinic acid, flucloxacillin, erythromycin, amitryptiline, phenytoin, chlorpromazine, trimethoprim–sulfamethoxazole	Cholestatic hepatitis (hepatocanalicular)
	Anabolic steroids, oestrogens	Canalicular
Granulomas	Diltiazem, allopurinol, hydralazine, carbamazepine, quinidine, quinine	Varying degrees of cholestasis/hepatitis
Fibrosis	Methotrexate	-
Vascular	Azathioprine, busulphan	Veno-occlusive disease
	Vitamin A, methotrexate	Non-cirrhotic portal hypertension

Mechanism of toxicity

Drugs may induce liver injury through 2 broad types of reaction (see Fig. 2.12).

- Dose-dependent, direct hepatotoxic effects. Toxic effects may relate to 'increased dose' (e.g. <u>paracetamol</u>) or 'cumulative dose'.
- Idiosyncratic effects. Reaction unpredictable, not dose-related. Likely to occur due to 'multihit' process involving genetic and immune mechanisms. Onset 5–90 days after ingestion, and usually damages hepatocytes, leading to a hepatitis (i.e. ↑ AST/ALT). Continued use or re-exposure to drug may be fatal.

Site of injury

Clues to the causative agent may be gained by the morphological pattern of liver injury (table on previous page). Hepatocellular injury may manifest as steatosis, hepatic necrosis, or acute/chronic hepatitis.

Clinical features

- No pathognomonic features of drug-induced liver injury.
- Fever, rash, lymphadenopathy may be present in allergic idiosyncratic reactions, and jaundice may be preceded by prodrome of nausea, vomiting, and anorexia (as with viral hepatitis).
- Cholestatic patterns of injury may mimic biliary obstruction (i.e. pruritis and jaundice).

Diagnosis/investigation

- Usually no specific diagnostic tests (except in <u>paracetamol overdose</u>), so diagnosis relies on clinical suspicion, careful drug history (including all prescribed, complementary, and recreational drugs/preparations), consideration of the temporal relationships between drug ingestion and liver disease, and exclusion of other disorders.
- 'Liver screen' of blood tests necessary to define pattern and severity of liver injury, and other causes (see <u>Approaches to recent-onset jaundice and well patient with abnormal liver tests</u>). Serum ALT > 1000 U/l strongly suggests drug injury, acute viral hepatitis, or hepatic ischaemia.
- Peripheral eosinophilia may point towards an allergic drug reaction.
- Liver U/S excludes biliary obstruction in patient with cholestasis.
- <u>Liver biopsy</u> findings are rarely specific for a drug reaction (although eosinophils and granulomas may suggest an allergic reaction).

Avoid diagnostic rechallenge with the suspected drug in almost all cases (risk of even more severe reaction), unless drug toxicity is highly questionable, or no alternative to suspected drug for a serious condition.

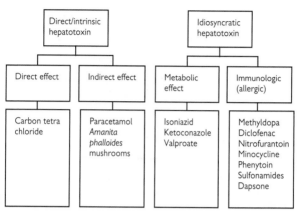

Fig. 2.12 Mechanisms of drug-induced liver injury, and common examples.

Management

- Stopping causative drug is fundamental intervention (failure to do so is associated with high mortality). In patients on combination of drugs, the one started most recently may be the likeliest culprit. Nevertheless, stopping all drugs is the wisest manoeuvre, if clinically possible. If patient improves, drugs least likely to be responsible may be carefully reintroduced.
- CORTICOSTEROIDS may be used for severe allergic-type reactions, and URSODEOXYCHOLIC ACID (UDCA) for cholestatic reactions, but no clear trial evidence of benefit.
- Patients with evidence of liver failure (e.g. INR >1.5, or hepatic encephalopathy) require transfer to a liver transplantation centre (also see Acute liver failure).

Drug-induced oesophagitis

- Many drugs have been reported to cause oesophageal injury. See box opposite. 90% of cases are due to NSAIDs, antibiotics (especially tetracyclines), antivirals, potassium chloride, iron, quinidine, and bisphosphanates.
- Patients with strictures, <u>oesophageal tumour</u>, <u>achalasia</u>, scleroderma should take pills upright with plenty of water.
- Chemotherapy oesophagitis: adriamycin, 5FU, <u>METHOTREXATE</u>, vincristine can all cause oropharyngeal mucositis and consequent dysphagia. Oesophageal damage is unusual in the absence of oral changes. Chemotherapy potentiates radiation damage to the oesophagus.

Dubin–Johnson syndrome

- Rare, autosomal recessive cause of conjugated hyperbilirubinaemia (see <u>Approach to recent-onset jaundice</u> and <u>bilirubin metabolism</u>). Impaired excretion of bilirubin, leading to mild jaundice (Bn < 120 µmol/l, 50% conjugated), but normal liver function. No specific treatment, but good prognosis.

Dukes staging system

Cuthbert Esquire Dukes, 1932. A classification of <u>colon cancer</u> invasion still in routine use because the relation of advancing stage to cancer mortality has been repeatedly demonstrated.

- **Stage A** tumours are mucosal (may invade into the submucosa but do not reach the muscularis propria). 5 year survival 95–100%.
- **Stage B1** tumours invade the muscularis propria, and **B2** lesions completely penetrate the smooth muscle layer to the serosa but without lymph node involvement. 5 year survival 80–85%.
- **Stage C** lesions are defined by regional lymph node involvement. They are further divided into primary tumours limited to the bowel wall (C1) and those that penetrate the bowel wall. 5 year survival 50–70%.
- **Stage D** lesions include all those with metastases. 5 year survival 5–15%.

The American Joint Commission on Cancer devised the TNM classification (see <u>tumour staging</u>), which has largely replaced the Dukes staging system, for randomizing patients into clinical trials. Comparison of Dukes with TNM yields the following: Dukes A = T1/2, N0, M0. Dukes B = T3/4, N0, M0. Dukes C = T1–4, N1 or N2, M0. Dukes D = M1.

Causes of drug-induced oesophagitis

NSAIDs: naproxen, ibuprofen, aspirin-containing pills
Antibiotics: tetracyclines, clindamycin, penicillins
Antivirals: AZT, ddC, foscarnet
Iron and **potassium** formulations
Cardiovascular medications: quinidine, nifedipine, verapamil, captopril
Other common drugs: bisphosphanates, phenytoin, oral contraceptive

Dumping syndrome

One of a number of <u>post-gastrectomy syndromes</u> (see also <u>Approach to surgically revised anatomy and stomas</u>), resulting from alteration in the storage function of the stomach and the pyloric emptying mechanism. Incidence relates to the extent of gastric surgery and may affect 20–25% of patients. Syndrome is much less common now because of decline in number of operations for peptic ulcer disease and lower incidence of problems with gastric emptying after newer operations such as proximal gastric vagotomy.

- **Early dumping** occurs 30–60 minutes after a meal and is thought to result from accelerated emptying of hyperosmolar gastric contents into the small bowel. This leads to fluid shifts from the intravascular compartment into the bowel lumen, resulting in **vasomotor symptoms**: tachycardia, vasodilatation, sweating, and light headednesss as well as **distension**, **crampy pain**, and **diarrhoea**. Postprandial release of gut hormones (enteroglucagon, peptide YY, pancreatic polypeptide, VIP, neurotensin) is increased in patients with dumping and some of these may play a part in the pathogenesis of dumping syndrome.
- **Late dumping** occurs 1–3 hours after a meal. The rapid delivery of a meal to the small intestine leads to rapid absorbtion of glucose and a hyperinsulinaemic response, causing subsequent hypoglycaemia. The diagnosis can be confirmed by an extended glucose tolerance test.

Postoperative dumping is common and tends to improve with time. Dietary manipulation with high protein/low carbohydrate meals can help. Inhibitors of gastric emptying can help, and there is some evidence to support the use of <u>OCTREOTIDE</u>. Acarbose interferes with carbohydrate absorption and may help with late dumping.

Duodenal diverticulum

- Peri-ampullary diverticula are a common finding at <u>ERCP</u>, and it is debated whether they are associated with common bile duct (CBD) stones, and biliary obstruction. Their presence may make CBD cannulation difficult (and occasionally impossible), and particular care during biliary sphincterotomy is essential, in order to avoid retroperitoneal perforation (see <u>endoscopic complications</u>). Food debris in diverticulum may be confused on U/S or <u>MRCP</u> as an intraductal filling defect.
- Large diverticula may occur elsewhere in small bowel (see <u>jejunal diverticulum</u>), where they may cause abdominal discomfort, diarrhoea, and features of <u>bacterial overgrowth</u>. Many are diagnosed incidentally during imaging.

Duodenal ulcer

Pathogenesis, epidemiology, treatment, and complications are discussed in section on peptic ulceration.

Management recommendations. Don't take biopsies routinely at endoscopy because malignancy is extremely rare. Take a CLO test or alternative test to establish *Helicobacter* status and treat if positive. Continue anti-secretory treatment with <u>PROTON PUMP INHIBITORS (PPI)</u> for at least 4 weeks. Although PPIs are the commonest drugs used, there is no clear evidence of superiority of PPI over other drugs for uncomplicated DU in patients not taking NSAIDs.

If symptoms resolve and compliance with treatment good, routine follow up endoscopy and confirmation of HP eradication is not necessary. However, follow up endoscopy is suggested for complicated ulcers that have bled or perforated. Studies on maintenance therapy for complicated ulcers are limited, and this issue remains disputed; consider maintenance if recurrence would be high risk (elderly, severe comorbidity).

Dye spraying

See: <u>chromoendoscopy</u>.

Dysentery

A clinical term: bloody mucoid diarrhoea, tenesmus, fever, cramps, and polymorphs in the faeces. It implies an invasive pathogen affecting the large bowel, commonly *Shigella*, enteroinvasive or enterohaemorrhagic *E. coli*, or amoebiasis (note: <u>amoebiasis</u> does not give leucocytes in the stool). See <u>Approach to acute diarrhoea.</u>

Dysplasia

> 'Britain and America—divided by a common language'
> George Bernard Shaw 1856–1950.

- A term that induces frustration and uncertainty into the hearts of gastroenterologists, particularly when they want a straight answer from the pathologists: 'is it cancer or not?'
- Dysplasia refers to **cellular and architectural changes that are associated with malignancy** (premalignant/adjacent to malignancy) but that, by definition, are not invasive. Differentiate from metaplasia, which refers to the conversion of one type of differentiated tissue into another specialist type (e.g. intestinal metaplasia in stomach related to *Helicobacter pylori*).
  - **Cellular changes** in dysplasia include an increase in cell nuclei size (↑ nuclear:cytoplasmic ratio), loss of nuclear polarity, and loss of cellular differentiation (e.g. mucin production).
  - **Architectural changes** include loss of normal glandular spacing, without intervening stroma.

- In practical terms, high grade dysplasia on mucosal biopsy suggests significant risk of invasive malignancy developing, or being present at other sites (in view of tiny area of tissue sampled). Unless confident that all affected area removed (e.g. excised polyp), high grade dysplasia requires consideration of radical intervention (e.g. colectomy in ulcerative colitis, oesophagectomy/photodynamic therapy in <u>Barrett's oesophagus</u>).
- Vienna classification of GI epithelial neoplasia (see box below) aims to standardize reporting of dysplasia/neoplasia.

Vienna classification of gastrointestinal epithelial neoplasia

Category	Histological assessment
1	Negative for neoplasia/dysplasia
2	Indefinite for neoplasia/dysplasia
3	Non-invasive low-grade neoplasia (low-grade adenoma/dysplasia)
4	Non-invasive high-grade neoplasia
4.1	High-grade adenoma/dysplasia
4.2	Non-invasive carcinoma (carcinoma in situ)
4.3	Suspicion of invasive carcinoma
5	Invasive neoplasia
5.1	Intramucosal carcinoma
5.2	Submucosal carcinoma or beyond

E

Eating disorders

See: <u>anorexia</u>, <u>bulimia</u>, <u>Approach to obesity</u>.

Ectopic mucosa

Refers to the presence of mucosal tissue in sites distant to their normal location. Examples include:
- Meckel's diverticulum (often harbouring gastric mucosa).
- Pancreatic rests (islands of pancreatic acinar tissue, lacking anatomic and vascular continuity with main pancreas). Found in 1–14% of autopsies. Most common in stomach and duodenum, where appear as yellowish subcutaneous nodules. Usually asymptomatic, requiring no treatment.
- Gastric heterotopia also most common in duodenum, (but described in all parts of GI tract) appearing as sessile/polypoid lesion. Usually asymptomatic finding on endoscopy, but histological diagnosis necessary to exclude other causes of lesion.
- Malignancy may rarely occur within ectopic mucosa.

Ehlers–Danlos disease

After Edward Ehlers, a Danish dermatologist, in 1901 and Henri Danlos, a French physician, in 1908.

A group of 10 rare (frequency approx 1 in 400 000) inherited disorders of collagen metabolism resulting in a decrease in the tensile strength and integrity of the skin, joints, and blood vessels. The classical types 1 and II involve defects in type 5 collagen. The most relevant to gastroenterologists is type IV, involving a defect in type III collagen (chromosome locus 2q31), which can present with spontaneous rupture of the bowel or medium-sized arteries. Patients have prominent venous marking easily visible through the skin. It is the only type with increased mortality (median life expectancy 50 years).

Elderly and the GI tract

GI disease is generally more common in the elderly than the young (e.g. colonic <u>diverticula</u> in > 50% people > 60 years). In most cases the patient's age has little effect over their management. A number of inter-linked factors contribute to the high rate of GI symptoms in the elderly.

Malignancy. All the major GI tract cancers increase in prevalence with age, with steep increases after the age of 60 (e.g. <u>gastric</u>, <u>oesophageal</u>, pancreatic, <u>colonic cancer</u>).

Comorbidity. E.g. <u>Parkinson's disease</u> (leads to constipation per se and secondary to anticholinergic drugs); motor neurone disease (dysphagia—see <u>Approach to mouth and swallowing</u>); Alzheimer's disease (poor nutrition, <u>faecal incontinence</u>).

Drug effects. Motility disorders, especially constipation, promoted by wide range of drugs: e.g. diuretics, <u>ANTICHOLINERGICS</u>, antidepressants, opiate analgesics (see index of drugs). NSAIDs for joint pain/disease contribute to <u>peptic ulceration</u>.

Immobility. Leads to GI motility problems due to range of reasons, including embarrassment at needing assistance, associated depression, and anti-physiological posture for defecation of being supine/semi-supine. Supine position may also encourage gastro-oesophageal reflux.

Nutrition. Malnutrition is prevalent in the elderly, particularly if hospitalized, socially isolated, or with mental//physical health problems. In those with severe dementia and inadequate nutrition, difficult ethical considerations surround use of artificial feeding (see <u>Approach to nutritional support</u>).

Specific considerations

Constipation

- 25% prevalence of constipation/straining in elderly living at home (increases to 50% in those in hospital/institutional care).
- Faecal impaction and incontinence in >10% of those >75 years.
- Poor fluid intake, immobility, and drugs all contribute.
- Laxatives used regularly by 20–30% of people > 65 years.
- In hospital patient stimulant/osmotic <u>LAXATIVES</u> (see index of drugs) more effective than fibre, which may encourage faecal impaction in immobile patients.

Dyspepsia. Common practice of performing endoscopy in all elderly patients with new-onset dyspepsia recently challenged by NICE guidelines. These advise that endoscopy should not be 'age-dependent', and that endoscopy for dyspepsia should be reserved for those with sinister symptoms (see <u>Approaches to dyspepsia and reflux</u>).

Acute abdominal pain. In elderly, usual peritonitic response to viscus perforation or other acute abdominal event (e.g. <u>intestinal ischaemia</u>) may be impaired, leading to usual presentation being masked, and hence late diagnosis.

<u>Gallstones.</u> ERCP with sphincterotomy and stone extraction, without subsequent <u>cholecystectomy</u>, has been advocated for elderly patients with <u>choledocholithiasis</u>. However, > 40% will get further biliary problems within 2 years with this approach. Although <u>cholecystectomy</u> is safe in elderly, long-term endobiliary plastic stenting may be appropriate if cholecystectomy/bile duct clearance not possible.

Electrocoagulation

The principle of using electrosurgical or diathermy currents in therapeutic endoscopy is to cause heat with resultant coagulation of blood vessels and to facilitate tissue transaction. There is a difference between cutting and coagulating current, and between monopolar and bipolar electrodes.

- **Cutting current** has an uninterrupted waveform of low voltage. It has relatively high power but because it is low voltage it is less able to cross dessicated tissue and does not penetrate deeply.
- **Coagulating current** has intermittent high voltage spikes with intervening off periods lasting 80% of the time. This allows deeper spread of current and less local tissue destruction.
- **Monopolar current** involves current flowing between the wire of a snare loop or the jaws of biopsy forceps and a patient plate.
- **Bipolar current** involves all current flowing from one side of the snare to the other, with the attraction of much more localized effect.
- Local current density is critically important and higher for bipolar electrosurgery, which is why bipolar current is favoured for local haemostasis, e.g. from bleeding peptic ulcers, while monopolar current with a 'slow cooking' effect (essential on an adequate length of polyp stalk) is favoured for polyp surgery.
- The heat produced relates directly to the power settings on the unit dial. Current recommendations are to perform polypectomy at a low power setting (15–25 W) to allow time to react to what is happening and to avoid 'cheese-wiring' the stalk.
- Monopolar electrocoagulation of upper GI bleeding lesions is uncommon, having been replaced by bipolar electrocoagulation or thermal coagulation using a heater probe, often in conjunction with adrenaline injection. See endoscopic haemostasis.

Elemental diets

- Originally designed for the US manned space programme, they were used in preparing some patients for surgery and a coincident benefit in <u>Crohn's disease</u> was noted. Possible modes of action include effect on endogenous flora or mucosal permeability. Their use is attractive in children where <u>CORTICOSTEROIDS</u> affect growth, and in pregnancy where drug usage is minimized.
- Several studies have purported to show equivalence between elemental diets and steroids in achieving short-term remission in Crohn's disease. Subsequent meta-analyses tend not to confirm this, but patients with small bowel disease may benefit. Those with perianal disease or who relapse quickly should avoid it. Efficacy is higher in children than adults.
- Dietary composition varies: elemental diets include polymeric feeds using whole protein and complex carbohydrate, peptide-based diets (containing di- and tripeptides, thought to be better absorbed than amino acids), and true elemental feeds containing amino acids, glucose, and short-chain triglycerides. Available data suggest little difference between elemental and polymeric feeds. There has been concern that the fat content of enteral diets may influence response, but there is little evidence to support this. Compliance is an issue: 85% can manage sip feeding but 15% require a nasogastric tube.

Embolization

- Radiological embolization of arteries leads to obstruction of flow more distally. Usually achieved through placement of intraluminal coils.
- Indications for embolization include acutely bleeding posterior duodenal ulcer (due to gastroduodenal artery (GDA)); pseudoaneurysm related to <u>pancreatic pseudocyst</u> (often splenic artery); colonic <u>angiodysplasia</u> or post-polypectomy bleed (branch of superior or inferior mesenteric arteries).
- Malignant tumours are often hypervascular, and so embolization may reduce tumour load due to ischaemia/infarction (e.g. embolization of branch of hepatic artery in patients with hepatocellular carcinoma).
- Selective ipsilateral portal vein embolization in patients with <u>hepatocellular carcinoma</u> or liver metastases from <u>colonic cancer</u> may produce compensatory hypertrophy of contralateral liver lobe, so providing sufficient liver reserve to allow hemihepatectomy and tumour resection.

Important complications of embolization include vascular compromise of surrounding tissue: duodenal ulceration/stricture following GDA embolization; liver infarction and <u>acute liver failure</u> following hepatic artery embolization (particular risk in patients with <u>portal vein thrombosis</u> and those with <u>Child–Pugh score</u> B/C.

Encephalopathy

See: <u>hepatic encephalopathy</u>.

Endocarditis

See: <u>antibiotic prophylaxis in endoscopy</u>.

Endometriosis affecting the GI tract

Endometrial tissue outside the uterus may occur, usually without symptoms, in 15% of menstruating women. In women undergoing surgery for endometriosis, 30% have intestinal involvement, usually of the rectosigmoid colon. Penetration of endometriomas into the bowel can cause partial obstruction with pain and constipation. Intestinal bleeding is rare: endometrial deposits do not usually invade the mucosa but are associated with muscular hypertrophy and fibrosis. Less than half of patients show cyclical symptoms associated with menses, but nearly all women with intestinal involvement have associated features of pelvic endometriosis.

Diagnosis can be difficult. Rectal biopsy is normal unless there is associated rectal bleeding. CT and MRI are usually non-specific because of the small size of endometrial deposits. Endorectal ultrasound may be useful but experience is limited. Laparoscopy can be diagnostic and allows tissue diagnosis.

Differential diagnosis includes <u>irritable bowel syndrome</u>, <u>Crohn's disease</u>, and even <u>colon cancer</u>. <u>Diverticular disease</u> usually occurs in older women and radiation-induced stricturing should be diagnosed from the history. Malignant degeneration of extra-ovarian endometriosis is rare but documented. Very rarely mucosal involvement by endometrial tissue can simulate adenomatous polyps.

Treatment. If medical treatment with hormonal control fails, surgical resection is usually recommended. If ovarian function is preserved, recurrence of symptoms is substantial.

Endoscopic complications

Endoscopy is an invasive procedure, carrying definite risk.
- Cardiorespiratory adverse events (aspiration pneumonia, hypoventilation, vaso-vagal attack, arrhythmias) account for >50% of complications: risk correlates with age and comorbidity.
- Respiratory depression is a particular risk with the widely used combination of sedative benzodiazepines and opiate analgesics.
- Risk in an individual patient relates to:
  - Patient factors (age, comorbidity, anaesthetic risks).
  - GI disease-related factors (large polyp, malignant stricture).
  - Endoscopic-technique issues (e.g. endoscopist experience, inherent risk of specific intervention).

Upper GI endoscopy

Diagnostic OGD: morbidity 0.1%, mortality of approximately 0.01%. Perforations in 0.01% (usually due to (unsuspected) anatomical abnormality, e.g. pharyngeal pouch, oesophageal stricture).

Certain **therapeutic procedures** are associated with specific risks.
- Oesophageal dilatation. Overall perforation rate 2.6%, mortality 1%, with increased risk in elderly and malignant strictures (see endoscopic dilatation and oesophageal rupture).
- Variceal banding ligation (VBL)/endoscopic sclerotherapy (EST). During acute variceal bleeding, endoscopy-related aspiration of blood/gastric contents is a serious complication (which may be avoided by prior endotracheal intubation—see Acute upper GI bleed). Complications of EST reported in 10–15%: fever, retrosternal discomfort, and dysphagia usually resolve in < 48 hours. EST-induced oesophageal ulceration is common, but oesophageal perforation, mediastinitis, broncho-oesophageal fistula, and stricture formation rarely occur. Bacteraemia may lead to endocarditis in patient with prosthetic/diseased heart valves (see antibiotic prophylaxis). VBL appears to carry a significantly lower risk of oesophageal ulceration, mediastinitis, and perforation than EST.
- Percutaneous endoscopic gastrostomy (PEG) insertion. 30 day mortality of 20% largely reflects the underlying disease (e.g. advanced dementia, stroke), and immediate PEG-related mortality <1%. Excoriation and infection of the skin around the stoma are common. Peritonitis and gastroenteric fistulae may arise from intra-abdominal migration of the intragastric bumper.

Colonoscopy

Diagnostic colonoscopy has a morbidity of approximately 0.25%, mortality 0.02%. Therapeutic procedures involve a morbidity of 1–7% with a mortality of 0.04%.

Perforation may relate to:
- Direct tip trauma (e.g. into colonic diverticulum) or endoscope looping during scope insertion. The rectosigmoid is the site of >60% of perforations: the splenic flexure is a relatively common site of injury; avulsion of the ligaments attaching the colon to the spleen can result in significant haemorrhage.
- Intervention (0.3–1% of polypectomies). A 4–5% perforation rate is associated with balloon dilatation of colonic strictures.
- Free perforation into the peritoneal cavity may occasionally be recognized during the procedure, but usually the diagnosis is suggested by marked persistent abdominal distension or pain after the procedure. Fever, and signs of shock and peritonitis may develop.
- Retroperitoneal perforation may present with subcutaneous emphysema.
- Management. Plain abdominal and erect chest X-rays should be performed, and may show pneumoperitoneum. If they are normal, but clinical suspicion remains, abdominal CT scan may give the diagnosis. Conservative management is sufficient for most small perforations (nil by mouth, IV fluids, IV antibiotics), but close in-patient review necessary, and surgery required in 25% of cases (particularly if perforation large).

Bleeding
- Immediate bleeding is the most common complication of polypectomy. Most cases of immediate bleeding resolve spontaneously. Management includes injecting 5–10 ml of 1:10 000 epinephrine (adrenaline) solution into the stalk/submucosa or haemoclip placement (see also <u>endoscopic haemostasis</u>). Angiography, and even laparotomy are occasionally required.
- Delayed bleeding can occur up to 2 weeks after colonoscopy.

Postpolypectomy coagulation syndrome presents with pain, peritonitis, and fever, and needs to be differentiated from perforation, as it invariably settles with conservative management.

Splenic rupture is rare, but may present with pain, peritonitis, and hypovolaemic shock, with bloods showing acute anaemia and raised white cell count. Diagnosis made on CT, and laparotomy often required.

ERCP

Overall complication rate about 5%. For severity grading, see table opposite.

- <u>**Pancreatitis**</u> is the most common complication of ERCP (3–5% of cases). A severe course is followed in 30%, with mortality rate from sphincterotomy-induced pancreatitis 0.5%. A number of risk factors are associated with post-ERCP pancreatitis (see box opposite). Careful patient selection for ERCP is vital, as ERCP is most dangerous for people who need it least (20–30% risk of pancreatitis in young woman with abdominal pain, normal bilirubin, and non-dilated bile duct).
- **Retroperitoneal perforation** occurs in <1% of sphincterotomies. It may present acutely with surgical emphysema, but pain in the absence of a rise in serum amylase may also provide a diagnostic clue. In those patients in whom the diagnosis cannot be made on a plain abdominal X-ray, CT scanning may be required. Most cases settle with IV antibiotics and a strict 'nil by mouth' policy, but close observation is required in view of the risk of retroperitoneal sepsis and abscess formation, which may require percutaneous or surgical drainage.
- **Bleeding** relating to sphincterotomy usually settles spontaneously, but <u>endoscopic haemostasis</u> techniques may be needed. Angiographic embolization, or surgery are rarely required.
- <u>**Cholangitis**</u> occurs in approximately 2% of patients following ERCP, usually when the intrahepatic ducts have been filled with contrast, but effective biliary drainage has not been obtained. It is managed with broad spectrum IV antibiotics, and further efforts to establish effective drainage (e.g. percutaneous transhepatic drain (PTD)).

ERCP complications and severity grading

	Mild	Moderate	Severe
Bleeding	Clinical evidence of bleeding, but Hb fall < 3 g/dl, and no transfusion required	Transfusion required, but < 5 units, and no angiographic or surgical intervention	> 4 units transfused, or angiographic/ surgical intervention
Retroperitoneal perforation	Possible, or only very slight leak, with < 4 days of treatment required	Proven perforation treated medically for 4–10 days	Medical treatment for > 10 days, or intervention (percu- taneous or surgical)
Pancreatitis	Amylase > 3 × ULN more than 24 hours after ERCP, with hospital stay extended by 2–3 days	Hospitalization for 4–10 days	Hospitalization for > 10 days, or haem- orrhagic pancreatitis, phlegmon, pseudo- cyst, or intervention (percutaneous or surgical)
Cholangitis	Temp > 38°C for 24–48 hours	Septic illness requiring > 3 days of hospital treatment, or endoscopic/ radiographic intervention	Septic shock or need for surgery

(Reproduced with permission from Cotton PB, Lehman G, et al. (1991) *Gastrointest Endosc.* **37**: 1383)

Risk factors for post-ERCP pancreatitis

- Young
- Female
- Suspected <u>sphincter of Oddi dysfunction</u> (SOD)
- Normal serum bilirubin
- Previous ERCP-related pancreatitis
- Difficult common bile duct (CBD) cannulation
- Pancreatic duct filling
- Pre-cut (needle–knife) sphincterotomy
- Pancreatic sphincterotomy
- Balloon sphincter dilatation

Endoscopic dilatation

Mechanical dilatation of GI tract obstruction has been attempted for hundreds of years. The most common site for endoscopic dilatation is the oesophagus, with indications including: benign peptic strictures (see Approach to dyspepsia and gastro-oesophageal reflux and caustic ingestion); oesophageal tumours; Schatzki's rings; achalasia. A course of dilatation provides good relief in > 85% of patients with benign strictures due to reflux, but less effective if stricture due to radiation or corrosives. Most gastric strictures occur at pylorus: causes include peptic ulceration, gastric cancer, and caustic ingestion. Duodenal strictures are usually due to external compression (e.g. pancreatitis, pancreatic cancer) and rarely due to duodenal carcinoma. The most common indication for small bowel or colonic endoscopic dilatation is Crohn's disease.

Types of dilator:

- Fixed diameter dilators ('bougies') have long been used to dilate oesophageal strictures. Most dilators (e.g. Savary–Gillard) are inserted over an endoscopically placed wire. May have 20 cm tapered tip, but gradually widen to 5–20 mm fixed diameter. For benign strictures usual dilatation to 16–18 mm, but wider dilatation may be needed for Schatzki's rings.
- Endoscopic dilatation in sites other than oesophagus almost exclusively performed using over-the-wire balloons. Balloons are more expensive than push dilators, in part because of their single use. They can be inserted over a wire and positioned either under imaging control or directly at endoscopy through the scope (TTS). Balloon diameters vary from 4 to 40 mm. Larger balloons (30–40 mm) reserved for treatment of achalasia. Balloons exert a direct circumferential pressure rather than the shearing force exerted by bougies. Radial force exerted is less than with bougies and very rigid fibrotic strictures may be difficult to dilate with balloons.

Practice points

- Fluoroscopic screening may be needed with both techniques if the stricture cannot be passed endoscopically. Balloons exert only radial force and probably are less effective than bougies. Both methods safe in hands of experienced endoscopist familiar with their use.
- Anticoagulation should be discontinued prior to endoscopic dilatation, either by discontinuing oral anticoagulants if low risk of thromboembolism, or transferring to intravenous heparin, and discontinuing this 4–6 hours prior to dilatation, if at high risk of thromboembolism. Aspirin not of significant risk. Antibiotics should be given to patients with higher risk of cardiac lesions (see antibiotic prophylaxis in endoscopy).
- Overall oesophageal perforation rate 2.6%, mortality 1%, with increased risk for malignant strictures (6.4% perforation, 2.3% mortality). Other complications include bleeding and pulmonary aspiration.

Endoscopic haemostasis

Endoscopic treatment reduces rebleeding and mortality in patients with significant upper GI bleeding, but must be used in conjunction with effective resuscitation and additional medical therapies (see emergencies: acute upper GI bleed). Range of haemostatic modalities used for different clinical indications.

Oesophageal varices

See emergencies and portal hypertension.

Variceal band ligation (VBL)

- a varix is sucked into a short plastic sleeve at tip of endoscope, and a tight rubber ring is applied around base (see Colour Plate 9).
- Varix thromboses and sloughs off in < 7 days. Up to 7 bands may be applied.
- Complications include 'banding ulcers', but fewer side-effects than sclerotherapy, and it is the endoscopic treatment of choice for gastro-oesophageal varices.

Injection sclerotherapy

- longer established than VBL.
- Involves injection of 1–4 ml of sclerosant (e.g. 5% ethanolamine) into or adjacent to varix.
- Like VBL, controls acute bleeding in 85–95% of cases, but risk of sclerotherapy ulcers, oesophageal stricture, mediastinitis, and perforation (see endoscopic complications).

Gastric varices

- VBL and standard sclerotherapy not effective.
- Injection of other tissue adhesives (e.g. 2-cyanoacrylate) or thrombin may be effective.
- If bleeding not controlled, Sengstaken–Blakemore tube insertion (see 'how to') and TIPSS (transjugular intrahepatic portosystemic shunt) may be necessary, as for oesophageal varices.

Bleeding peptic ulcers

Endoscopic therapy is required for patients with: active bleeding, a visible vessel in ulcer base, or adherent clot. Techniques include:

- Injection: approx 4–10 ml adrenaline 1:10 000 injected around and then into bleeding point. Thrombin or fibrin injection also effective, but not widely used. Another modality, in addition to injection, gives best haemostatic results.
- Heat: options include heater probe, multipolar coagulation (BICAP; see electrocoagulation), or argon plasma coagulation (APC). Heater probe includes powerful water jet to clear blood clot, and achieves haemostasis via combination of compression of bleeding point and heat.
- Mechanical clips: range of products available, and may be very effective at clipping clearly visible vessels.

Post-polypectomy bleeds

As with ulcers, injection of adrenaline into the base of polyp stalk, followed by heater probe, may be effective, as may clip placement.

Angiodysplasia/vascular malformation/<u>gastric antral vascular ectasia (GAVE)</u>

Application of heat, with <u>heater probe</u> or <u>argon plasma coagulation (APC)</u>, may be effective.

Endoscopic retrograde cholangiopancreatography (ERCP)

Technique

Side-viewing duodenoscope allows selective cannulation of biliary system, and insertion of cannulae into pancreatic/common bile ducts, with biliary system delineated with contrast injection and X-ray imaging.

Indications

Less role now for ERCP as a primarily diagnostic technique, because of risks of procedure, and alternative less invasive modalities to investigate pancreaticobiliary system (MRI/MRCP, CT scanning, transabdominal and endoscopic ultrasound). Indications include relief of biliary obstruction with endoscopic stenting (e.g. for pancreatic carcinoma, cholangiocarcinoma), removal of stones from common bile duct, and biopsy or cytological brushing of biliary strictures/lesions. ERCP is required to perform biliary manometry in patients with suspected sphincter of Oddi dysfunction.

Complications

Higher complications in units doing < 200 ERCPs/year, and endoscopists doing < 40/year, but 'patient-related' factors probably even more important. Post-ERCP pancreatitis rate 3–5%, with highest rates (> 20%) in 'those who need procedure least' (e.g. young female patient without jaundice, a non-dilated bile duct, and intermittent right upper quadrant pain—also see sphincter of Oddi dysfunction). Post-sphincterotomy bleeding and retroperitoneal perforation less common. Also see endoscopic complications.

Endoscopic ultrasound (EUS)

EUS is becoming more important in diagnosis and management of GI disorders. Echoendoscopes use sound waves for imaging tissue consistency and interfaces between tissue planes, and typically use higher frequencies than those used in transabdominal ultrasound (this results in better definition, but reduced penetration). 3 main types of echoendoscope are in use.

- **Radial echoendoscope** has a rotating ultrasound probe integrated into its tip, and 270° or 360° images obtained in a circumference perpendicular to the endoscope tip. Fine needle aspiration (FNA) not currently possible with radial EUS. Main indications include staging of GI tract tumours in terms of local invasion and regional lymphadenopathy (especially <u>oesophageal</u>, <u>gastric</u>, and <u>rectal cancer</u>); and diagnosis in pancreaticobiliary disease (exclusion of <u>choledocholithiasis</u>, characterization of pancreatic lesions not seen on CT, and assessment of <u>neuroendocrine tumours</u>). In experienced hands, EUS for detecting mediastinal lymphadenopathy in oesophageal cancer has sensitivity 80%, specificity 90%.
- **Linear array echoendoscope** also has an ultrasound probe in tip, but images are obtained along a plane parallel to the endoscope axis. FNA, and even Trucut biopsies, may be obtained using linear EUS, allowing therapeutic functions in addition to the diagnostic uses of radial EUS, including: mediastinal lymph node sampling in lung cancer; FNA of submucosal GI tract lesions, and particularly pancreatic masses and <u>pancreatic cystic tumours</u>; endoscopic drainage of <u>pancreatic pseudocysts</u>; EUS-guided coeliac plexus nerve block in patients with pain due to <u>chronic pancreatitis</u> or <u>pancreatic cancer</u>. Doppler ultrasound capability allows vascular structures to be missed by the needle, and blood flow to be assessed (e.g. <u>portal vein thrombosis</u>).
- **Ultrasound probes** are thin and need to be advanced through the channel of a regular endoscope. These probes generally provide a high-resolution circumferential view along the same plane as the radial echoendoscope. Miniprobe U/S may be used in the assessment of <u>biliary strictures</u>.

Endoscopy in anticoagulated patients

- The GI tract is the most common site of bleeding in patients on anticoagulants and anti-platelet drugs.
- Previous GI bleeds are a risk factor (30% incidence at 3 years therapy in those with a history of bleeding compared to 5% in those with no bleeding history).
- The risk of bleeding caused by the endoscopic procedure has to be balanced against the risk of a thrombo-embolic event related to stopping anticoagulation.

Recommendations (see tables opposite)

1. Low-risk procedures

No adjustments to anticoagulation needed whatever the underlying condition. Avoid elective procedures when the level of anticoagulation is above the therapeutic range.

2. High-risk procedures in patients with low-risk conditions

Stop warfarin 3–5 days before the procedure. There may be a need to obtain a pre-procedure INR.

3. High-risk procedures in patients with high-risk conditions

Stop warfarin therapy 3–5 days before procedure. There may be a need for IV heparin once the INR is subtherapeutic. If used, discontinue heparin 4–6 h pre-procedure and restart 2–6 h after procedure. Restart warfarin on the night of the procedure (but note risk of major bleed post-biliary sphincterotomy 10–15% if anticoagulation restarted within 3 days).

Aspirin and other NSAIDs

Cyclo-oxygenase inhibition by NSAIDs results in suppression of thromboxane A2-dependent platelet aggregation. Limited data suggests aspirin and other NSAIDs do not increase the risk of significant bleeding after endoscopy, polypectomy, or sphincterotomy.

Patients on anti-platelet therapy

Currently anti-platelet therapy includes:
- Antagonists of the adenosine diphosphate receptor (P2T) such as ticlopidine and clopidogrel.
- IIb/IIIa receptor antagonists such as abciximab and tirofiban.

Both classes are associated with increased bleeding risk, particularly in association with aspirin. Recurrent GI bleeding is more common with clopidogrel than aspirin plus a PPI (Chan, FKL *et al.* (2005) *N. Engl J. Med.* **352**: 238).

Data regarding GI bleeding after endoscopy in these patients are not adequate to make recommendations. For elective high-risk procedures temporary discontinuation, especially if the patients is also on aspirin, is desirable.

Procedure risks

High-risk	Low-risk
Colonoscopic polypectomy (1–2.5%)*	Diagnostic OGD and enteroscopy
Gastric polypectomy (4%)*	Flexible sigmoidoscopy and colonoscopy with or without biopsy
Laser ablation and coagulation (< 6%)*	Diagnostic ERCP
Endoscopic sphincterotomy (2.5–5%)*	Biliary stent without sphincterotomy
Pneumatic dilatation, PEG placement, EUS-guided needle aspiration or biopsy	Endoscopic ultrasound (EUS)

*bleeding risk without anticoagulation

Condition risk

High-risk	Low-risk
AF and valvular heart disease (risk is 5–7% annually, higher in dilated cardiomyopathy or after recent thrombo-embolic events)	DVT
Mechanical valve in the mitral position	Uncomplicated or paroxysmal non-valvular AF
Mechanical valves of any type in patients with prior thrombo-embolic event	Bioprosthetic valve. Mechanical valve ion the aortic position

Reversing anticoagulation
- The degree of reversal needs to be individualized.
- Supra-therapeutic INR may be treated with fresh frozen plasma.
- Correcting the INR to 1.5–2.5 allows successful endoscopic diagnosis and therapy at rates comparable to those in non-anticoagulated patients.
- If vitamin K is used, give small aliquots (0.5–1 mg) intravenously. **Do not give large intramuscular doses of vitamin K** unless permanent reversal of anticoagulation is the goal: the onset of action of vitamin K is delayed and prolongs the time needed to re-establish effective anticoagulation.

It is generally safe to restart warfarin on the evening of the procedure, **but** the benefits of immediate anticoagulation must be balanced against the risks (risk of bleeding is > 10% if anticoagulation restarted within 3 days of sphincterotomy).

Enteral feeding

In patients who need supplemental feeding, enteral feeding has many advantages over parenteral nutrition—see box opposite. Also see Approach to nutritional support

Enteral feeding regimens use defined **liquid formula feeds**. Although pure sources of protein, carbohydrate and lipid are available (so-called feeding modules), these are rarely used in our experience.

Monomeric feeds contain nitrogen as free amino acids, carbohydrates as glucose polymers (providing most of the calories), and minimal amounts of fat as long chain triglycerides (LCT). These feeds are often unpalatable and expensive. There are theoretical disadvantages (dipeptides and tripeptides are absorbed more efficiently than free amino acids) and controlled trial evidence does not show a clear benefit in many situations.

Oligomeric feeds contain hydrolysed proteins as small peptides together with simple sugars or starch and fat as LCT or a mix of LCT and medium chain triglycerides (MCT). The protein is theoretically better absorbed than free amino acids or whole protein. While there is some support of this from clinical studies, no clinical benefit has been demonstrated in outcome studies, apart from some reduction of diarrhoea and GI side-effects in patients receiving cytotoxic chemotherapy.

Polymeric feeds contain nitrogen as whole protein, carbohydrates as glucose polymers, and fat as LCT or a mix of LCT and MCT. They can be made from blenderized food (e.g. beef or milk as protein source, cereal fruit and vegetables as CHO source, and corn oil or soy oil as a fat source) or made from milk as a source of protein and fat with addition of corn oil solids and glucose as a source of carbohydrate. Most polymeric feeds however are lactose-free formulas containing casein or soy as a protein source. Fibre is not present in most lactose-free formulas.

Why is enteral feeding better than parenteral nutrition?

- Fewer complications of line sepsis
- Enteral feeding can supply gut preferred fuels such as glutamine and short chain fatty acids that are often absent from TPN preparations
- Enteral feeding can prevent mucosal atrophy, preserves mucosal and pancreatic enzyme function, maintains GI IgA secretion
- Enteral feeding prevents cholelithiasis by stimulating gallbladder motility
- Less expensive

Enteroclysis

- A radiological method of examining the small intestine that involves intubation of the duodenum or proximal jejunum, usually combined wtth metaclopramide to accelerate small bowel transit. 200–250 ml of barium is injected into the small bowel , followed by 1.5–2 l of 0.5% methycellulose.
- Enteroclysis provides better luminal distension than a small bowel meal and there is less flocculation of barium. However, intubation is not pleasant for the patient, and the technique requires extra time and expertise from the radiologist. Enteroclysis can be helpful in diagnosing small bowel obstruction (especially intermittent obstruction), mucosal irregularities (e.g. lymphangiectasia or scleroderma), the anatomical extent of small bowel <u>Crohn's disease</u>, and small bowel tumours such as <u>carcinoid</u>.
- CT enteroclysis is a similar technique using cross-sectional imaging instead of barium radiology: there is some evidence that this is particularly helpful in diagnosing high-grade intestinal obstruction from abdominal tumour recurrence.
- In general enteroclysis has poor diagnostic yield in cases of suspected small intestinal bleeding: emerging evidence suggests that combination of endoscopic and video capsule enteroscopy is significantly superior.

Enteroscopy

There are three endoscopic methods currents available to image the 5 m of the human small intestine.

- The least used is **sonde enteroscopy**, which uses a 2.75 cm dedicated instrument to examine the whole of the small intestine. The instrument is carried down by peristalsis so that the examination takes several hours to perform. Biopsy and therapy are not possible. Patient discomfort, expense, and time taken have all prevented wide-spread use of this technique.
- **Push enteroscopy** is a useful method of examining the upper small intestine but its range is limited to the proximal 50–75 cm of jejunum. Biopsy and therapy are possible through a standard size operating channel and the technique is carried out using a dedicated 240 cm enteroscope or often a paediatric colonoscope that approximates to the enteroscope in length and handling characteristics.
- **Capsule endoscopy** ('wireless enteroscopy') has been a significant advance in recent years, providing the possibility of visualizing areas of the bowel inaccessible to conventional flexible endoscopy (i.e. most of small bowel). The 11 × 26 mm capsule is swallowed, and video images are transmitted to a data recorder worn on patient's belt for approximately 8 hours. Precise role relative to other diagnostic modalities is being investigated, but diagnostic yield of capsule endoscopy is superior to push enteroscopy for defining obscure small bowel bleeding in those with negative endoscopy and colonoscopy

(68% compared to 32%). Detailed comparisons of capsule endoscopy with a combined approach of push enteroscopy and radiological examination of the small bowel are still awaited (see Swain, P and Fritscher-Ravens, A. (2004) *Gut* **53**: 1866), and further developments in flexible enteroscopy (e.g. double-balloon enteroscopy (DBE)) may also influence relative merits of techniques. Capsule carries disadvantage of not allowing biopsy, and technique is contraindicated in patients with suspected significant intestinal strictures, as capsule may precipitate mechanical obstruction.

Eosinophilia and the GI tract

The differential diagnosis of a peripheral blood eosinophilia in association with GI symptoms includes:

- **Drugs** (aspirin, sulphonamides, penicillin, cephalosporins, azathioprine, carbamazepine).
- **Vasculitis** (e.g. Churg–Strauss syndrome).
- **Lymphoma.**
- **Connective tissue disorders (scleroderma/dermatomyositis).**
- **Addison's disease.**
- **Parasites** are an important cause. Invasive helminths are classically the causal group. Hook worm (see <u>roundworms</u>) and pinworms may cause eosinophilic infiltration. *Giardia* can cause eosinophilic infiltration of the jejunum without peripheral blood eosinophilia. People who eat raw fish may be infected with anisakis. <u>Schistosomiasis</u>, *ascaris*, *tricuris* can cause eosinophilia and abdominal pain *Fasciola* can cause right upper quadrant pain, fever, hepatomegaly.
- **Asthma and allergic rhinitis** are common and can cause peripheral eosinophilia.
- <u>Eosinophilic gastroenteritis</u> (see below).

Eosinophilic gastroenteritis

Rare disease, usually presenting at age 30–50 years with following diagnostic criteria.

- Presence of GI symptoms.
- Eosinophilic infiltrate of one or more areas of the GI tract on biopsy.
- Absence of involvement of organs outside the GI tract.
- Absence of parasitic infestation or other cause of peripheral blood eosinophilia.

Pathogenesis is poorly understood but involves damage to the gut wall through degranulation of eosinophil granules. The trigger for this is unknown but may involve type 1 allergy or parasitic causes.

Clinical features. Stomach and small intestine are most commonly affected but any part of the GI tract may be involved. Most commonly the disease affects mucosa and submucosa and this leads to colicky pain, nausea, vomiting, diarrhoea, and weight loss. If the muscle layer is mainly affected presentation can be with pyloric or upper GI obstruction. Very rarely serosal disease can cause eosinophilic ascites.

Investigation. 80% have a peripheral blood eosinophilia. Serum iron and albumin may be low. The IgE may be raised, especially in children. Stool studies are necessary to exclude parasitic infestation. Histological samples from affected areas are needed for diagnosis.

Treatment

- If there is no muscle or serosal involvement, dietary manipulation is reasonable, especially if there is a history suggestive of food intolerance. Children often respond well to diet—milk protein is the most often implicated allergen.

- If there is a history of travel or residence in high-risk areas a trial of anti-parasitic therapy such as mebendazole 100 mg bd for 3 days is reasonable.
- CROMOGLYCATE (200 mg tds–qds) is often tried; it stabilizes mast cells and can reduce antigen absorption by the small intestine.

CORTICOSTEROIDS are used in patients who fail to respond to the above measures or in those with obstructive symptoms or eosinophilic ascites. 90% of patients respond to oral steroids in a dose of 20–40 mg/day. The dose can be tapered over several weeks and 30–50% will relapse on stopping steroids. The use of second-line immunosuppressives as steroid-sparing agents in patients who are steroid-dependent has not been examined systematically.

Eosinophils in the GI tract

- Eosinophilic infiltration of the GI tract by itself does not indicate eosinophilic gastroenteritis. The diagnosis requires full thickness infiltration of the gastrointestinal mucosa and exclusion of known causes including drugs and parasites
- Causes include:
  - IgE-mediated food allergy
  - Gastro-oesophageal reflux disease
  - Allergic colitis and inflammatory bowel disease
  - Cow's milk allergy
  - Gastric cancer
  - Hypereosinophilic syndrome.

Erythema nodosum (EN) (see Colour Plate 10)

Red, well demarcated, raised 1–6 cm lesions usually limited to the extensor aspects of the lower legs. Wide range of causes, including infection (e.g. *Streptococcus*, *Campylobacter*, TB, *Yersinia*, fungal infection), drugs (e.g. sulphonamides, sarcoidosis, Behçet's syndrome. EN occurs in approximately 2% of patients with IBD (Crohn's disease > ulcerative colitis), and usually parallels disease activity. Histology of lesions shows a panniculitis. Individual lesions usually spontaneously resolve in 6 weeks, but others may occur. Nonsteroidal anti-inflammatories may help, as may control of underlying activity of IBD.

Escherichia coli

A major component of the normal intestinal microflora. There are 6 types of pathogens.

- **Enteropathogenic *E. coli* (EPEC)**. Produces watery diarrhoea in children and neonates. Virulence is via localized adherence to enterocytes. Infection is usually self-limiting.
- **Enterotoxigenic *E. coli* (ETEC)**. Affects children in developing countries and travellers. Bacteria bind to enterocytes, produce heat labile or heat stable toxin leading to watery diarrhoea that can be mild or severe. Antibiotics usually not needed, although effective therapy given early (quinolone, septrin, tetracycline) can shorten duration of diarrhoea.
- **Enteroinvasive *E. coli* (EIEC)**. Rare cause of dysentery. Resembles *Shigella*.
- **Enterohaemorrhagic *E. coli* (EHEC):** An important invasive pathogen responsible for 15–35% of haemorrhagic colitis: *E. coli* 0157 associated with haemolytic–uraemic syndrome (especially in children) and thrombotic thrombocytopenic purpura. Commonest vehicle is hamburger meat. Incubation period 1–14 d, can produce marked colitis. AXR can show submucosal oedema (thumbprinting). Laboratory studies can reveal *E. coli* 0157 serotypes or characteristic shiga-like toxins (Stx I and II). **Antibiotics do not help and may increase risk of HUS**.
- **Entero-aggregatory *E. coli* (EAggEC)**. Pathogenicity uncertain but may be associated with diarrhoea in HIV-positive people who seem to respond to ciprofloxacin.
- **Diffusely adhering *E. coli* (DAEC)**. Pathogenicity uncertain, virulence factors unknown.

Exclusion diets

Systematic exclusion of different foods and the use of a food/symptom diary can help identify foods to which a patient may be intolerant or allergic (also see <u>food allergy</u>). A true elimination diet is difficult to pursue and should ideally involve the help of an experienced dietician. It involves a 'washout period' of taking bland food such as boiled rice, fish, and chicken followed by the re-introduction of a favorite food every day. About 30% of patients with irritable bowel can identify foods that aggravate symptoms.

Extracorporeal shock-wave lithotripsy (ESWL)

ESWL utilizes ultrasound shock waves to fragment stones. In gastro-enterology the main (but rare) indications are for gallstones, bile duct stones, or pancreatic duct stones that require dissolution, which cannot be achieved endoscopically and when surgery is not an option.

- Gallstone destruction with ESWL requires a patent cystic duct and single < 2 cm radiolucent stone. <u>URSODEOXYCHOLIC ACID</u> is given after fragmentation to aid dissolution.
- In patients with <u>choledocholithiasis</u> and impacted common bile duct stone, ESWL (and endoscopic laser lithotripsy) may induce sufficient fragmentation to allow endoscopic stone removal. Biliary stent/ nasobiliary drain may improve localization of stone for ESWL.
- Pancreatic duct stones that cannot be removed endoscopically may be treated with ESWL, followed by further attempts at stone fragment clearance.
  Complications include biliary colic and <u>acute pancreatitis</u>.

F

Fabry's disease

An X-linked disorder of glycolipid metabolism due to deficiency or absence of α-galactosidase A. Sphingolipid deposition occurs in all tissues. GI manifestations include impaired motility leading to recurrent cramping abdominal pain and watery stools. <u>Bacterial overgrowth</u> and delayed gastric emptying can occur. Electron microscopy show lipid-filled vacuoles in ganglion cells of Meissner's plexus and endothelial cells: lipid deposition in small vessels can lead to vasculitis and thrombosis. Mucosal enterocytes are normal.

Faecal incontinence

See: <u>Approach to faecal incontinence</u>.

Faecal occult blood tests (FOBT)

- Qualitative tests that rely on oxidation of a colourless compound to a coloured one in the presence of pseudoperoxidase activity of haemoglobin and a developer solution of hydrogen peroxidase in alcohol. Cheap, readily available, and convenient, but distasteful for patients to carry out. Relatively high incidence of both false positives and false negatives (see box). Most tests become positive when about 2 ml blood is lost per day.
- Positive predictive value of FOBT is about 20% for adenomas and 5–10% for cancers. Rehydration of slides with a drop of water before processing results in an increase of positivity and sensitivity but a fall in specificity and positive predictive value.
- New tests that decrease the false positive rates of FOBT while maintaining sensitivity include Hemeselect (an immunochemical test for human haemoglobin), HemoQuant (quantitative assay based of fluorescence of haem-derived porphyrins), and Haemoccult SENSA, a guaiac-based test with greater sensitivity. There is emerging evidence that screening strategies using an immunochemical test rather than a guaiac-based test may be most effective.
- See also <u>colorectal cancer screening and surveillance.</u>

Familial adenomatous polyposis (FAP)

Aetiology + pathogenesis. FAP is the most common adenomatous polyposis syndrome (others include <u>juvenile polyposis</u>, <u>Peutz–Jeghers</u>, <u>Gardner's</u>, and <u>Turcot's syndromes</u>). Autosomal dominant inheritance, with prevalence 1:7500, and 80–100% disease penetrance. APC (adenomatous polyposis coli) gene located on chromosome 5 encodes for a protein that functions as a tumour suppressor protein, probably through interaction with β-catenin. If APC protein mutated, β-catenin no longer downregulated, allowing it to upregulate target genes that then promote adenoma formation.

Limitation of faecal occult blood tests and recommendations for correct use

False positive tests

- Endogenous peroxidase (e.g. vegetable peroxidase in broccoli, turnips, cauliflower, radishes, melon)
- Non-human haemoglobin: red meat
- Any source of GI bleeding (epistaxis, gingival bleeding, haemorrhoids)
- Aspirin and NSAIDs, which increase upper GI bleeds
  - **Recommendation:** patients should avoid red meat, peroxidase containing vegetables and vitamin C and NSAIDs for three days before and during testing. Avoiding iron preparations is also recommended, although the evidence for this is weak.

False negative tests

- Haemoglobin degradation by storage or faecal bacteria
  - **Recommendation:** develop slides within 4–6 days. Do not rehydrate slides for average risk screening
- Ascorbic acid (vitamin C) interferes with indicator dye
- Lesion not bleeding at time of sampling
  - **Recommendation:** Two samples of each of three consecutive stools should be tested.

Clinical features. Patients may present with rectal bleeding and diarrhoea, but many identified for screening/surveillance on basis of a careful family history from an affected index case (nevertheless, 20% of patients with FAP have no family history, suggesting germline mutations).

Colonic disease. Hundreds to thousands of adenomatous <u>colon polyps</u> develop after puberty, and diagnosis is usually made at age 20–30 years. <u>Colonic cancer</u> is an inevitable part of the disease course, approximately 10 to 15 years after the onset of the polyposis. 90% of cases of FAP are diagnosed < 50 years.

Gastroduodenal disease. Duodenal adenomas occur in 60–90%, and duodenal/periampullary cancers develop in 5–12% (see Colour Plate 11). Following the widespread use of prophylactic colectomy, duodenal cancer is now the major cause of cancer death in FAP. Spigelman classification assesses duodenal FAP according to number, distribution, and histology of polyps. Endoscopic assessment (with duodenoscope, not gastroscope, in view of peri-ampullary involvement) is advised every 1–3 years following colectomy or > 20 years of age. Very poor prognosis following radical surgery in FAP patients with duodenal carcinoma, and >30% risk of developing cancer in those with 'Spigelman IV' disease has led most specialist units to advise prophylactic <u>Whipple's resection</u> for extensive premalignant duodenal FAP. <u>Gastric polyps</u> are common, but <u>gastric cancer</u> occurs rarely.

Cancer in other sites. Although less common than luminal GI cancers, other associations with FAP include pancreatic cancer, hepatoblastoma, diffuse mesenteric fibromatosis (desmoid tumours), and cancers of the thyroid and brain.

Investigation. In an affected individual with no family history, diagnosis is suggested by finding hundreds of adenomatous polyps on colonoscopy/sigmoidoscopy. Most polyps are < 1 cm, and individually are identical to adenomatous polyps found in general population.

Management
- Where diagnosis is established, there is no specific merit in waiting before advising colonic resection in the post-pubertal patient, in view of near certainty of developing malignancy.
- Colectomy with ileorectal anastomosis maintains continence, but cancer recurrence occurs in rectal stump in 15%, even with regular surveillance, and carries a dismal prognosis. Colectomy with ileoanal anastomosis, or total colectomy with ileostomy are usual advised.
- Polyp regression has been shown with sulindac (which may act through COX-2 inhibition), but reliable prevention of progression to malignancy has not been shown, and medical management cannot be used in place of surgery. It has been used to reduce development of new polyps in rectal stump. Its role in inducing regression of gastroduodenal polyps is under assessment.

Screening. A genetic diagnosis of APC mutation can be made in > 98% of patients using exhaustive genetic techniques. The commercially available 'truncated protein test' for APC mutations will be positive in 80% of FAP families. Where it is in a family member, gene carriage of other family members can be demonstrated with near 100% accuracy. A negative test in a family member removes need for regular surveillance, but in those tested positive, sigmoidoscopy should be performed yearly from age 10–12 years. If affected family member is negative for genetic test, screening relies on clinical assessment (i.e. sigmoidoscopy). Genetic counselling is a vital component of screening.

Familial mediterranean fever

Epidemiology + pathogenesis. Autosomal recessive disease, affecting up to 1:200 in high prevalence populations (e.g. Sephardic Jews, Armenians). Mutations of MEFV gene on chromosome 16 encode for Pyrin, expressed in neutrophils.

Clinical features. Symptoms begin at < 20 years in > 95% of cases. Recurrent episodes of fever, peritonitis (mimicking acute abdomen), pleurisy, arthritis, and rash. Episodes last 24–72 hours. Amyloid A deposition may lead to renal failure. Presentation to gastroenterologists with unexplained recurrent attacks of pain (often with 'negative' laparotomies). See Acute abdominal pain

Investigations. Diagnosis never made unless considered!
- ↑ Acute phase response (ESR, CRP) and neutrophilia.
- ↑ IgD in 13%.

Genetic analysis for common MEFV mutations allows definitive diagnosis, so less role for 'trial of colchicine'.

Management. Colchicine 600 μg BD PO markedly effective in > 95% of cases, and may prevent development of amyloidosis.

Familial pancreatitis

See: hereditary pancreatitis.

Fat malabsorption

See: Approach to malabsorption and steatorrhoea.

Fatty liver

- A spectrum characterized by the presence of fat deposition within hepatocytes. May range from fatty liver alone (steatosis) to fatty liver associated with inflammation (steatohepatitis). It can occur with the use of alcohol (see <u>alcoholic liver disease</u>) or in its absence (<u>non-alcoholic fatty liver disease</u>—NAFLD). Non-alcoholic steatohepatitis (NASH) increasingly considered as part of the spectrum of NAFLD, but associated heptatocyte inflammation and cell death in NASH may lead to fibrosis and cirrhosis.
- Steatosis affects > 20% of US adult population, with most common associations including alcohol, obesity, and diabetes mellitus. Steatosis also found on <u>liver biopsy</u> in 50% of patients with chronic <u>hepatitis C</u>. Prognostic factors in developing fibrosis include age > 45 years, diabetes mellitus, and high <u>body mass index</u> (BMI).
- Most patients asymptomatic. Hepatomegaly is common, but splenomegaly and ascites suggests cirrhosis.
- In <u>liver function tests</u>, AST-to-ALT ratio of > 2 suggests alcohol use, whereas ratio < 1 more consistent with NAFLD.
- On U/S liver is hyperechogenic, or bright. Steatosis is detected only when > 30% fatty change present.
- Diagnosis of fatty liver only definitively established with <u>liver biopsy</u>. Histologic findings include steatosis, which is usually macrovesicular, and neutrophil/mononuclear cell infiltrate. Fibrosis or cirrhosis may be present in advanced cases.
- Management depends on addressing the cause (e.g. weight reduction, diabetic control, abstinence from alcohol, drug cessation), but specific treatments for <u>non-alcoholic fatty liver disease</u> show promise. Fatty liver may completely resolve, with no residual architectural damage.

Felty's syndrome

First 5 cases described in 1924 by American physician Augustus Felty in *Johns Hopkins Medical Bulletin*.
The clinical combination of rheumatoid arthritis, splenomegaly, and leucopenia. Occasional relevance to gastroenterologists as > 50% have abnormal liver histology ranging from portal fibrosis to <u>nodular regenerative hyperplasia</u>. This can cause <u>portal hypertension</u> and variceal bleeding.

Fibre

Refers to residue of food, usually from structural and matrix components of plant cell walls, that is resistant to hydrolysis by human digestive enzymes. Some fibres can bind ions (calcium, iron, magnesium, zinc) and also adsorb bile salts, proteins, and bacterial cells. Fermentation of fibre by bacteria generate short chain fatty acids, which are a preferred energy source for colonocytes. Although water insoluble fibres have a greater effect on stool mass than water soluble fibres, ingestion of degradable fibre stimulates bacterial growth and generates a faecal mass largely composed of bacteria.

Effects on GI tract. Fibre affects GI motility: gums and pectins slow gastric emptying, while particulate fibres like wheat bran appear to increase it. Effect on intestinal transit time depends on particle size and bulk forming capacity: large particle size (e.g. coarse bran) is more effective than small particle size in speeding colonic transit. Increased fibre intake has been proposed to reduce the incidence of various diseases including <u>colonic cancer</u>, <u>diverticular disease</u>, <u>appendicitis</u>, <u>cholelithiasis</u>, constipation, haemorrhoids. The bulk of evidence supports a high fibre diet but a direct protective effect against colon cancer or in preventing adenoma recurrence has not been proven.

Fissures

See: <u>anal fissure</u>.

Fistulae

See: <u>anorectal fistulae</u>.

Flukes (flatworms, trematodes)

The three common **intestinal flukes** are *Fasciolopsis*, *Heterophyes*, and *Echinostoma*. They tend to be geographically restricted (Asia, Indonesia). People get infected by eating fish or freshwater plants infected with metacercariae. *Fasciolopsis* can be up to 7.5 cm long; *Heterophyes* and *Echinostoma* are only a few mm long. Symptoms are often minimal but may include abdominal cramps, and mild diarrhoea. Diagnosis in all cases involves finding eggs in the stool. Treatment with praziquantel, 25 mg/kg every 8 hrs for 1 day.

Liver flukes include <u>Clonorchis</u>, *Opisthorcis*, *Fasciola*.

- *Clonorchis* and *Opisthorcis* are endemic to Southeast Asia (1 species found in Russia/Ukraine). Infection occurs by eating metacercariae in undercooked fish. The worms grow into adults in the biliary tree and can cause <u>cholangitis</u>, <u>biliary strictures</u>, and <u>liver abscesses</u>. The most important complication is <u>cholangiocarcinoma</u>.
- *Fasciola* is similar to <u>Clonorchis</u> and *Opisthorchis* but has a worldwide distribution, is larger (up to 7 cm long), and is frequently asymptomatic. They migrate from the intestine into the liver across the peritoneal cavity and can cause abdominal pain and hepatomegaly in this phase. They can cause intermittent biliary obstruction and cholangitis. They release few eggs, so stool analysis is insensitive: diagnosis is by an ELISA test on serum. They are resistant to praziquantel and triclabendazole is the drug of choice.

Blood flukes include <u>schistosomiasis</u>.

Focal nodular hyperplasia (FNH)

- Most commonly found in women < 40 years, and incidental finding in majority.
- Non-specific abdominal pain in 15%, and spontaneous haemorrhage is rare. No clear link with oral contraceptive, in contrast with hepatic adenomas. FNH is thought to arise as hyperplastic response to pre-existing vascular malformation (and condition linked to cavernous haemangiomas elsewhere.
- On CT, central hypodense scar, and vascular enhancement with IV contrast, is characteristic. Most lesions < 5 cm, with histology resembling cirrhosis (but with surrounding normal parenchyme), and central stellate scar often containing thick-walled blood vessels.
- Surgical resection may be indicated if significant symptoms are clearly attributable to FNH, if complication has occurred (e.g. haemorrhage), or if there is doubt about the diagnosis.

Folic acid (vitamin B9)

- A complex pterin molecule conjugated to glutamic acid. Found in spinach, liver, peanuts, and beans. Destroyed by prolonged cooking.
- Functions as a carrier of one-carbon groups; necessary for synthesis of nucleic acid, proteins, acetylcholine, and methionine.
- Recommended intake is 200 mg/day. Uptake is by a specific carrier-mediated process that involves a hydrolase. This enzyme is inhibited by exposure to alcohol, which may contribute to the folate deficiency seen in chronic alcoholics. Folate deficiency is seen in small intestine mucosal diseases such as coeliac and Whipple's disease.
- Folate metabolism is affected by methotrexate, pyrimethamine, trimethoprim, and triamterene. Salazopyrine inhibits folate transport. Phenytoin and carbamazepine lower folate levels and may produce a megaloblastic anaemia.
- The risk of children born with neural tube defects is reduced by pharmacological doses of folate (4 mg/d) given periconceptually.

Food allergy (food intolerance)

- Food allergy implies an immune-mediated reaction to certain foods; food intolerance is a better term for non-immune reactions. Food intolerance can be enzymatic (e.g. lactose intolerance due to congenital or acquired lactase deficiency), pharmacological (e.g. sensitivity to vasoactive amines such as tyramine in cheeses), or idiopathic.
- The prevalence of true food allergy can be up to 8% in children < 3 years, with perhaps 2.5% infants under 2 years having cow's milk allergy. The rate falls to 2.5% of the population after the first decade.
- Risk factors include an immature mucosal immune system, early introduction of solid food, IgA deficiency, and inadequate challenge of the mucosal immune system with commensal flora.
- Pathogenesis of true food allergy in most cases is thought to involve failure of tolerance mediated by gut-associated lymphoid tissue. Both IgE- and cell-mediated process can occur.
- Food allergy is the commonest cause of anaphylactic reactions; peanut allergy has a prevalence of 0.5 to 7% of adults in the USA and UK. Other common causes are cow's milk, eggs, seafood, and fish.
- IgE-mediated hypersensitivity reactions.

Food poisoning

Can be caused by parasites (_Giardia_, _Cryptosporidium_, trichinosis), viruses (e.g. hepatitis A), chemicals (e.g. mushrooms) but approximately 75% are caused by bacteria. The common organisms are shown in the table: most are discussed under separate entries.

- Immediate (within minutes to 2 hours of consumption). This includes **oral allergy syndrome and gastrointestinal anaphylaxis.** There may be contact hypersensitivity with angio-oedema, allergic rhinitis, wheezing. Diagnosis can be established by history; skin-prick testing is widely used as a diagnostic aid but the correlation with intestinal symptoms and skin sensitivity is poor.
- Eosinophilic gastroenteritis may in some cases be a manifestation of cell-mediated hypersensitivity to food antigens.

Fundoplication

See: anti-reflux procedures.

Bacterial causes of food poisoning

Salmonella	Over 50% confirmed cases
Enterotoxigenic *E. coli* (ETEC)	Usually food borne, short (< 4 h)
Staphylococcus aureus	Transmitted to food by humans. Outbreaks often happen when food is kept warm so organisms can multiply. Toxins are heat stable and if ingested produce symptoms in 2–6 h. Growth is favoured in food with high salt or sugar content
Clostridium perfringens	Spores in meat, 8–22 h
Shigella	
Clostridium botulinum	
Vibrio cholerae and V. parahaemolyticus	
Bacillus cereus	2 different syndromes caused by different toxins **Diarrhoea syndrome** has incubation period 6–14 h, lasts approximately 24 h and probably depends on bacterial division *in vivo*, after ingestion from variety of contaminated food **Vomiting syndrome** has short incubation period (2 h); diarroea in only 30%. Illness lasts 9 h, classically comes from contaminated rice in Chinese restaurants
Campylobacter, Yersinia, Listeria	

G

Gallbladder cancer

Epidemiology. Rare malignancy, usually affecting elderly patients. Associated with <u>gallstones</u> in 70–90% of cases, calcified ('porcelain') gall-bladder (gallbladder cancer in 25%), and <u>gallbladder polyps</u> > 1 cm in diameter (malignant in 23–88% of patients). Prophylactic <u>cholecystectomy</u> should particularly be considered for the last 2 risk factors. Tumour found in fundus in 60%, body in 30%, neck in 10%.

Clinical features. Right upper quadrant discomfort, weight loss, and jaundice. A hard, tender mass is sometimes felt in region of the gallblad-der. Occasionally condition is asymptomatic, with diagnosis made follow-ing 1–3% of cholecystectomies performed for gallstones.

Investigations. CT and U/S may show thickened gallbladder wall and mass within gallbladder lumen. Local spread well shown with CT. ERCP may show obstructed cystic duct, and mid-common bile duct stricture. Percutaneous biopsy may make histological diagnosis.

Management. Surgical resection rarely curative unless diagnosis made incidentally at time of <u>cholecystectomy</u>, as cancer spreads early to sur-rounding structures, including liver. Radical surgery (including right hepatectomy) rarely of benefit, and no clear role for systemic chemo-therapy or radiotherapy. Palliative approaches include biliary stenting to relieve jaundice, and <u>photodynamic therapy</u> may find a role in maintaining bile duct patency. Overall mean survival rate 6 months, and the 5-year survival rate < 5%.

Gallbladder empyema

Refers to the presence of pus within the gallbladder. It usually develops following acute <u>cholecystitis</u>, but cystic duct obstruction due to tumour (e.g. <u>cholangiocarcinoma</u>) may also occur. Infection may arise from <u>cholangitis</u>. Usually presents with right upper quadrant pain and signs of sepsis. Gallbladder perforation with subsequent peritonitis is an impor-tant complication if left untreated. CT or U/S may show a distended, fluid-filled gallbladder, with pericholecystic fluid. Treatment is with IV antibiotics (e.g. 3rd generation <u>CEPHALOSPORIN</u> and <u>METRONIDAZOLE</u>) and percutaneous gallbladder drain insertion (cholecystectomy is usually delayed because of high rate of post-operative septic complications).

Gallbladder polyps

- Refers to any mucosal projection into lumen of gallbladder. Prevalence 1–4%. More than 90% not neoplasms at all (e.g. cholesterol 'polyp' aris-ing from wall of gallbladder), and < 5% are true adenomas. Difficult to accurately define different types on imaging (usually ultrasound), but malignant change very rare in any gallbladder polyp < 10 mm.

- Usually asymptomatic, or found in association with symptomatic gallstones.
- Prudent management is to perform cholecystectomy if polyp > 10 mm (and certainly if > 18 mm, as these polyps carry significant risk of invasive adenocarcinoma). In those with polyps < 10 mm, 6–12 monthly ultrasound may be considered to exclude an increase in size.

Gallstones

Epidemiology + pathogenesis

Present in 10–20% of the world's adult population. Increased prevalence in women, first-degree relatives of sufferers, obesity, and pregnancy. Terminal ileal disease, including <u>Crohn's disease</u>, and surgical resection associated with increased risk (possibly due to reduced bile acid absorption, increased cholesterol:bile acid secretion, and supersaturated bile). High carbohydrate, low fibre diet may be linked. Pigment stones linked with haemolysis (e.g. sickle cell anaemia) and chronic biliary infection (e.g. *Clonorchis* infection). Cholesterol-predominant stones account for 75% of cases; pigment stones (calcium bilirubinate, mucin glyocoprotein, bacterial products) account for 25%.

Clinical feature. Range of clinical scenarios in patients with gallstones, and pattern determines specific investigation and management. Symptoms develop in 1–3% of patients per year with gallstones.

Asymptomatic gallstones. Up to 80% of gallstone carriers remain asymptomatic, with incidental diagnosis made on imaging.

Symptomatic gallstones
- Bilary colic refers to 1–5 hours of constant severe, dull, or boring pain, most commonly in the epigastrium or right upper quadrant. Pain may radiate to right scapular region. Severe biliary colic occurs in 1–8%/year, and other complications (e.g. <u>acute pancreatitis</u>, <u>cholecystitis</u>) in 1–3%/year.
- Acute <u>cholecystitis</u> presents with biliary colic-type pain, except that it lasts hours–days, and is commonly associated with nausea, vomiting, and fever.
- Jaundice ± right upper quadrant suggests <u>choledocholithiasis</u>, or more rarely <u>Mirizzi's syndrome</u>, and evidence of sepsis points to <u>cholangitis</u>.
- <u>Acute pancreatitis</u>.

Investigations

Imaging
- Transabdominal <u>ultrasound</u> is > 92% sensitive, and 99% specific for gallbladder stones > 2 mm, and is usually the only modality required. It is much less sensitive (approximately 50%) at detecting common bile duct (CBD) stones.
- AXR rarely of use as only 10% of gallstones are radiolucent.
- <u>CT scanning</u> may miss 20% of gallbladder stones, but is better at detecting complications of cholecystitis (e.g. perforation, empyema).
- <u>Endoscopic ultrasound</u> is highly accurate in detection of gallbladder stones or sludge, but is invasive and rarely necessary in uncomplicated cases.

Blood tests
- In patients with asymptomatic gallstones or biliary colic all blood tests should be normal.
- See also <u>cholecystitis,</u> <u>choledocholithiasis,</u> <u>cholangitis</u>.

Management

<u>Cholecystectomy</u> rarely indicated for asymptomatic gallstones (but needless and ineffective surgery often erroneously performed upon finding them), but indicated for symptomatic disease (see <u>cholecystitis</u>, <u>choledo-cholithiasis</u>).

Gardner's syndrome

A familial disease consisting of gastrointestinal polyposis and osteomas associated with several benign soft tissue tumours such as desmoids, epidermoid cysts, fibromas, lipomas, dental impactions, and congenital hypertrophy of the retinal pigment epithelium. It is a variable manifestation of a mutation in the APC gene.

Gastrectomy/gastroenterostomy

- Elective peptic ulcer surgery (see <u>Billroth</u>) is now rare and most often applied to patients with gastric outlet obstruction due to longstanding <u>peptic ulceration</u>. Emergency surgery is still needed, largely when perforation or catastrophic bleeding is the first manifestation of disease. Subtotal gastrectomy to remove the source of gastrin and parietal cell mass has a high rate of complications and is now reserved for treatment of uncontrollable haemorrhagic gastritis and gastric cancer.
- Surgery is the only curative procedure for <u>gastric cancer</u> and is also useful for palliation of symptoms, especially of obstruction. There is controversy about the necessary extent of surgery, with some groups advocating total gastrectomy in all 'curative' cases, and also the extent of lymph node re-section.
- Gastroenterostomy (loop of jejunum anastomosed to stomach) may be performed without partial gastrectomy. Indications include malignant duodenal invasion/stenosis (e.g. due to <u>pancreatic cancer</u>). Long afferent limb makes endoscopic access to duodenal papilla at ERCP difficult, occasionally impossible, and may predispose to a range of complications (see <u>afferent loop syndrome</u>).

Complications of gastrectomy. Peptic ulcer surgery has mortality of 0.3%–1%, higher if emergency surgery is required. Morbidity includes postoperative haemorrhage, leakage from anastomoses with abscess formation, <u>post-gastrectomy syndrome</u>, <u>biliary reflux</u>, and <u>afferent loop syndrome</u> (e.g. following Billroth II gastrectomy). See <u>Approach to surgically revised anatomy and stomas</u>.

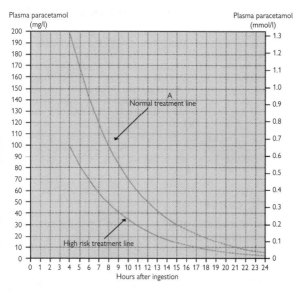

Fig. 2.13 Partial gastrectomies. Left, Billroth I. The duodenum is divided distal to the pylorus. 40–60% of the stomach is removed, and the gastric remnant is anastomosed directly to the duodenum. Right, Billroth II. The duodenal stump is closed. The gastric stump is anatomosed to a loop of jejunum about 15 cm distal to the ligament of Treitz. This creates afferent (duodenum to stomach) and efferent (stomach to distal bowel) loops.

Gastric antral vascular ectasia (GAVE)

Vascular lesion of gastric antrum, characterized by tortuous dilated blood vessels radiating proximally from pylorus GAVE (also called 'watermelon stomach').

Most commonly seen in middle-aged–elderly women, with auto immune disease (e.g. Sjögren's syndrome, atrophic gastritis). Association with portal hypertension in 30% of patients. Focal capillary thrombosis, with dilated submucosal venous channels, and fibromuscular hyperplasia of the muscularis mucosa found histologically, but diagnosis made on endoscopic appearance. May cause acute upper GI bleeding, or chronic iron deficiency anaemia. Iron therapy and transfusions may be required. Endoscopic therapy with laser photocoagulation, argon plasma coagulation, and heater-probe therapy increasingly used. GAVE is not a recommended indication for TIPSS.

Gastric cancer

Definition and epidemiology

Adenocarcinoma accounts for > 90% of gastric neoplasms (others include gastric lymphoma, gastrointestinal stromal tumour (GIST), carcinoid). Two broad types of gastric adenocarcinoma: **diffuse form** has the same frequency worldwide, is more common in women, occurs at younger age, and carries a particularly poor prognosis. More common **intestinal form** closely linked to environmental factors. Early gastric cancers ('EGC') mainly reported in Japan (accounting there for approximately 35% of cases), and are defined as tumour not extending beyond mucosa. Despite fall in incidence over the last 30 years (particularly in the West), gastric adenocarcinoma remains the second most common cancer worldwide. Large geographical variation, with highest incidence in Far East. Majority of patients > 60 years.

Aetiology and pathogensis

- Combination of genetic and environmental factors important. 10% of cases of gastric cancers exhibit familial clustering. Mutations of p53 tumour suppression gene and APC gene appear to be important in tumour development.
- **Risk factors** include: _Helicobacter pylori_ (probably predisposes to cancer by inducing atrophic gastritis, and classified by World Health Organization as class 1 carcinogen); smoking; high intake of salted and/or preserved foods; familial adenomatous polyposis (x10 risk of gastric cancer, related in part to gastric adenomas (found in >30% of cases); hereditary non-polyposis colorectal cancer (11% chance of gastric cancer); Ménetriér's disease; pernicious anaemia/atrophic gastritis/post-partial gastrectomy; high grade dysplasia on biopsy. Gastric adenocarcinoma develops in < 1% of gastric polyps, usually in those > 1.5 cm.

- Distribution of cancer within stomach: 40% in antrum, 35% in body, 15% in fundus/cardia, and 10% diffuse (i.e. linitus plastica). Decline in gastric cancer particularly relates to distal tumours, but proximal lesions may be increasing (see also <u>oesophageal tumours</u>). Metastases commonly to liver (40%), lung, bone marrow, peritoneum.

Clinical features

Gastric cancer usually presents late, with epigastric discomfort, weight loss, anorexia, nausea, upper GI bleeding, or symptoms of anaemia. Symptoms may be indistinguishable from those of <u>peptic ulceration</u>. Vomiting may relate to pyloric obstruction, and tumour bulk may give early satiety. On examination palpable epigastric mass may be found.

Investigation

- Blood results non-specific (no reliable tumour markers), but iron deficiency anaemia may be present.
- Upper GI endoscopy is the most frequently used diagnostic tool. Tumour may have appearance of benign gastric ulcer (repeat endoscopy and biopsies until resolution of even 'benign-looking' gastric ulcers is essential), polypoid mass, or diffuse gastric wall involvement (linitis plastica).
- <u>Endoscopic ultrasound</u> (EUS) allows depth of invasion to be determined with 80% accuracy (gastric cancers usually staged according to TNM classification (see <u>tumour staging</u>)). EUS > 90% accurate at distinguishing between stage T1 and T2, so is best modality at determining early from advanced cancer.
- Barium studies are widely used in Japan for detecting EGC.
- <u>CT scanning</u>. Main role in detecting distant metastases and as complement to EUS for determining depth of invasion.
- <u>PET scanning</u> may have an increasing role in detecting lymph node metastases.

Management and prognosis

- Surgery provides only hope of cure for locally advanced gastric cancer. The optimal surgical approach (e.g. total gastrectomy/subtotal gastrectomy/gastrectomy + splenectomy/extent of lymph node resection) is debated.
- Endoscopic mucosal resection (EMR) of early cancers confined to the mucosa (particularly common in Japan). EMR should be limited to those with solitary small tumours (< 2 cm), with no evidence of extension beyond mucosa on imaging, including EUS.
- Gastric adenocarcinoma is poorly responsive to chemotherapy or radiotherapy, but chemoradiotherapy as adjuvant to surgery has recently been shown to provide survival benefit. A range of chemotherapy regimens has been used (e.g. 5-fluorouracil and leucovorin).
- EGC have a 90% 5 year survival, but overall, 5 year survival in the United States is approximately 20%.

Gastric emptying

A major function of the stomach is to act as a food reservoir and to control food delivery to the intestine. A delay in emptying produces postprandial fullness, bloating, nausea, and vomiting: causes are outlined in the box.

Diagnosis. Mechanical obstruction is best excluded with endoscopy or barium studies. Non-invasive scintigraphic techniques are the principal clinical tools for assessing gastric motor function: different isotopes can be used to study emptying of solids and liquids. Some reports of abnormal electrical rhythms studied with electrogastrography (EGG) and found to be associated with abnormal gastric emptying and its symptoms have recently appeared: clinical application requires further clarification.

Vagotomy impairs receptive relaxation of the stomach and the resulting rapid emptying of hyperosmolar liquids contributes to early <u>dumping</u>. Later phases of solid emptying are impaired.

Diabetic gastroparesis (see <u>Diabetes and the GI tract</u>) can cause disabling and difficult to treat symptoms.

Gastric emptying and functional dyspepsia. Many studies report disturbed motility in a substantial proportion of patients (<u>ca.</u> 40%) with functional dyspepsia. The relation to symptoms and also therapeutic response to prokinetics is imperfect. There is some evidence that viral infection with CMV and HSV results in impaired emptying (Bityutskiy, LP et al. (1997) Am.J. Gastroenterol. **92:** 1501–4.)

Therapy

Gastric dysmotility can be difficult to treat. Available classes of <u>PROKINETIC DRUGS</u> include <u>DOPAMINE RECEPTOR ANTAGONISTS (METACLOPRAMIDE</u>, domperidone) and <u>MACROLIDES</u> (erythromycin). Cholinergic agonists or <u>ANTICHOLINESTERASES</u> are not widely used, and cisapride, an effective prokinetic belonging to the group of substitute benzamides, has been withdrawn because of concerns about it causing cardiac arrhythmias. Novel agents undergoing evaluation include prucalopride and tegaserod.

Gastric lymphoma

(See <u>lymphoma in GI tract</u>)

Causes of delayed gastric emptying

Mechanical obstruction
- Pyloric stenosis
  - Adult hypertrophic pyloric stenosis
  - Chronic benign peptic ulceration
  - Gastric cancer
  - Bezoars
- Duodenal tumour
- Pancreatic disease (e.g. pancreatic cancer, chronic pancreatitis)

Impaired motility
- Autonomic neuropathy
  - Diabetes
  - Shy–Drager syndrome
- Infiltrative
  - Amyloidosis
- Collagen vascular disease:
  - Scleroderma
- Post-surgical
  - Vagotomy
  - Roux-en-Y anastomosis
- Drugs
  - Anticholinergics
  - Opiates
  - Tricyclic antidepressants
- Other
  - Postviral (e.g. CMV)
  - Trauma (e.g. head injury)
  - Dermatomyositis
  - Pregnancy
  - Myotonic muscular dystrophy
  - Parkinson's disease
  - Hypothyroidism
  - Anorexia nervosa

Gastric polyps

Uncommon (found in 1% autopsies). Usually asymptomatic and benign. Some authorities recommend biopsy of polyps over 5 mm to exclude neoplasia. Polyps can be snared using electrocautery: bleeding can occur as a complication in about 5%.

Histology. Most common type is the hyperplastic polyp (75% of all polyps). Multiple fundic gland polyps can occur (in the fundus) and are not significant. Adenomas account for 10–20% of gastric polyps, may progress to adenocarcinoma, and may occur in pernicious anaemia. The risk of cancer relates to size of polyp and is low in polyps less than 2 cm diameter. Patients with adenomatous polyps require follow up because of the risk of malignancy.

Gastric ulcers

Pathogenesis, epidemiology, treatment, and complications are discussed in section on peptic ulceration.

Management recommendations. Take 6 biopsies from the edge of the ulcer and a biopsy remote from the ulcer to look for *Heliobacter pylori* (HP). Eradicate HP if present. Continue anti-secretory therapy for a total of 8 weeks. Healing rates are higher with a PROTON PUMP INHIBITOR than a H2 RECEPTOR ANTAGONIST. Follow up endoscopy is widely practised but current recommendations suggest that this is not necessary if ulcer is clearly benign on histology. Gastric brushings add expense and also provide a small increase in diagnostic accuracy. Follow up endoscopy is suggested for complicated ulcers (i.e. those that have bled or perforated).

Gastrinoma

Background

- One of the commonest types of neuroendocrine tumour. Incidence approximately 1/million; > 90% of gastrinomas occur in pancreas or duodenum (equal distribution). Unlike other pancreatic endocrine tumours, majority of gastrinomas are malignant. At presentation, pancreatic gastrinomas more likely to be > 2 cm, and to have metastasized, than duodenal lesion. Multiple endocrine neoplasia (MEN) in 30%.
- Zollinger–Ellison syndrome (ZES) refers to triad of severe peptic ulcer disease (PUD), gastric acid hypersecretion, and gastrinoma.

Clinical features

- Upper abdominal/epigastric pain in 75%, related to peptic ulceration. ZES accounts for 0.1% of cases of peptic ulceration.
- Chronic diarrhoea (± steatorrhoea) in >70%.
- Large pancreatic primary/liver metastases may present with abdominal pain/palpable mass.

Investigation

- Consider diagnosis in 'unusual' PUD (e.g. recurrent multiple ulcers, *Helicobacter pylori*, and NSAID-negative PUD, jejunal ulcers).
- Endoscopy may show single/multiple duodenal ulcers, and prominent gastric folds (may mimic <u>Ménétrier's disease</u>).
- Fasting serum gastrin level >1000 pg/ml highly specific for ZES (in absence of achlorydia and chronic atrophic <u>gastritis</u>). Gastrin 115–1000 pg/ml due to range of causes, including gastrinoma (see table and <u>Gut hormone profile</u>).
- Secretin provocation test performed if equivocal fasting gastrin (>200 pg/ml increase in serum gastrin after secretin injection is diagnostic).
- Gastric pH less than 2.0, with large gastric fluid volume (>140 ml over 1 h) confirms hypersecretion (but rarely performed in practice).
- Serum hypercalcaemia suggests possibility of MEN-1.
- To localize primary and metastases, scintigraphy (e.g. Octreoscan) sensitive (most gastrinomatos are somatostatin receptor positive). CT scan useful for identifying gastrinomas >1 cm. <u>Endoscopic ultrasound</u> increasingly used for small lesions.

Management

- Management in specialist units advised. Aim to control acid secretion and resect primary tumour.
- High dose <u>PROTON PUMP INHIBITORS</u> (e.g. Omeprazole 40–80 mg/day, pantoprazole 80–160 mg/day) effectively control hyperacidity in most patients.
- If localized pancreatic head/duodenal gastrinoma, curative surgical resection possible in majority of cases.
- Management of metastatic disease (often to liver) similar to that of other <u>neuroendocrine tumours</u>. Following resection of liver metastases 5-year survival of 85% reported, but cure in < 30%.

Cause of serum gastrin 115–1000 pg/ml	
Gastrinoma	Vagotomy
Proton pump inhibitors (stop for >1 week prior to test)	Small bowel resection
Atrophic gastritis	Renal failure (impaired gastrin excretion)
Primary hyperparathyroidism (?linked to MEN-1)	Hyperlipidaemia (may interfere with gastrinassay)
<u>Gastric cancer</u>	<u>Pyloric stenosis</u>

Gastritis

Histological inflammation of the stomach correlates poorly with endoscopic appearances and clinical symptoms. Some erosive and hyperplastic disorders may not be associated with much inflammation. Diagnosis requires endoscopic biopsy: indications and biopsy protocol are shown in the box.

Classification. There is no universally accepted system: The Sydney system is the best but is apparently too complicated for widespread use. A general classification is shown in the box.

Viruses

Cytomegalovirus (CMV) may affect oesophagus and stomach. Biopsy specimens reveal enlarged cells with CMV 'Owl eye' inclusion bodies. Herpesvirus can (rarely) produce multiple small raised ulcers. Biopsies show intranuclear inclusion bodies surrounded by haloes.

Bacteria

- Acute necrotizing gastritis is rare and dangerous. There is an association with alcohol binges, respiratory infections, AIDS, and infected peritoneal shunts. The mucosa appears thickened with a greenish black exudate. Treatment involves extensive resection and penicillin.
- Very rarely the stomach may be infected with TB (usually associated with pulmonary TB), actinomyces, and syphilis.
- Reactive gastropathy (acute erosive gastritis).
- Inflammation is not a major feature. Causes are shown in the box.

Gastroenteritis

See: entries under causative organisms.

Gastrograffin

A water soluble contrast medium. Safer than barium in radiological contrast examinations especially where there is a suspicion of peritonitis if examining the lower bowel or mediastinitis if performing a contrast swallow.

Gastro-oesophageal reflux (GORD)

See: Approach to dyspepsia and gastro-oesophageal reflux.

When and how to take gastric biopsies

Indications for biopsy
Gastric erosion or ulcer, thickened folds, gastric polyps or masses, possible *Helicobacter*, possible diffuse of chronic gastritis.

Biopsy protocol
Take 5 biopsies: Antrum (greater and lesser curve) incisura, and gastric body (greater and lesser curve).

Classification of gastritis

Inflammation associated
- <u>Atrophic gastritis</u>
- Infectious: viral, bacterial, *H. pylori*, fungal, parasitic
- Granulomatous: <u>Crohn's</u> <u>sarcoid</u>, TB, foreign bodies
- Distinctive: <u>eosinophilic</u>, lymphocytic
- Graft versus host.

Minimal inflammation
- Aspirin/NSAIDs
- Alcohol, cocaine
- Radiation
- <u>Bile reflux</u>
- Ischaemia
- Hiatus hernia
- Hyperplastic: <u>Ménétrier's disease</u>, Zollinger–Ellison syndrome.

Gastrostomy

The commonest method of nutritional support in patients requiring tube feeding for over 2 weeks. Can be placed endoscopically (see <u>percutaneous endoscopic gastrostomy (PEG)</u>), radiologically, or (rarely) surgically.

Complications of both percutaneous and radiological endoscopy can be major (leakage with peritonitis, necrotizing fasciitis, and haemorrhage) in about 3% or minor (minor leaks, wound infection, ileus, fever) in about 20%. Peristomal infection is reduced by a single dose of IV <u>CEPHALOSPORIN</u>.

Giardiasis

Giardia lamblia is a protozoan with flagella and a common cause of malabsorptive diarrhoea. Worldwide, infects children more than adults; infection can be waterborne, food borne, or person–person.

There is a cyst form and a motile trophozoite. Cysts can survive for weeks in cold water. If they are swallowed the cyst wall is dissolved by stomach acid and the trophozoites are released and adhere to small bowel enterocytes.

Clinical signs can include diarrhoea, fatigue cramps, bloating, weight loss, and fever. The signs vary and may depend on host immune response; common variable immunodeficiency is associated with severe disease—but no increase in severity has been reported in AIDS.

Diagnosis. Stool exam is only 50% sensitive. Duodenal biopsy is better (ca. 80%) but testing stool by ELISA or direct fluorescence antibody microscopy is probably first choice.

Treatment. Tinidazole 2 g single dose or <u>METRONIDAZOLE</u> 250 mg tds for 5 days. In pregnancy, use paromomycin (25–35 mg/kg/day in 3 divided doses for 7 days). Treatment may fail and need higher doses of metronidazole but confirm persistent infection before retreating, look for immune deficiency (check immunoglobulins for common variable immune deficiency), and remember the high incidence of <u>lactose intolerance</u> after *Giardia* infection.

Gilbert's syndrome

> Described by Nicolas Augustin Gilbert, 1858–1927, French physician, so 'soft' G in pronunciation.

Gilbert's syndrome is the commonest of the disorders of hyper-bilirubinaemia (see <u>bilirubin metabolism</u>), and is found in 5–10% of Caucasian populations. Diagnosis often made on routine blood testing (raised bilirubin (usually < 65 µmol/l), with all other liver tests entirely normal; or occasionally when intercurrent illness leads to transient clinical jaundice (see <u>Approach to recent-onset jaundice</u>). Prolonged fast may down-regulate bilirubin uridine diphosphate glucuronosyltransferase (UGT)-1 enzyme, so precipitating jaundice, but test has low sensitivity in making diagnosis. <u>Liver biopsy</u> is rarely needed, or the risks justified. Life expectancy normal, and no specific treatment.

GIST (gastrointestinal stromal tumours)

Aetiology and pathogenesis. Subset of mesenchymal GI tumours, previously classified as leiomyomas, leiomyosarcoma. Represent 3% of GI tumours. Intramural, well-demarcated spherical masses arising from muscularis propria. They may project intraluminally, with overlying mucosal ulceration (see Colour Plate 12). Malignancy not reliably predicted by tumour size (may be > 30 cm), and 10–30% are malignant, with > 40% of malignant GISTs metastasized by the time of presentation. GISTs usually arise from upper GI tract (stomach 70%, small bowel 20%).

Clinical features. May be found incidentally, but common presentations include abdominal pain, gastrointestinal bleeding, or a palpable mass. Rarely present with obstruction, and perforation occurs in 20%.

Investigation

- Endoscopy may show smooth mass with central ulceration.
- <u>Endoscopic ultrasound</u> (EUS) allows accurate assessment of GIST, including demonstration that tumour arises from muscularis propria.
- CT scanning and barium meal/follow-through may also delineate mass.
- Histologically graded as benign, borderline, or malignant, with histology showing diffuse sheets of spindle cells. Immunohistochemical staining of biopsy specimens is important, with expression of surface markers CD117 and CD34 characteristic, and vimentin expression in > 90%. Correlates with malignancy include tumour size of > 4 cm, irregular extraluminal border, and cystic spaces and echogenic foci within GIST. Presence of two or three of these features predicts malignancy with 80–100% confidence.

Management

- Surgical resection is treatment of choice (but complete resection may not be possible due to tumour size).
- Significant recent advance in treatment of metastatic or non-resectable GIST is development of Gleevec (imatinib mesylate), a tyrosine kinase inhibitor. In patients with unresectable GIST, 2 year survival increases from 26% with conservative treatment, to 76% with Gleevec. Tumours often become unresponsive after 2 treatments with Gleevec, and additional treatments are now in development. In patients with malignant GIST, 5 year survival post-surgery is 30–35%.

Globus

A feeling of a lump or tightness in the throat. Not accompanied by dysphagia or odynophagia, may be worsened by dry swallowing and emotional stress. It is a common symptom in patients with somatization disorder.

There is no documented association with abnormalities of the upper oesophageal sphincter. 90% report coincident heartburn but oesophagitis or significant GORD on pH testing is rare. Perception of oesophageal stretch may be increased in globus patients.

Gluten sensitivity

See: <u>coeliac disease</u>.

Graft versus host disease (GvHD)

- Can affect any part of the GI tract. Most common after bone marrow transplants, it is caused during by 'foreign' (allogeneic) immune cells.
- Acute GvHD occurs during post-transplant days 21–100; chronic GvHD occurs after day 100. Usually affects small and large intestine, less commonly the stomach and oesophagus.
- Gastric involvement often causes nausea, vomiting, upper abdominal pain. Endoscopy and gastric biopsies are necessary. Histology shows necrosis of single cells in large and small intestinal crypts.
- Jaundice due to cholestasis is a feature of severe acute GvHD. <u>Liver biopsy</u> may show bile duct damage and eventually ductopenia. Hepatocellular necrosis is rare.
- Acute GvHD is treated with high dose <u>CORTICOSTEROIDS</u>. First-line treatment of chronic GvHD is with <u>CYCLOSPORIN</u> and <u>CORTICOSTEROIDS</u>; but further treatment is ineffective and difficult.

Granulomas

A focal process composed of macrophages and other inflammatory cells, granuloma formation can be triggered by foreign bodies, infectious agents, or antigens that can cause delayed hypersensitivity. Granulomas are found in 3–10% of livers at autopsy. See <u>hepatic granulomas</u> as separate entry.

Granulomas in the intestine are most commonly associated with <u>Crohn's disease</u> and <u>lymphoma</u>: <u>tuberculosis</u> is an important differential diagnosis.

Gut hormone profile

- Measurement of serum gut hormones (see table) can be an invaluable part of investigation of patients with suspected <u>carcinoid</u> and <u>neuroendocrine/pancreatic endocrine tumours</u>. However, completely invalid results may be obtained if sample not taken, and handled, correctly.
- <u>Serum chromogranin A</u> correlates quite well with tumour burden in neuroendocrine tumours, but may also be elevated in prostatic cancer.

Patient preparation

- <u>H2 RECEPTOR ANTAGONISTS</u> blockers should be stopped for 72 h, and <u>PROTON PUMP INHIBITORS</u> for 12 weeks, before blood is taken.
- After an overnight fast, take blood (10 ml) using a syringe and needle.

Sample preparation

- Inform the analysing laboratory that you are taking the sample and when. Inform lab of patient's serum calcium and urea, list all drugs currently administered, clinical question, and details of any gastric surgery (also see <u>gastrinoma</u>).
- Transfer 10 ml of blood into a heparin tube (containing aprotinin, 0.2 ml, 2000 kIU). Mix by inversion. Place on ice and transfer immediately to the laboratory. Plasma separated in a refrigerated centrifuge, and frozen at $-20°C$ within 15 min of venepuncture, for subsequent analysis.

Gut hormone profile

Hormone	Normal range	Disease association
Chromogranin A	0–38 ng/l	Carcinoid
Gastrin	0–40 pmol/l	Gastrinoma
Vasoactive intestinal polypeptide (VIP)	0–30 pmol/l	VIPoma
Somatostatin	0–150 pmol/l	Somatostatinoma
Pancreatic polypeptide (PP)	0–300 pmol/l	
Neurotensin	0–100 pmol/l	

Haemangioma

- Benign vascular liver lesion, with reported prevalence of 1–20% of adult population. More common in women (may get larger in pregnancy), and usually identified at age 30–50 years. Range from < 1 cm to > 20 cm (most < 5 cm), and usually asymptomatic (rarely present with pain, haemorrhage, or rupture).
- Diagnosis on transabdominal <u>ultrasound</u> suggested by sub-liver capsule, well-defined hyperechoic lesion. <u>CT scan</u> classically shows low density lesion with delayed filling with contrast. Appearance on <u>MRI</u> of hyper-intensity on T2-weighted images. Angiography occasionally necessary.
- Surgery indicated if haemangioma very large, getting larger (e.g. on 6–12 monthly U/S), or diagnosis uncertain (misdiagnosis of malignant liver tumours as haemangiomas is well recognized).

Haemobilia

- Bleeding into the biliary tree is an unusual cause of <u>acute upper GI tract bleeding</u>. Causes include blunt or penetrating trauma, instrumentation (e.g. <u>liver biopsy</u>, <u>ERCP</u>, <u>TIPSS</u>), <u>gallstones</u>, hepatic artery aneurysms, bile duct ('peridochal') varices, <u>liver abscesses</u>, and tumours (e.g. <u>hepatocellular carcinoma</u>).
- May be associated with right upper quadrant discomfort and jaundice (due to intraluminal blood clot or underlying disease, such as tumour).
- Making diagnosis often requires consideration of possibility (e.g. in patients with ↓ BP and Hb post-liver biopsy). At endoscopy, finding of blood in second part of duodenum without clear bleeding point should be followed by close inspection of ampulla with duodenoscope ± ERCP, if any risk factors for haemobilia. Source of bleeding may be suggested on CT, and bleeding point may be defined by angiography.
- Management involves correcting any coagulopathy and biliary decompression with endoscopic stent if obstructed. Haemobilia usually settles spontaneously, but may require angiographic embolization and rarely surgery.

Haemochromatosis

Epidemiology + pathogenesis

- Haemochromatosis denotes <u>iron</u> overload, and may be 'primary' (genetic haemochromatosis (GH)), or 'secondary' (repeated transfusions, excess dietary iron). Usual total body iron is 3–4 g; in GH it may be > 20 g.
- 90% of GH cases are due to substitution of tyrosine for cysteine at position 282 of the HFE gene located on chromosome 6 (C282Y mutation). It shows autosomal recessive inheritance, with 10% of northern European populations heterozygous (+/–) and 1% homozygous (+/+) for C282Y mutation. There is low penetrance of clinical disease, partly due to menstruating iron loss in pre-menopausal women.

- Understanding of mechanism of iron overload is incomplete, but may involve reduced expression of HFE gene product at cell surface, increasing affinity of transferrin receptor for transferrin. Cellular iron may induce tissue injury through oxidant injury.
- Relationship between alcohol and iron overload is complex. In patients with GH (C282Y +/+), cirrhosis is 9 times more common in those drinking > 60 g of alcohol/day than in those taking less. Reasons for this are unclear, but likely due to cofactor effect of alcohol and GH on oxidative stress, hepatic stellate cell activation, and hepatic fibrogenesis. Hepatic iron overload may also occur in <u>alcoholic liver disease</u> *per se*, independent of GH (but C282Y mutation should be excluded in alcoholic patients with any evidence of iron overload—see below).
- C282Y+/– has been linked with a number of clinical scenarios (<u>porphyria</u> cutanea tarda, increased fibrosis in <u>hepatitis C</u>, <u>alcoholic liver disease</u>, non-alcoholic steatohepatitis (see <u>non-alcoholic fatty liver disease</u>), but evidence for clinical iron overload in compound heterozygotes (C282Y+/–, H63D+/–) is more convincing.

Clinical features

- Abdominal: hepatomegaly, cirrhosis, <u>hepatocellular carcinoma</u> (15% of untreated cases), splenomegaly.
- Cardiovascular: cardiomyopathy.
- Endocrine: diabetes mellitus, hypogonadism, panhypopituitarism, testicular atrophy.
- Skin: pigmentation ('bronze diabetes'), <u>porphyria</u> cutanea tarda (vesicular rash, back of hands), loss of axillary/pubic hair (secondary to hypopituitarism).
- Skeletal: chondrocalcinosis (often affecting knees), arthritis in 2nd and 3rd metacarpophalangeal joints.

Investigations

- Serum ferritin (upper normal limit males: > 300 µg/l, females: > 200 µg/l). In absence of other causes of elevated ferritin (e.g. inflammatory disease), serum ferritin > 1000 µg/l strongly suggests GH.
- Transferrin saturation: > 45% suggestive of iron overload.
- <u>Liver biopsy</u>. Gold standard for diagnosis, with assessment of severity and pattern of Perl's haemosiderin stain (grade I–IV siderosis), and measurement of hepatic iron index (HII; µmol iron per g dry weight of liver/age in years). HII > 1.9 suggests GH.
- C282Y gene analysis useful, but incomplete penetrance of C282Y+/+ and fact that GH also occurs in C282–/– patients necessitate full biochemical tests in those with features suggestive of GH.
- <u>MRI</u> scanning has high specificity for demonstrating liver iron overload, but poor sensitivity, and has not replaced need for biopsy in most cases.
- <u>Liver function tests</u>. Often normal or minimally deranged.
- Fasting glucose.
- LH/FSH. May be reduced, with impaired response to gonadotrophin-releasing hormone.

Management

- Venesect one unit of blood (450 ml; 0.25 g of iron) every 1–3 weeks, with measurement of ferritin and Hb every 4–6 sections. Aim for Hb lower end of normal range, and ferritin < 50 µg/l. May take 2 years, but when achieved can reduce venesection rate to 3–6 monthly.
- Iron chelation (desferrioxamine infusion 2 g × 3/week) occasionally needed when venesection not tolerated (e.g. patients with heart failure), but less effective, and rarely first-line treatment.
- Excluded <u>hepatocellular carcinoma</u>, especially if cirrhotic, with 3–6 monthly <u>alpha fetoprotein</u> + <u>ultrasound</u>.
- Refer to endocrinologist for management of hypogonadotrophic hypogonadism. Hormone replacement often required.
- Strongly advise stopping/minimizing alcohol (no clear safe lower limit defined).
- Screening of relatives for GH is vital. If index case has C282Y+/+, screen using genetic analysis, transferrin saturation, and serum ferritin. If index case does not have genetic mutation demonstrated, screen biochemically.

Haemolytic–uraemic syndrome (HUS)

- Acquired and inherited forms exist, but particular interest for gastro-enterologists is in the association (in 90% of cases) with verocytotoxin-producing <u>E. coli</u> (VTEC), and the commonest strain E. coli 0157:H7 (also see <u>food poisoning</u>). Other enteric pathogens associated with HUS including <u>Shigella</u>, <u>Salmonella</u>, <u>Yersinia</u>, and <u>Campylobacter</u>. E. coli 0157 commonly acquired from unpasteurized milk or uncooked meat, but only 5% of these infections lead to HUS. Children < 5 years and elderly most susceptible to disease.
- Condition characterized by thrombocytopenia, microangiopathic haemolytic anaemia, and renal failure. Usually presents with acute illness characterized by abdominal cramps, bloody diarrhoea, nausea, and vomiting. <u>Acute pancreatitis</u> may rarely occur. Bruising, bleeding, CNS effects, and renal failure generally develop about a week later.
- Diagnosis made on clinical suspicion, blood results showing renal failure, haemolytic anaemia and ↓ platelets, and stool culture showing E. coli 0157.
- Treatment of the acute diarrhoeal illness with antibiotics or anti-diarrhoeal agents has been linked to an increased risk of developing HUS. 70% with VTEC–HUS recover completely, 30% require long-term renal dialysis, and 5% die of the disease.

Haemorrhoids

- Dilated vascular channels located in left lateral, right posterior, and right anterior positions within anal canal. A normal part of human anatomy, when diseased can lead to prolapse, bleeding, and itching (very common: 10–25% adult population). External haemorrhoids are covered with squamous epithelium, while internal haemorrhoids are classified into 4 groups (see box).
- Exact pathogenesis is not clear, but may be due to failure of supporting structures: upright posture and prolonged time straining at stool do not help.

Treatment is based on grade (see box).

Grade 1 and 2 usually repond to diet: increase fibre and fluid intake to ensure soft, easy to pass stool. Over-the-counter preparations often contain lubricants, astringents, vasoconstrictors, and antiseptics. Important constituents in prescribed preparations are steroids and local anaesthetics to reduce inflammation and provide relief from painful defecation. Don't use topical steroids for longer than a few days and beware of the possibility of perianal candidasis, which should be treated with oral and topical nystatin.

If these fail and patient does not have grade 4 haemorrhoids (which usually need surgical haemorrhoidectomy) aggressive non-surgical treatments include sclerosing agents, band ligation, cryotherapy, electrocoagulation, and use of heater probe. Only first two in common use.

- Sclerosing agents. Aim is to inject irritant (e.g. arachis oil containing 5% phenol) into submucosa above haemorrhoid to create fibrosis and prevent prolapse. Pelvic sepsis is rare, but usually occurs 3–5 days post-procedure, and can be life-threatening.
- Band ligation. Widely used for second and third degree haemorrhoids. Stop aspirin and NSAIDs for 5 days before and after treatment. Immediate pain signifies too close placement to the dentate line: band needs to be removed. Complications include bleeding (usually controlled by balloon tamponade with a Foley catheter balloon, but sometimes needing adrenaline injection or even a small suture) and sepsis.
- External haemorrhoids are visible and palpable on wiping, but cause few symptoms apart from slight interference with personal hygiene. However they may thrombose, causing rapid appearance of a lump and pain. This usually subsides after a few days.

Heater probe

Useful for treating actively bleeding ulcers in the GI tract within reach of an endoscope and also for lowering risk of bleeding of high-risk lesions. Keys to successful use include direct probe pressure to tamponade the vessel, use of 25–30 Joule setting, and repeated applications.

Classification of internal haemorrhoids

Grade 1 Bleeding with defecation
Grade 2 Prolapse with defecation but return naturally to their normal position
Grade 3 Prolapse at any time, especially with defecation, and can be replaced manually
Grade 4 Permanently prolapsed

Heavy chain disease

Rare neoplastic disorders of B cells with abnormal monoclonal heavy chains. The least uncommon is <u>alpha chain disease</u>, usually found in Mediterranean regions. Infiltration of small intestine produces abdominal pain, masses, weight loss, malabsorption, steatorrhoea, hypocalcaemia, with complications including obstruction, intussusception, and perforation. Diagnosis is by small bowel biopsy.

Helicobacter pylori (HP)

- A slow growing microaerophilic Gram-negative spiral rod that is causally linked with <u>gastritis</u>, <u>peptic ulceration</u>, <u>gastric cancer</u> (adeno-carcinoma), and <u>gastric lymphoma</u>.
- Usually acquired in childhood, prevalence varies with age, country, and social class. Transmission is usually person to person.
- Acute infection can occur, causing a neutrophilic gastritis that can lead to epigastric discomfort with nausea and vomiting.
- Infection in adults is usually chronic, producing non-atrophic superficial gastritis. The physiological effect of this process on acid and gastrin secretion depends in part on the area of stomach affected: gastritis in the body of the stomach tends to reduce acid output (although there is rebound hypergastrinaemia), while antral predominant gastritis is associated with increased acid output and also with duodenal ulceration.
- Progression to atrophic gastritis may occur and may explain in part the association with gastric cancer.

Diagnosis

Tests not requiring mucosal biopsy

- These include serology, urea breath tests, and stool antigen tests. Tests on saliva, buccal scrapes, or urine are at present unreliable. Serum tests are useful to confirm infection but unreliable in confirming eradication, as antibody titres do not always fall.
- Urea breath tests use urea labelled with ^{13}C or ^{14}C. The more commonly used ^{13}C method requires a mass spectrometer for analysis involving a delay of at best several days. The test requires the patient to be off PPI therapy for 14 days, H2 antagonists for 3 days, and at least 14 days after eradication therapy. Accurate method of demonstrating ongoing HP infection.
- Stool antigen testing appears to show comparable sensitivity and specificity for diagnosis to urea breath testing, but the test may need to be delayed for 3 months after therapy to confirm eradication.

Tests requiring mucosal biopsy

- Biopsy generally unnecessary unless culture and antibiotic sensitivity testing required. Routine H&E histology will show HP if large numbers are present: a special (e.g. silver) stain is more sensitive for smaller number of organisms. In patient undergoing diagnostic upper GI endoscopy, mucosal biopsies may be tested for urease by agar gel slide tests such as <u>CLO test</u>.

Treatment

- Cure requires combinations of at least two antibiotics and non-antibiotics such as <u>PROTON PUMP INHIBITORS</u> (PPI). Pre-treatment sensitivity testing is not performed so the proportion of failed treatments due to resistant organisms is not known.
- Standard therapeutic strategies include triple therapy as first-line treatment, consisting of a PPI with two antibiotics for 7 days. Failure of eradication is dealt with by changing antibiotics, increasing the length of treatment to 10–14 days, or adding in a fourth agent, usually bismuth, either as subcitrate (De-Nol) or as subsalicylate (Pepto-Bismol).

Accuracy of diagnostic tests for *Helicobacter pylori*

Parameter	Percentages			
	Sensitivity	Specificity	PPV	NPV
Serum IgG	91	97	95	85
Urea breath test	90	96	98	84
CLO test	90	100	100	84

PPV= positive predictive value; NPV= negative predictive value.

Recommended regimens to treat *Helicobacter pylori*

PPI triple therapy: PPI twice daily plus amoxycillin 1 g bd plus clarithromycin 500 mg bd **or** metronidazole 500 mg bd

Quadruple therapy
PPI twice daily plus bismuth 2 tabs bd plus metronidazole 500 mg bd plus tetracycline 250–500 qds

- Choice of antibiotic regimen.
  - *H. pylori* is sensitive to amoxicillin and resistance is rare, but concomitant antisecretory therapy is essential for activity.
  - Tetracyclines are usually effective and resistance is low in Western countries. Contraindicated in children.
  - <u>METRONIDAZOLE.</u> Usually effective against *H. pylori*, but the incidence of metronidazole resistance varies widely and is increased in urban areas.
  - Clarithromycin. Incidence of resistance is approximately 15%.
  - Other antibiotics. There is some empirical evidence on the efficacy of furazolidone but it is not considered a first-line antibiotic for eradication of *H. pylori*.

Follow-up after eradication
- Although routine follow up testing is not performed, failed therapy in an ulcer patient is very often associated with recurrence of the ulcer. Certainly in patients with complicated peptic ulcer disease (i.e. bleeding or perforation) documentation of eradication is advised before maintenance anti-secretory therapy is stopped.
- Confirmation of HP eradication usually performed with urea breath tests 6 weeks after completing course of eradication therapy.

HELLP syndrome

Background
- HELLP syndrome (**h**aemolysis, **e**levated **l**iver **e**nzymes, **l**ow **p**latelets) is a microangiopathic disease, and one of the liver conditions specifically related to pregnancy (see also <u>acute fatty liver of pregnancy</u>, <u>obstetric cholestasis</u>).
- Occurs in 20% of patients with pre-eclampsia, and associated with significant fetal and maternal morbidity/mortality.

Clinical features
- Presentation usually weeks 27–36 of pregnancy, but after delivery in 30%.
- Classic features include malaise, right upper quadrant pain, nausea, vomiting, and symptoms/signs of pre-eclampsia (thirst, headache, blurred vision, proteinuria, hypertension, peripheral oedema). May develop in absence of pre-eclampsia. Clinical jaundice in only 5%.
- Maternal complications include disseminated intravascular coagulation (in 20%), placental abruption, subcapsular haematoma.
- Maternal mortality 1%; perinatal mortality up to 30%.

Investigations
See also <u>Approach to liver problems in pregnancy</u>.
- ↓ Hb (usually < 9 g/dl), fragmented cells on film, and serum lactate dehydrogenase (LDH) level > 600 IU/l suggest haemolysis. Platelets < 100 × 10^9/l.

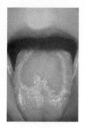

Plate 1 Geographic tongue.

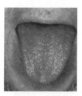

Plate 2 Glossitis. Reproduced with permission from Echenique-Elizondo M *et al.* (2004). *Journal of the Pancreas* online. **5**,179–85.

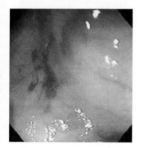

Plate 3 Angiodysplasia in the caecum. Reprinted with permission from William B. Silverman.

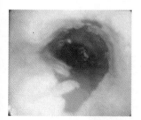

Plate 4 This figure shows an irregular and abnormal junction between oesophageal squamous (white) mucosa and gastric (pink) mucosa. This is Barrett's oesophagus but it is impossible to accurately define the extent from this picture because the gastro-oesophageal junction (point of disappearance of the gastric rugal folds) is not clearly seen.

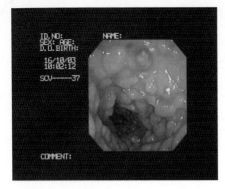

Plate 5 Endoscopic image of pseudomembranous colitis caused by *C. difficile*.

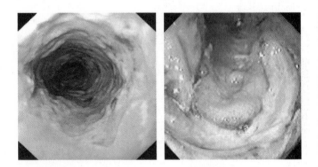

Plate 6 CMV oesophagitis (left) and colitis (right). Reproduced with permission from Wilson Jackson, Jackson Gastroenterology, and from Yamada T *et al.* (2005). *Handbook of Gastroenterology* Lippincott Williams and Wilkins respectively.

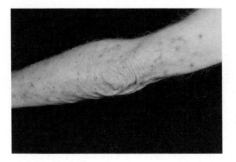

Plate 7 Dermatitis herpetiformis

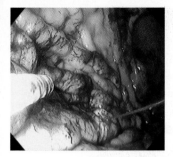

Plate 8 Endoscopic image of spurting Dieulafoy lesion. Reproduced with permission from Klaus Mönkemüller and Walter Curioso. www.giatlas.com

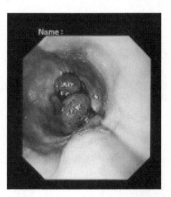

Plate 9 Variceal band ligation. 2 rubber bands are seen applied to a varix in the 5 o'clock position. Reproduced with permission from Yamada T *et al.* (2005). *Handbook of Gastroenterology.* Lippincott Williams and Wilkins.

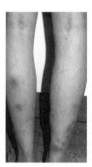

Plate 10 Erythema nodosum. Reproduced with permission from Dokyo University School of Medicine, Japan.

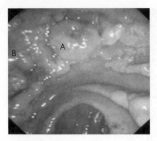

Plate 11 Duodenal familial adenomatous polyposis. View with duodenoscope showing a carpet of polyps involving ampulla (A) and peri-ampullary region (B).

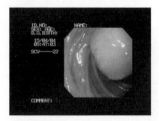

Plate 12 Endoscopic view of gastrointestinal stromal tumour (GIST) in duodenum.

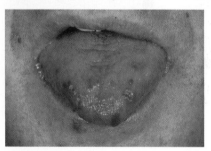

Plate 13 Hereditary haemorrhagic telengectasia.

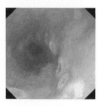

Plate 14 Endoscopic view of herpes simplex vesicles in the oesophagus. Reproduced with permission from Yamada T et al. 2005. *Handbook of Gastroenterology*. Lippincott Williams and Wilkins.

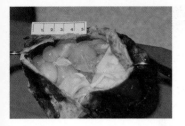

Plate 15 Hydatid cyst. Right hepatectomy specimen showing multiple daughter cysts.

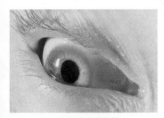

Plate 16 Kayser–Fleischer rings, found around edge of iris.

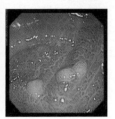

Plate 17 Melanosis coli

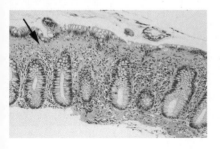

Plate 18 Collagenous colitis. The arrow shows a thickened subepithelial collagen band.

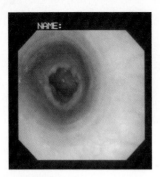

Plate 19 Oesophageal web on endoscopy.

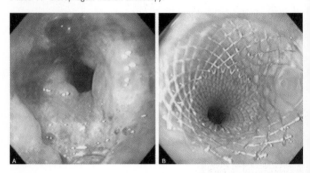

Plate 20 Figure showing stenosing oesophageal carcinoma before (left) and after (right) insert of a self-expanding metal stent. Reproduced from Feldman M, Friedman LS, and Sleisenger MH (2003). *Sleisenger and Fordtran's Gastrointestinal and Liver Disease*, with permission from Elsevier.

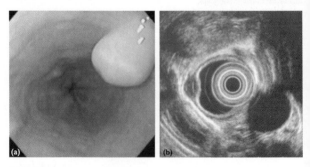

Plate 21 Oesophageal GIST (leiomyoma). (a) Endoscopic image. (b) EUS shows the lesion as a hypoechoic mass arising from the muscularis propria. Reproduced from Feldman M, Friedman LS, and Sleisenger MH (2003). *Sleisenger and Fordtran's Gastrointestinal and Liver Disease*, with permission from Elsevier.

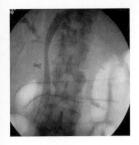

Plate 22 Endoscopically placed biliary and duodenal mesh metal stents in patient with inoperable pancreatic cancer.

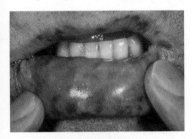

Plate 23 Brown macules on lips in patient with Peutz-Jeghers syndrome.

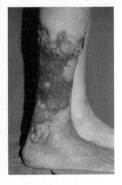

Plate 24 Pyoderma gangrenosum.

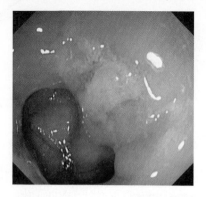

Plate 25 Solitary rectal ulcer on endoscopy. Reproduced with permission from Yamada T *et al.* (2005). *Handbook of Gastroenterology*. Lippincott Williams and Wilkins.

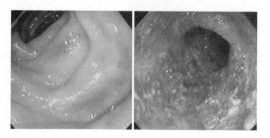

Plate 26 Mild (left) and severe (right) ulcerative colitis. Reproduced from Feldman M, Friedman LS, and Sleisenger MH (2003). *Sleisenger and Fordtran's Gastrointestinal and Liver Disease*, with permission from Elsevier.

- Serum aminotransferase (AST, ALT) levels × 2–15 ULN (mean approx 250 U/l), and bilirubin ×2 ULN (i.e. approx 40µmol/l). Massive elevation of AST/ALT (e.g. > 2000 U/l) suggests liver infarction/haematoma.
- ↑ D-dimers may predict severity.
- <u>Liver biopsy</u> demonstrates periportal haemorrhage/necrosis and fibrin deposition, but rarely warranted, as findings correlate poorly with laboratory tests and outcome, and there are increased risks of procedure.
- <u>U/S</u> or <u>CT scan</u> may show subcapsular haematoma/infarction.

Management

- Delivery as soon as possible (ideally beyond 32 weeks, by vaginal delivery), usually leads to prompt resolution. <u>CORTICOSTEROIDS</u> are often given prior to delivery (largely for speeding fetal lung maturity), but no clear evidence of improvement in outcome of HELLP.
- <u>Liver transplantation</u> has been successful in those with acute liver failure.
- Recurrence of HELLP in future pregnancies of < 5%.

Helminth infection

Parasitic worms (helminths) are classified into <u>roundworms</u> (nematodes) <u>tapeworms</u> (cestodes), and <u>flukes or flatworms</u> (trematodes). Travel, migration, and exotic cuisine allow helminths to appear in any locale. They are complex and often well adapted to their host—so much so that light infection may cause no symptoms, only heavy infestation resulting in disease. They almost never cause diarrhoea but are a potent cause of <u>eosinophilia</u> or <u>eosinophilic gastroenteritis</u>. They often induce a Th2 response (Il-4 mediated): this may limit multiplication but also impairs excessive Th1 responses. Diseases mediated by Th1 such as <u>Crohn's disease</u> and multiple sclerosis are rare where helminths are common: it may be that parasitic infection offers some protection against immune mediated disease.

Henoch–Schönlein purpura

Edward Henoch, nineteenth century. German paediatrician. Should really be called Schönlein–Henoch, as it was first described by Henoch's teacher, Schönlein.

A clinical syndrome of palpable non-thrombocytopenic purpura, arthritis, glomerulonephritis together with abdominal pain. Common in children, but can occur in adults. The main lesion seems to be an IgA nephropathy but blood levels of IgA and complement are variable.

GI symptoms include pain, nausea, and vomiting. Bleeding can occur in 40%, which can be small or large intestinal in origin. Less common complications include intramural haematomas, intussusception, cholecystitis, appendicitis, bowel infarction, and peritonitis.

Hepatic drug metabolism

- Phase 1 metabolism usually involves oxidation reaction, with insertion of a hydroxyl group, catalysed by the cytochrome p450 family of enzymes. There are 20 cytochrome p450 members falling into three groups. Some are inducible and some not.
- Phase 2 metabolism involves conjugation to polar ligands (glucuronide, sulphate, glutathione, amino), which generally enhances water solubility.
- Effects on drug metabolism (e.g. induction of cytochrome p450) underlie some types of <u>drug-induced hepatotoxicity</u>.

Hepatic encephalopathy

Background

- Hepatic encephalopathy (HE) encompasses a spectrum of neuropsychiatric disturbances observed in patients with significant liver dysfunction. It may also occasionally occur in patients with large portosystemic shunts in the absence of intrinsic liver disease.
- May develop in Acute liver failure or in patients with chronic liver disease and portal hypertension. In the latter, HE may be acute and episodic, related to a precipitant, or chronic and persistent, due to the combination of portosystemic shunting and liver dysfunction (see Approach to cirrhosis and chronic liver disease).
- Debate remains as to the most important toxins contributing to HE, but there is consensus that it develops due to reduced hepatic metabolism of gut-derived metabolites, as a result of impaired liver synthetic function and portosystemic shunting. Ammonia appears to be important, but hypotheses have also implicated the role of opiates, manganese, false neurotransmitters, and tryptophan.

Clinical features

- HE is a clinical diagnosis that should be considered in any patient with liver disease and confusion or altered consciousness (see Approach to agitation and confusion in the GI patient).
- Subclinical HE may be difficult to diagnose, but may have a significant effect on the lives of > 30% of patients with cirrhosis. Diagnosis may require electroencephalography or psychometric testing. A clinical grading system is applied to overt HE (first table). Overt HE in chronic liver disease carries a poor prognosis, with a 1 year survival of < 50%.

Assessment

In the history, ask about increased sleepiness and reversal of normal sleep pattern. Has patient or friends/family noted any change in personality or intellect?

Investigations

- In the patient with suspected HE, in whom a diagnosis of liver disease has not previously been made, the extent and cause of liver injury need to be established (see Approach to recent onset jaundice, and Approach to well patient with abnormal liver tests).
- Laboratory findings that suggest underlying liver disease include ↑prothrombin time, ↑bilirubin, ↓albumin (the 3 tests most indicative of poor liver function), ↑liver enzymes (AST/ALT/ALP/GGT), ↓platelets (?splenomegaly/hypersplensim in portal hypertension), ↓serum Na^+.

Grade of hepatic encephalopathy

Grade	Features	Liver flap (asterixis)
1	Impaired higher functions (e.g. arithmetic), but no effect on conciousness	Usually absent
2	Disorientation and personality change with inappropriate behaviour	Usually present
3	Confusion and gross disorientation with increased somnolescence	Present
4	Coma	Usually absent

Precipitants of HE and hepatic decompensation

Progressive liver injury	Dehydration (may be secondary to diuretics)
Additional liver insult (e.g. alcohol, hepatitis A)	Constipation
Upper GI bleeding	Renal failure
Hepatocellular carcinoma	Drugs (e.g. opiates)
Infection (e.g. spontaneous bacterial peritonitis)	Non-compliance with treatment
Increased portosystemic shunt (e.g. new TIPSS formation)	Large protein meal
Zinc deficiency	

- In patients with known cirrhosis, HE in association with worse liver function requires a search for an additional liver insult (e.g. alcohol binge, acute viral hepatitis, ischaemia.
- Abdominal U/S or CT scan may show evidence of portal hypertension.
- Tests for HE per se are relatively non-specific. Raised serum ammonia levels are elevated in patients with portal hypertension, but correlation with HE is poor. Sensory evoked potentials remain a research tool. On EEG, normal waveform may be replaced in HE by slower, higher amplitude delta waves. Although similar changes seen in renal or respiratory failure, their appearance may predate overt HE, and so EEG has a role.
- Seek a precipitant, including septic screen (culture of blood, urine, sputum, acites), exclusion of GI bleed (? ↓Hb, melaena on examination, serum urea disproportionately elevated with respect to creatinine), or renal impairment.

Management

- **Supportive care** for the patient in coma is essential. ITU assessment and admission is necessary for patients with grade 3/4 HE, with consideration of endotracheal intubation if safe airway not maintained.
- **Treatment** of precipitants alone leads to resolution of HE in > 60% of cases. Give antibiotics for overt sepsis, as well as for patients with variceal bleeding, in view of an association of sepsis with bleeding (see Acute upper GI bleeding), and the potentially additive effects of sepsis and high protein gut load leading to HE. Obsessive care of potential new sites of sepsis, such as IV cannulae, pressure areas, is vital. Precipitant drugs should be stopped. Renal impairment should be treated by controlling sepsis and ensuring adequate plasma expansion (also see hepatorenal syndrome).
- **Diet**. There is little evidence for the time honoured role of protein restriction in patients with HE and, as these patients are often malnourished, it may exacerbate problems. Protein intake should be maintained at 1–1.5 g/kg/day, with a transient reduction to 0.5 g/kg/day only if overall treatment fails. Vegetable-based protein diets may be more effective than animal-based ones.
- **Bowel cleansing** helps to reduce ammoniagenic substrates from the gut. Give lactulose 30–50 ml qds orally or via NG (no evidence that fine-bore NG tubes precipitate bleeding in patients with varices), aiming to ensure 2–4 soft stools passed daily. Improvement in HE is expected in 24–48 hours.
- **Antibiotics** against urease-producing gut bacteria are rarely used as first-line treatment, but may have a role in patients unresponsive to standard therapy e.g. neomycin 1–2 mg/day; metronidazole 250 mg tds PO. Antibiotics should not be given long term in view of toxicity.
- **Newer treatments** may gain an established role. Sodium benzoate 10 g/day PO improves ammonia clearance by increasing nitrogen excretion, and may be used with lactulose. Metabolic substrates for the conversion of ammonia to urea (e.g. ornithine aspartate 9 g/day PO) have been shown to reduce clinical period of clinical HE. Conversion of ammonia to urea is zinc-dependent, and zinc acetate 600 mg daily has been shown to improve HE, compared to placebo.

Hepatic granulomas

- Granulomas are found in 4–10% of <u>liver biopsies</u>, and there is a wide range of causes, although autoimmune liver disease, <u>sarcoidosis</u>, and TB probably account for most (see box). They are frequently found in patients with <u>HIV</u>, often related to underlying infection (*M. tuberculosis*, *M. avium intracellulare*, *Cytomegalovirus*, *Toxoplasma*), lymphomatous infiltration, or drug reaction. Hepatic granulomas may develop as part of a lupus-like drug reaction.
- The classical presentation is varied (reflecting the wide range of underlying causes). but hepatomegaly is found in only 20% of cases. Granulomatous hepatitis presents with 'pyrexia of unknown' origin in 50% of cases, and there is debate as to whether it is a variant of sarcoidosis.
- LFTs often show ↑ALP/GGT. Range of diagnostic tests may needed to identify cause (e.g. CXR and serum angiotensin-converting enzyme (SACE) for sarcoidosis).
- Treatment depends on the cause. Corticosteroids may improve fever and LFTs in hepatic sarcoid/idiopathic granulomatous hepatitis. Drug-related granulomatous reaction usually responds to cessation.

Hepatitis A

Epidemiology

Hepatitis A virus (HAV) infection remains the cause of 50% of reported cases of acute viral hepatitis in the UK. Transmission is through faecal–oral route, infected water supply, and ingestion of uncooked shellfish. It is the most common vaccine-preventable infection in travellers to areas of high endemicity (e.g. N. Africa, S. America, where > 95% of children by 10 years have been exposed).

Clinical features

- HAV only causes acute, never chronic, hepatitis. Likelihood of developing jaundice increases with age (79% in patients > 15 years), and this occurs 3–5 weeks after infection, often preceded by a prodrome of malaise, anorexia. Adults often feel unwell for 6 weeks.
- Prolonged cholestasis may occur in 5% of cases. <u>Acute liver failure</u> reported in < 0.1% of cases, but may be more common in conjunction with chronic <u>hepatitis C</u>.

Investigation

<u>Liver function tests</u> demonstrate markedly ↑ ALT (often > 1000 U/l) during acute icteric phase. Diagnosis usually confirmed by HAV IgM Ab in serum, which appears 5–8 weeks after onset of symptoms. <u>Liver biopsy</u> rarely indicated.

Management

- No specific treatment of acute hepatitis A is necessary.
- Prednisolone 40 mg PO daily, and tapering off over 2–4 weeks, may speed resolution of prolonged cholestasis. See <u>Acute liver failure</u> for very rare severe hepatitis A.

Causes of hepatic granulomas

Drugs
- Sulphonamides
- Hydralazine
- Procainamide
- Allopurinol
- Isoniazid
- Carbamazepine
- Chlorpropramide
- Phenylbutazone
- Quinidine
- Tolbutamide

Infection
- Myco bacterium <u>Tuberculosis</u>
- M. avium intracellulare
- Brucella
- Syphilis
- Leprosy
- <u>Schistosomiasis</u>
- <u>Whipple's disease</u>
- Q fever
- Coxiella burnetii
- <u>HIV</u>/AIDS

Industrial
- Berylliosis

Neoplasia
- Hodgkin's lymphoma
- Non-Hodgkin's lymphoma

Immunological disease
- <u>Inflammatory bowel disease</u>
- <u>Sarcoidosis</u>
- Systemic lupus erythematosis
- Granulomatous hepatitis
- <u>Primary biliary cirrhosis</u> (PBC)
- PBC/autoimmune hepatitis <u>overlap syndrome</u>
- <u>Polyarteritis nodosum</u>
- Wegener's granulomatosis

- 'Prevention is better than cure'. HAV vaccine is very effective, and should be offered to: travellers to areas of increased risk; IV drug users; men who have sex with men; patients with haemophilia or chronic liver disease (including <u>hepatitis C</u>, who may have increased risk of acute liver failure); those at occupational risk (e.g. child care centre workers). 1 ml of vaccine given initially, and then at 6–12 months, provides 95% protection for > 5 years.
- Passive immunization, with human normal immunoglobulin (HNIG) has few indications, due to the rapid efficacy of HAV vaccine (even post-exposure), and worries about transmission of prion disease (HNIG manufactured from pooled serum).

Hepatitis B

Epidemiology

- More than 300 million people worldwide are infected with hepatitis B virus (HBV), with chronic infection in 0.1–2% in Western Europe and USA, and up to 20% in areas of Southeast Asia.
- Most common route of transmission is perinatally (90% infection rate in infants born to HBeAg+ve mothers), but blood inoculation through unclean needles remains important. Sexual transmission accounts for 30% of infections in developed countries.

Clinical features

Acute hepatitis B. Jaundice, malaise, and right upper quadrant pain may develop 1–4 months after infection. Although acute liver failure may develop in 2% of cases, acute hepatitis results in viral clearance in > 95% of infected adults.

Chronic hepatitis B. Defined by HBsAg+ve in serum > 6/12. Age at infection strongly determines chronicity, reflecting host immunity (> 90% in neonates, 20–50% age 1–5 years, < 5% in adults). Different patterns of chronic infection correlate with serological markers (see table). Highest rate of complications in highly replicating disease (i.e. HBeAg+ve, or precore mutant infection). Spontaneous clearance of infection (i.e. becoming HbsAg–ve) occurs in 1% of chronically infected patients/year. **Complications** include:

- **Cirrhosis.** Once develops (usually 30–40 years after perinatal infection, but very variable), 5 year survival of approximately 80%, but this falls to 35% after episode of decompensation (see Approach to cirrhosis and chronic liver disease).
- Hepatocellular carcinoma. Nearly 100-fold increased risk in chronic hepatitis B. Annual incidence 2–6% in those with cirrhosis, 0.4–0.6% in non-cirrhotics.
- Membranous glomerulonephritis.
- Polyarteritis nodosum.

Investigations

- HBV serology: HBsAg (indicates ongoing infection); HBeAg (presence confirms high viral replication, but may be negative in HbeAg–ve chronic hepatitis B ('pre-core mutant'); anti-HBe (reciprocal of HBeAg); anti-HBc IgM (acute infection); anti-HBc IgG (previous or ongoing infection); anti-HBs (resolved infection or vaccinated).
- HBV DNA by PCR: Essential if HBsAg+ve, HbeAg–ve, in order to exclude precore infection (HBeAg+ve, HBV DNA > 10^5 copies/ml, ↑ALT).
- Liver function tests. AST/ALT usually > 1000 U/l in acute hepatitis. LFTs may fluctuate in chronic infection, but ALT < 80 U/l strongly predicts lack of HBeAg seroconversion (loss of HBeAg, development of serum anti-HBe) in response to antiviral therapy (i.e. a lack of sustained treatment response).
- Alpha fetoprotein. Perform 6 monthly with liver ultrasound, especially in cirrhotics, in view of hepatocellular carcinoma risk.

Patterns of HBV infection and serology

Clinical state	HBsAg	HBeAg	Anti-HBc IgM	Anti-HBc IgG	Anti-HBs	Anti-HBe	HBV DNA	Serum ALT	Comments
Acute infection	+	+/–	+	+/–	–	+/–	+/–	↑↑	HBsAg may be –ve at presentation
Chronic low replication	+	–	–	+	–	+	+	N	
Chronic high replication	+	+	–	+	–	–	+++	N/↑	ALT may be > 1000 U/l, and anti-HBcIgM+ve in flare of disease
HbeAg–ve chronic hepatitis B ('pre-core mutant')	+	–	–	+	–	+	++	↑	Common in S Europe
Vaccinated	–	–	–	–	+	–	–	N	
Resolved infection	–	–	–	+/–	+	+/–	–	N	Anti-HBc IgM+ve if recently resolved

Practice points in interpreting HBV serology

- HBsAg may rarely be negative at presentation in acute hepatitis B (and particularly in severe/fulminant disease, due to profound immune-mediated response to infection, and associated liver damage). However, anti-HBc IgM will be positive
- HBeAg positive confirms high level of HBV DNA (measurement of absolute level of virus rarely changes management in this setting). In contrast HBV DNA quantification is essential in all cases of HBeAg-negative chronic infection, to exclude 'pre-core mutant' infection
- Anti-HBc IgM may occasionally be positive in acute flares of chronic infection. Differentiation from acute primary infection often difficult, but chronic infection may be suggested by knowledge of prior positive serology, and subsequent lack of HBsAg seroconversion (as occurs in > 95% of cases of acute infection). Liver biopsy may be needed to confirm chronic disease

- <u>Liver biopsy</u>. Rarely needed in acute hepatitis B. Indicated in chronic infection, when treatment is considered (see management algorithm).
- HIV testing should be considered in all with chronic hepatitis B, especially if lamivudine planned for HBV infection (as lamivudine monotherapy for undiagnosed HIV infection may promote HIV treatment-escape mutants).

Management
- ***Acute hepatitis B***. No definitive evidence that antiviral therapy effects disease course, but lamivudine has been given for fulminant hepatitis B.
- ***Chronic hepatitis B***. Usual goal of treatment is to suppress HBV replication, induce HBeAg seroconversion (clearance of HBeAg, appearance of anti-HBe), and reduce liver injury. Ultimate goal is to clear HBsAg and prevent cirrhosis and HCC. Treatment is indicated for those with replicative disease (i.e. HBeAg+ve, or pre-core infection) and liver injury. Rate of HBeAg seroconversion with present antivirals closely related to pre-treatment ALT (<10% if ALT < ×2 ULN, >50% if ALT > ×5 ULN). See index of drugs for further information.
  - <u>INTERFERON ALPHA</u> (IFN-α) (e.g. 6 MU ×3/week for 6 months) induces HBeAg seroconversion in 30% at 1 year, and HBsAg loss in 5–10%, after 4/12 course. Standard IFN increasingly being replaced (in trials and clinical practice) by pegylated (PEG) IFN, with recent trials showing 30–36% HBeAg seroconversion following 1 year course of treatment (Lau, GKK et al. (2005). *N. Engl. J. Med.* **352**: 2682; Janssen, HL et al. 2005) *Lancet* **365**: 123). Range of important side effects of IFN (see index of drugs and <u>hepatitis C</u>), and contraindicated in decompensated cirrhosis.
  - <u>LAMIVUDINE</u> has few side-effects and is easy to take. Induces HBeAg seroconversion in 25% after 1 year of use, 56% after 3 years, but treatment-resistant YMDD variants may develop in > 40% after 3 years of use. Conflicting trial results on merit of combination <u>LAMIVUDINE</u> + PEG IFN therapy, but recent large trials of HBeAg+ve infection (see above) suggest no additional benefit of adding <u>LAMIVUDINE</u> to PEG IFN. Lamivudine remains drug of choice in patients with decompensated cirrhosis, and prior to <u>liver transplantation</u> to control replication.
  - <u>ADEFOVIR</u> depixol. Main indication at present as additional therapy in patients on maintenance <u>LAMIVUDINE</u> who develop YMDD variants, especially post-transplantation.
  - Newer antiviral therapies, including other nucleoside/nucleotide analogues, are in final stage of development, and combination therapy is the likely future for treatment.

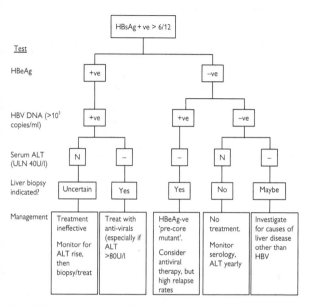

Fig. 2.14 Management algorithm for chronic hepatitis B.

Note. Consider surveillance for hepatocellular carcinoma in all chronically infected patients (e.g. 6 monthly AFP and U/S).

Indications for HBV immunization

Active (hepatitis B vaccine)	Passive (HBIG)
Family contacts of individual with HBV infection	Post-exposure prophylaxis
Babies born to infected mothers (± HBIG if mother HBsAg+ve, HBeAg+ve)	Newborns of mothers who are HBsAg+ve, HBeAg+ve (with vaccine)
IV drug users	
Regular receivers of blood (e.g. haemophilia)	Newborns of mothers with acute hepatitis B in 3rd trimester
Patients with chronic renal failure	
Health care workers	
Sexual contacts of infected individual	
Travellers to areas of high endemicity	

- HBeAg-ve chronic infection ('pre-core mutant'). Need for effective treatment, as disease is often more progressive than HBeAg+ve disease. However, whilst antivirals may control HBV DNA during treatment (e.g. LAMIVUDINE, IFN, PEG IFN, combination), viral replication increases again after cessation.
- Other disease groups. LAMIVUDINE indicated in patients co-infected with HIV, in combination with other antiretroviral therapy. Antiviral therapy leading to control of replication may improve membranous glomerulonephritis and polyarteritis nodosum. LAMIVUDINE given to control replication prior to transplantation, and (± hepatitis B immunoglobulin (HBIG) peri-transplant) may reduce infection of new graft.
- Hepatitis B vaccination. In UK vaccination is not universal, and there are recommendations for temporary passive immunization with hepatitis B immunoglobulin (HBIG) and active immunization (see table on previous page). HBIG contains high titre of anti-HBs and is given at 0.1 ml/kg body weight after exposure (or birth to chronically infected mother). Active vaccination with 10 or 20 µg HBsAg given at 0, 1, and 6 months.

Hepatitis C

Epidemiology

- More than 150 million people worldwide are infected with hepatitis C virus (HCV), an RNA virus of the flavivirus family. Up to 2% of people have been exposed to HCV, with higher rates in Asia and Africa.
- Transmission mainly through injection-drug use (> 60% of cases in UK) or blood-product transfusion (virtually eliminated in developed countries now due to screening of donated blood). Use of non-disposable needles during treatment of schistosomiasis may have contributed to the high prevalence of HCV in Egypt (15% of population). Skin piercing procedures of proven risk. Rate of HCV transmission in monogamous heterosexual relationships appears low (< 6%). Transmission from mother to infant occurs in about 5% of cases, but increased to 18% if mother co-infected with HIV. Breastfeeding transmission not reported. No risk factors reported in 10–20% of cases.
- 6 main HCV genotypes, with subtypes (a–c). Geographical variation in predominant genotype: e.g. 1,2,3 in Europe, USA; genotype 4 in Egypt, Middle East.

Clinical features

- Less than 15% of patients develop acute icteric hepatitis (although spontaneous viral clearance may then occur in up to 50%).
- Chronic infection follows infection in 50–85% of cases, as defined by persistence of HCV RNA in the serum. Infection usually clinically silent, with liver damage occurring over many years. Studies suggest that 20% of patients will develop severe fibrosis/cirrhosis after 20 years of infection, but recent data suggest a lower rate in the absence of cofactors (e.g. alcohol). Risk factors for disease progression include high circulating virus level, long duration of disease, male sex, older age at acquisition, alcohol excess, and co-infection with HIV/hepatitis B.
- Up to 4% of patients per year with HCV cirrhosis develop hepatocellular carcinoma.
- Non-specific complaints, including fatigue, headache, and poor concentration, are commonly reported. HCV may have direct CNS effects.
- Extraintestinal manifestations have been associated with chronic HCV (See box), the pathogenesis of which remains uncertain.

Investigation

- Anti-HCV antibody. Positive ELISA test (and particularly RIBA test) confirms exposure to HCV, but not persistence of infection. May be negative in early phase of acute infection.
- HCV RNA by PCR. HCV RNA positivity confirms ongoing infection, with cut-off variable, but usually 100–1000 viral copies/ml.
- HCV genotype. Essential to determine this in patients considered for treatment, as influences regimen/treatment response.
- Liver function tests. ALT/AST ↑ approximately ×1.5–2.5 ULN in chronic hepatitis C, but fluctuations throughout the course of disease are common, and there is a poor correlation between the level of ALT and either level of viraemia or severity of histological disease. Other liver disease may also need to be excluded.

Extrahepatic associations of hepatitis C

- Cryoglobulinaemia
  - Detectable in 36–54% of chronic patients
  - Most patients asymptomatic
  - Arthralgia and pruritis in 18%
  - Neuropathy and glomerulonephritis in 2%
- Membranous glomerulonephritis
- Sjögren's syndrome
- Lichen planus
- Autoimmune hepatitis
- Thyroiditis
- Polyarteritis nodosum
- Polymyositis
- Porphyria cutanea tarda

- Liver biopsy. Only definitive method of assessing the degree of inflammation (grade) and fibrosis (stage), and may guide a decision concerning need for treatment. Should be considered in all HCV RNA+ve patients, especially if AST/ALT persistently abnormal.
- Additional blood tests. Anti-smooth muscle antibodies as, although they may be an epiphenomenon in chronic HCV, true autoimmune hepatitis is a disease association (see box overleaf), which can be exacerbated by antiviral therapy. Thyroid function tests and anti-thyroid autoantibodies, as abnormalities more common in hepatitis C, and thyroid abnormalities may occur with interferon therapy, particularly in the presence of anti-thyroid antibodies. HBsAg should be tested for as chronic hepatitis B is associated with more progressive histological disease in those with HCV. HIV testing should also be considered, in view of shared modes of acquisition.
- Abdominal U/S prior to liver biopsy, and to identify features of cirrhosis and portal hypertension. Repeat 6 monthly (with alpha fetoprotein) in patients with proven cirrhosis, in view of risk of hepatocellular carcinoma.

Management (see Fig. 2.15, p.381)

- Crucial to ensure that patient is aware of natural history of the disease, as many believe that progression to end-stage liver disease is inevitable, and that treatment is ineffective. Progression usually seen in those who drink excess alcohol, and no safe lower limit of alcohol known.
- Patients should be advised not to donate blood, and the risks of shared needles by drug users should be reiterated. Avoid sharing razors and toothbrushes. Sexual transmission is unusual, but condoms should be used during casual sexual contacts, to lower the risk of a range of transmitted infections (e.g. HIV). It is prudent to test regular sexual partners of patients, but to advise that the risk of transmission is low.
- Vaccinate against hepatitis A and hepatitis B, as co-infection may lead to disease progression (hepatitis B), or fulminant liver failure.

Antiviral therapy

- Treatment has advanced significantly over last 10 years.
- NIH consensus statement declared that treatment is indicated in a patient with positive anti-HCV antibody, positive HCV-RNA, raised liver enzymes (AST, ALT), and moderate–severe hepatitis on liver biopsy, but studies may confirm that treatment benefits all viraemic patients, even if minimal liver injury. Interferon is contraindicated in decompensated cirrhosis.
- Long-acting pegylated-αINTERFERON (PEG-IFN) + RIBAVIRIN has replaced standard αIFN alone as treatment of choice.
- 'Gold standard' for assessing treatment response is sustained virological response (SVR), defined as negative HCV RNA 6 months after completing treatment. Contraindications and side-effects of treatment should be discussed (see table).

Acute hepatitis C. Rare clinical diagnosis, but > 95% SVR with 6 months of INTERFERON ALPHA (IFN-α) monotherapy has been shown (Jaeckel, E. *et al.* (2001). *N. Engl. J. Med.* **345**: 1452). In practice, most experts would use PEG-IFN + RIBAVIRIN in this setting, in view of superior efficacy of this combination in chronic infection (although not as yet proven to be better than standard IFN for acute infection)

Chronic hepatitis C

- Standard IFN-α + RIBAVIRIN for 12 months leads to overall SVR of 38%, with a number of factors influencing treatment response (see second table on previous page).
- For HCV-genotype 2/3, PEG-IFN/RIBAVIRIN gives SVR of 80% on 6 months course (can even reduce to 4 months if HCV RNA negative at 6 weeks). Genotype 1 is less responsive, with 45–55% SVR after 12 month course (discontinue drug if HCV RNA positive at 3 months, as response unlikely).
- Special clinical scenarios in which treatment may be effective, but which require expert involvement include:
  - Patients with HIV/HCV co-infection.
  - Adults who have relapsed following a previous response to treatment.
  - Children with chronic hepatitis C.
- End-stage liver disease due to chronic hepatitis C is now the commonest indication for orthotopic liver transplantation. Recurrence of HCV in the grafted liver is almost universal, with cirrhosis sometimes occurring at an accelerated rate in these immunocompromised patients (up to 10% of patients within 5 years of transplantation).

Side-effects of hepatitis C treatment (also see index of drugs)	
Alpha interferon	
Influenza-like symptoms	Depression (even suicidal ideation)
Nausea	Myelosuppression
Lethargy	Hypersensitivity
Weight loss	Hypo/hyperthyroidism
Autoimmune reactions	Hair loss
Ribavirin	
Haemolysis (2 g fall in Hb usual)	Teratogenicity

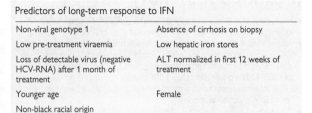

Predictors of long-term response to IFN

Non-viral genotype 1	Absence of cirrhosis on biopsy
Low pre-treatment viraemia	Low hepatic iron stores
Loss of detectable virus (negative HCV-RNA) after 1 month of treatment	ALT normalized in first 12 weeks of treatment
Younger age	Female
Non-black racial origin	

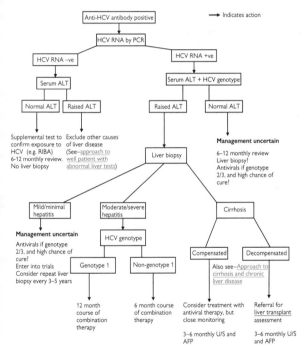

Fig. 2.15 Management of hepatitis C.

Hepatitis D virus (HDV)

- RNA virus that requires <u>hepatitis B</u> virus (HBV) for complete virion assembly (5% of HBV carriers co-infected with HDV).
- As with HBV infection, HDV may cause acute hepatitis (even <u>acute liver failure</u>), asymptomatic viral carriage, or progressive chronic liver disease with cirrhosis and <u>portal hypertension</u> (more aggressive course of HDV/HBV co-infection than HBV alone). For uncertain reasons, HDV infection associated with lower risk of <u>hepatocellular carcinoma</u> than HBV infection alone.
- Presence of HBsAg necessary for diagnosis of hepatitis D. Anti-HDV IgM present in acute infection, and IgG antibodies appear in resolved or chronic infection. In contrast to hepatitis B, IgM antibodies persist at high titre in chronic infection. Serum HDV RNA detectable by PCR in acute infection and chronic disease, but test not widely available.
- Vaccination against <u>hepatitis B</u> protects against hepatitis D.
- Treatment with standard IFN (9 MU × 3/week) for 48 weeks has been associated with reduced HDV RNA, but most studies show increased viral replication following cessation of a range of treatments, and antiviral therapy remains disappointing.
- <u>Liver transplantation</u> may be required in decompensated HDV/HBV cirrhosis (again, post-transplant survival better for HDV/HBV co-infection than for HBV alone, possibly related to inhibitory effects of HDV on HBV).

Hepatitis E virus (HEV)

- RNA virus that is endemic in India, Pakistan, Middle East, and Southeast Asia (accounts for > 90% of major hepatitis outbreaks in India).
- Virus spread by faecal–oral route, in association with poor sanitation (with epidemics often during monsoon season, on 10 year cycle).
- Incubation period 15–65 days, followed by acute icteric hepatitis (jaundice, malaise, nausea, anorexia). Cholestatic hepatitis more common than for hepatitis A or hepatitis B. Chronic hepatitis never occurs, and usually settles clinically within 6 weeks.
- Acute liver failure may occur, with a reported maternal mortality in those infected in 3rd trimester of > 20%.
- Diagnosis made by excluding other causes of acute hepatitis (see Approach to recent-onset jaundice), and IgM anti-HEV in the serum confirms recent infection (may be performed in specialist laboratories).
- Treatment is supportive, with liver transplantation considered for those with acute liver failure.

Hepatitis G virus (HGV)

HGV, and closely related GB virus, appear to be parenterally transmitted viruses, and were originally thought to be cause, in some cases, of non-A–E hepatitis. However, no clear evidence that they cause liver disease.

Hepatobiliary scintigraphy (e.g. HIDA scan)

Hepatobiliary iminodiacetic acid (HIDA) scan employs radioactive tracer that is excreted by liver into bile. Sequential scanning over 2 hours performed. Main uses include the diagnosis of:
- Acute cholecystitis (95% accuracy reported).
- Bile duct leak post-cholecystectomy.
- Cystic duct patency (e.g. blocked due to stone, tumour).
- Hepatic dysfunction (impaired excretion into bile).
- Sphincter of Oddi dysfunction.

In practice, HIDA scanning largely replaced by other imaging modalities.

Hepatocellular carcinoma (HCC)

Epidemiology

- 6th commonest cancer worldwide.
- 75–90% of patients with HCC have cirrhosis, and this complication develops in 4% of cirrhotics per year (less common if cirrhosis due to autoimmune hepatitis, primary biliary cirrhosis). Chronic hepatitis B increases risk of HCC 100-fold. Rare in hepatitis C in the absence of cirrhosis. Other risks include aflatoxins produced by fungi on nuts stored in damp conditions (e.g. common aetiology of HCC in North Africa, China).

Clinical features

- Pain, weight loss, anorexia, malaise are common symptoms.
- Hepatomegaly common; hepatic bruit sometimes found.
- HCC may be the precipitating cause of hepatic decompensation and hepatic encephalopathy.
- 10% of patients present with variceal bleeding, which may be linked to portal vein thrombosis.

Investigations

- Alpha fetoprotein (AFP) elevated in 70% of cases, with levels > 400 ng/ml strongly suggestive of HCC (normal range < 20 ng/ml). However, high levels also seen during hepatitis flares (i.e. in association with ↑↑ALT). > 60% HCCs < 4 cm have AFP < 200 ng/ml.
- Ultrasound widely used in screening/surveillance, and first modality if ↑AFP (sensitivity 95% for 1.5–3 cm HCCs). See box for differential diagnosis.
- CT or MRI may be necessary, particularly for multifocal HCC in cirrhotic liver.
- Angiography (± lipiodol) indicated if clinical suspicion (e.g. ↑↑AFP), but no mass on U/S, CT, MRI.
- Liver biopsy confirms histological diagnosis, but avoided if resection an option, because of risk (albeit < 2%) of needle track seeding.

Management

- Range of options for HCCs confined to the liver, determined by number, size, distribution of tumours, and underlying liver histology/function, but ongoing debate on optimal treatment. Without treatment, 3 year survival for small HCC in non-cirhotic liver 45%.
- Hepatic resection if HCC confined to single lobe of non-cirrhotic liver (liver biopsy of non-tumourous lobe indicated prior to surgery), with 45–60% 5 year survival. Resection also indicated in well-compensated cirrhosis (Child–Pugh score A), but risk of decompensation.
- Liver transplantation effective for decompensated cirrhotic with solitary HCC < 5 cm, or no more than 3 lesions all < 3 cm.
- In non-surgical candidates with localized HCCs local ablation (e.g. percutaneous alcohol injection or radiofrequency ablation) may provide good palliation, and survival comparable with hepatic resection, with mortality largely correlated with underlying liver function.

- Transcatheter chemoembolization (TACE) relies on engendering ischaemia in HCC, and targeting chemotherapy, but is contraindicated in decompensated cirrhosis and multifocal HCC.
- Systemic chemotherapy regimes disappointing to date.

Surveillance for HCC (probably with 6 monthly U/S and AFP) indicated for all patients with cirrhosis (although rate of HCC appears lower for auto-immune aetiologies, such as primary biliary cirrhosis); haemochromatosis; and chronic hepatitis B (irrespective of presence of cirrhosis).

Causes of mass lesions in liver

- Hepatocellular carcinoma
- Fibrolamellar carcinoma
- Metastases (commonest cause, due to e.g. colon, pancreas, gastric cancer, neuroendocrine tumour)
- Intrahepatic cholangiocarcinoma
- Gallbladder carcinoma
- Focal nodular hyperplasia
- Nodular regenerative hyperplasia
- Hepatic adenoma
- Haemangioma
- Liver abscess*
- Hydatid disease*
- Lymphoma
- Angiosarcoma
- Benign regenerative nodule
- Simple cyst*

* Cystic lesions.

Hepatorenal syndrome (HRS)

Background

- HRS is defined as development of renal failure in patients with severe liver disease (acute or chronic), in absence of other cause of renal pathology.
  - **Type 1 HRS** occurs acutely, often in conjunction with acute liver disease or decompensation of cirrhosis. Often in association with marked jaundice and coagulopathy.
  - **Type 2 HRS** is more chronic, usually in patients with refractory ascites and relatively mild jaundice.
- Common clinical mistake is to assume that any 'liver' patient with renal impairment has hepatorenal syndrome. Wide range of other causes (see table opposite).
- Pathological process in HRS is that of profound renal arteriolar vaso-constriction leading to renal hypoperfusion in setting of haemodynamic changes of decompensated liver disease (↑ heart rate, ↑ cardiac output, ↓ systemic vascular resistance, ↓ mean arterial pressure).

Diagnosis

- Clinical diagnosis based around major diagnostic criteria:
  - Acute or chronic liver disease with advanced hepatic failure.
  - Serum creatinine > 200 µmol/l, or creatinine clearance < 40 ml/min.
  - Other causes of renal impairment excluded (hypovolaemia, bacterial sepsis, nephrotoxic drugs).
  - No sustained improvement with 1.5 l plasma expansion.
  - Proteinuria < 0.5 g/day.
  - Normal renal tract U/S.
- Note that low urinary Na^+ no longer major criterion for diagnosis.

Management

- Stop all potentially nephrotoxic drugs (e.g. diuretics).
- Correct hypovolaemia (give 1.5 l crystalloid or colloid—and more if clearly volume depleted (see also <u>albumin (use in liver disease)</u>).
- Consider terlipressin.
- Search for and treat sepsis (common precipitant of liver decompensation). Send blood, sputum, urine, ascitic fluid.
- Drain ascites if tense (see <u>paracentesis</u>).
- Consider renal support (usually haemofiltration) if likely improvement in liver function/liver transplantation. (HRS rarely resolves unless liver function improves. HRS has 50–95% mortality dependent on aetiology.)

Hereditary angio-oedema

See: <u>angio-oedema</u>.

Causes of renal dysfunction in patient with liver disease

Hepatorenal syndrome	Leptospirosis
Hypovolaemia (e.g. over diuresis)	Amyloidosis
Nephrotoxic drugs (e.g. NSAIDs, aminoglycosides, paracetamol)	Membranous glomerulonephritis (e.g. due to hepatitis B)
Sepsis	Renal tubular abnormalities
Polycystic disease	Acute fatty liver of pregnancy

Hereditary haemorrhagic telangiectasia (Osler–Weber–Rendu syndrome)

Rendu was first to describe the condition in 1896: should really be Rendu–Osler–Weber.

- Autosomal dominant disorder characterized by telangiectasia of the skin and mucous membranes. see Colour Plate 14.
- Commonest presentation is epistaxis at puberty: the cutaneous telangiectasia can appear later, usually before 20 years. Severe GI bleeds occur, usually after age of 40. Melaena is most common manifestation. The telangiectasia are easily seen at endoscopy. Angiography may show the arteriovenous (AV) malformations. Pathologically the disease affects capillaries, venules, and less commonly arterioles. Pulmonary AV malformations occur in 20%, especially those families with HHT1, caused by a mutation in the endoglin gene on chromosome 9: this can lead to high output cardiac failure. Arteriovenous malformations occur less commonly in the cerebral and hepatic circulations. HHT2 maps to chromosome 12 where mutations have been identified in the ALK-1 gene.
- Treatment is difficult; options include oestrogens, aminocaproic acid, endoscopic ablation, and bowel resection. Endoscopic ablation including the use of <u>argon plasma coagulation</u> and thermal contact devices is probably the most promising.

Hereditary non-polyposis colon cancer (HNPCC)

- An autosomal dominant condition, causing about 5% of <u>colon cancers</u>. Cancer arises in discrete adenomas but polyposis does not occur. About 80% are caused by germline mutations in genes involved in repair of DNA damaged during replication (this tends to occur at repetitive DNA sequences called microsatellites). These genes are called mismatch repair genes and include hMSH2 on chromosome 2 (40–50%) and hMLH1 on chromosome 3 (20–30%).
- The best known criteria for defining HNPCC are the 'Amsterdam' criteria (see box). However these criteria do not account for the frequent occurrence of non-colonic cancers in these families. There may be early onset of endometrial, ovarian, upper urinary tract, small intestinal, and stomach cancer.
- **Clinical features** of HNPCC compared with sporadic cancers are shown in the table. There is a high incidence of synchronous and metachronous tumours (mean annual rate of about 3%).
- **Diagnosis** of HNPCC is still made on clinical grounds, but identification of the responsible genes suggests that genetic testing will become available.
- **Screening**. Lifetime risk for colorectal cancer is about 1 in 2: start colonoscopy screening at 25 years old or 5 years before earliest colon cancer in family; repeat every 2 years (upper GI screening also required).

Hereditary pancreatitis

- Hereditary pancreatitis displays autosomal dominant pattern due to specific genetic defect. Familial pancreatitis is more generic term when more members in family affected with pancreatitis than expected, but without obvious cause.
- Range of mutations in hereditary pancreatitis (e.g. in cationic trypsinogen gene (PRSS1), secretory trypsin inhibitor gene (SPINK1)). Trypsinogen converts to trypsin, which then activates pancreatic proenzymes to enzymes (except <u>amylase</u> and lipase). Trypsinogen conversion is tightly controlled; hence trypsinogen gene mutations associated with excess enzyme production, autodigestion, and pancreatitis.
- Genetic testing available, and 80% with PRSS1, R122H, or N29I mutations will develop pancreatitis (80% penetrance). Negative test in family with known mutation eliminates risk.
- Recurrent episodes of pancreatitis begin < 40 years (mean 10 years), with chronic pancreatitis developing in 50%. Standard management for <u>acute</u> and <u>chronic pancreatitis</u> applies.
- Cumulative risk of <u>pancreatic cancer</u> may be > 40% by 70 years. No effective cancer screening programme established for gene carriers.

Amsterdam II criteria for hereditary non-polyposis colorectal cancer

At least three relatives with HNPCC-associated cancer (colorectal cancer, cancer of the endometrium, small bowel, ureter, or renal pelvis) plus all of the following:
1 One affected patient is a first-degree relative of the other two
2 Two or more successive generations affected
3 One or more cases of colon cancer diagnosed before age 50
4 FAP excluded
5 Tumours verified by pathological examination

Clinical features of HNPCC compared with sporadic colon cancer (Reproduced with permission from Feldman M, Friedman LS, Sleisenger MH, and Scharschmidt BF (1998). *Sleisenger and Fordtran's gastrointestinal and liver disease*, 7th edn. W.B. Saunders, Philadelphia)

	HNPCC	**Sporadic cancer**
Mean age at diagnosis (years)	45	65
Multiple cancers	35%	4–11%
Proximal location	72%	35%
Excess malignancy at other sites	Yes	No
Mucinous tumours	Common	Rare
Prognosis	Favourable	Variable

Hereditary polyposis

Inherited polyposis may be broadly considered in terms of adenomatous and hamartomatous syndromes.

Adenomatous polyposis syndromes

Range of inherited adenomatous polyposis syndromes characterized by the development of large numbers of adenomatous polyps in the colon, and high risk of <u>colon cancer</u>.

- <u>Familial adenomatous polyposis</u> (FAP).
- <u>Gardner's syndrome</u>. Similar intestinal polyp pattern to that of FAP, with additional thyroid/adrenal tumours, fibromas, desmoid tumours, and bone tumours. Associated with APC gene.
- <u>Turcot's syndrome</u>. Colonic adenomas (usually fewer than in FAP), with medulloblastoma.

Hamartomatous polyposis syndromes

Hamartomas are of mesenchymal origin, and carry lower risk of malignant change than adenomas. However, increased cancer risk (GI and non-GI seen in these conditions).

- <u>Peutz Jeghers syndrome</u>.
- <u>Juvenile polyposis syndrome</u>.
- <u>Cowden's disease</u>.

See also <u>hereditary non-polyposis colon cancer</u> (HNPCC).

<u>Cronkite–Canada</u> syndrome is a rare, non-inherited cause of polyposis.

Herpes simplex

A DNA virus, causing painful vesicles with erythematous bases in squamous epithelium of skin, mouth, oesophagus. Resolution of infection is followed by latency in roots and ganglia supplying affected regions.

90% of cases of primary herpetic gingivostomatitis occur in people before puberty. Recurrent orolabial herpes simplex is common and precipitated by illness, sunlight, or stress. Topical <u>ACICLOVIR</u> speeds healing and reduces severity. Immunosuppression predisposes to infection but the symptoms may be milder (e.g. just nausea and vomiting, while immunocompetent people may have acutely painful swallowing). Also see <u>HIV and the gut</u>.

Diagnosis usually made at endoscopy (see Colour Plate 14). 1–3 mm vesicles appear in mid–distal oesophagus: the centres slough to form 'volcano' lesions. Biopsies for diagnosis should include epithelium. Virus can be detected by culture or immunostaining within 24 hours. Treatment is with <u>ACICLOVIR</u>, although resistant strains are beginning to emerge. Complications of untreated disease include mucosal necrosis, oesophageal perforation, haemorrhage, strictures, HSV pneumonia, <u>tracheo-oesophageal fistulae</u>. Perianal infection can occur, especially in AIDS patients, usually with HSV type 2. This causes painful ulcers, tenesmus, and occasional bleeding. Treatment is with <u>ACICLOVIR</u> and topical anaesthetics: avoid steroid ointments.

HSV can also infect the colon and is a cause of bloody diarrhoea in immunocompromised patients; sigmoidoscopy shows characteristic vesicles.

Herpes zoster

Zoster can cause severe <u>oesophagitis</u> in immunocompromised people (see <u>HIV and the gut</u>), although oesophageal involvement is relatively mild compared with that seen in encephalitis, pneumonitis, and hepatitis). Zoster can be distinguished from simplex by culture or immunostaining but much more practically by the presence of skin lesions (rare with HSV). Gastric involvement is rare. T7 through L1 nerve involvement can cause abdominal pain before lesions appear. Sacral nerve root involvement can give constipation and pain with defecation.

Treatment with <u>ACICLOVIR</u>, and foscarnet as second-line treatment.

Hiatus hernia

Two types: a **sliding hernia**, when the gastro-oesophageal junction and some part of the stomach are displaced above the diaphragm (the commonest type, accounting for about 95%; usually small and of no clinical significance), or **para-oesophageal**, when the stomach protrudes through the oesophageal hiatus alongside the oesophagus.

Most sliding hernias are small but can predispose to gastro-oesophageal reflux (see also <u>Approach to dyspepsia and gastro-oesophageal reflux</u>). Large hernias may develop Cameron ulcers, usually on the lesser curve at the level of the hiatus: they can cause upper or lower GI bleeding or be a cause of iron deficiency anaemia.

Treatment. Simple sliding hiatus hernias do not need treatment. Giant or para-oesophageal hernias may require surgery (see <u>anti-reflux procedures</u>).

Hirschsprung's disease

Harald Hirschsprung (1830–1916)—the first paediatrician to be appointed in Denmark.

An important cause of congenital <u>megacolon</u>. Hirschsprung's occurs in 1:5000 live births. Autosomal dominant or recessive inheritance, with low penetration (30%). Absence of ganglion cells from myenteric and submucosal plexuses, extending proximally from internal anal sphincter, is characteristic.

Clinical features. Usually presents after birth with failure to pass meconium, and later in childhood with recurrent faecal impaction, constipation, and malnutrition. May be complicated by enterocolitis in infancy. Overflow rarely occurs. Associated with multiple endocrine neoplasia (MEN)-2 and <u>Down syndrome</u>.

Investigation

- Barium enema may show a narrowed distal rectum free of faeces, with proximal colonic dilatation.
- Procto-sigmoidoscopy normal, with deep rectal biopsy showing absence of ganglion cells in submucosa.
- Anorectal manometry may show that resting internal anal sphincter pressure is normal/elevated, and that, in response to rectal distension, internal anal sphincter contracts (rather than relaxes, with compensatory external sphincter contraction, as in normal 'rectal inhibitory reflex').

Management

Primary treatment is surgery, aimed at excising the aganglionic segment. Colostomy prior to definitive surgery may be required. Persistent problems with soiling may occur in approximately 10%.

HIV and the gut

Background and aetiology

- All areas of GI tract may be affected (also see <u>HIV and the liver</u>).
- Before development of highly active antiretroviral therapy (HAART) opportunistic infections associated with immunocompromise were major cause of GI problems. Now, drug-induced side-effects and other non-opportunistic diseases are more common (see table).

Clinical feature

Broad categories of presentation include:

- **Oesophageal disease**: dyspepsia/dysphagia/odynophagia (pain on swallowing: suggests oesophageal ulceration (e.g. <u>cytomegalovirus</u> (CMV), <u>herpes simplex virus</u> (HSV)).
- **Abdominal pain.** Any cause of this in the non-HIV patient can, of course, be the culprit in the patient with HIV. Inflammation, ulceration, perforation of any point in GI tract may be caused by range of pathogens, including CMV. <u>Acute pancreatitis</u> due to HAART, CMV, or infiltration by Kaposi's sarcoma.
- **Diarrhoea** occurred in 90% of patients in pre-HAART era. Still common; now related to side-effects of HAART (20% in patients taking protease inhibitor nelfinavir), and causes not related to opportunistic infection/malignancy.
- **Anorectal disease:** most common in homosexual men with HIV, with increased risk of anal squamous cell carcinoma related to HPV.

Investigation

- CD4 count guides investigation and differential diagnosis (opportunistic infections unlikely if CD4 > 200/µl).
- 3 stool samples for microscopy and culture essential in patients with diarrhoea.
- Upper GI endoscopy in oesophageal disease, and colonoscopy necessary if diarrhoea persistent, stool samples negative, and CD4 > 200/µl. Classic appearances may suggest diagnosis endoscopi- cally (e.g. large deep oesophageal ulcers due to CMV), but histology necessary. Vital that pathologists provided with details re HIV status, CD4 count, and suspected diagnosis. Check with referring clinicians re special requirements (e.g. biopsies into viral culture medium).

Management

- Effective treatment depends on making a specific diagnosis.
- In patient presenting with opportunistic infection, commencement of HAART, with subsequent immune reconstitution, may negate necessity of antimicrobials for opportunistic infection (e.g. <u>Cryptosporidium</u>).
- Candidal oesophagitis treated with fluconazole 100 mg od for a week, but maintainance often required. Active CMV disease treated with 2–3 week course of ganciclovir IV. Idiopathic ulceration responds well to oral or intralesional steroids.
- Treatment of diarrhoea depends on isolating cause. Enteric pathogens (e.g. <u>Salmonella</u>, <u>Shigella</u>) treated with standard antibiotics, but treat- ment for protozoal infections (e.g. <u>Cryptosporidium</u>) less effective, particularly if low CD4.

Common GI problems in HIV patients and their causes

Cause	Comment
Oesophageal disease (dysphagia/odynophagia)	
Candida albicans	<u>Oesophagitis</u> usually linked with oral thrush. Suggests CD4 < 200/µl
<u>Cytomegalovirus</u> (CMV)	Large deep ulcers
Idiopathic ulcers	Small aphthous ulcers. Usually when CD4 < 200/µl
<u>Herpes simplex virus</u> (HSV)	Diffuse, shallow ulcers
Kaposi's sarcoma, lymphoma	Often develops in oral cavity
Diarrhoea	
Bacterial: <u>Salmonella</u>, <u>Shigella</u>, <u>Campylobacter</u>, <u>Clostridium difficile</u>. <u>Mycobacterium</u> TB (MTB)/*avium* complex (MAC) <u>Bacterial overgrowth</u>	*Salmonella*, *Shigella* more common in HIV patient, even on HAART. MAC most common identified GI opportunistic infection if low CD4. Acid-fast staining of biopsies
Protozoal: *Cryptosporidium*, *Micros-poridium*, *Entamoeba* (see <u>hydatid</u>)	Oocytes of *Cryptosporidium* found on faecal smears. Treatment difficult, but may improve with HAART
Fungal: *Histoplasma*, *Cryptococcosis*	Diffuse colitis with histoplasmosis. Treatment with amphotericin B
Viral: <u>Cytomegalovirus</u>, <u>Herpes simplex virus</u>, <u>adenovirus</u>	CMV colitis in 5–10% with AIDS. Mucosal ulceration with inclusion bodies on histology Treatment IV ganciclovir.
'AIDS enteropathy'	Chronic diarrhoea in AIDS, where no cause found. Increasingly uncommon with more intensive investigation
Drugs: e.g. protease inhibitors	Diarrhoea mild/mod, no weight loss
Kaposi's sarcoma (KS), lymphoma	KS may cause ulceration and chronic diarrhoea, but usually asymptomatic
<u>Pancreatic insufficiency</u>	
Anorectal disease	
Chlamydia trachomatis, *Neisseria gonorrhoeae*	Most common in homosexual men
<u>Herpes simplex virus</u>	Perianal ulceration and proctitis
Human papilloma virus	Cause of anal warts, linked to anal Ca
Idiopathic ulcers	Usually when CD4 < 200/µl

HIV and the liver

Background and aetiology

Liver test abnormalities occur in 80% of patients with HIV, due to:

- Coexistent liver disease. <u>Hepatitis B</u> and <u>hepatitis C</u> common, due to similar modes of acquisition, and run more aggressive course than in non-HIV patient. Acute exacerbation of liver disease may occur following start of anti-HIV treatment due to enhanced immunity against hepatitis B.
- Immunosuppression-related infection (e.g. CD4 < 50μl): e.g. *Mycobacterium avium intercellulare* (MAI), *M. tuberculosis* (MTB), fungal infection (e.g. *Histoplasma capsulatum*), *Pneumocystis carinii*.
- Treatment. Highly active retroviral therapy (HAART) frequently associated with LFT derangement (see table). Acute liver failure may occur, with syndrome of hepatomegaly, steatosis, lactic acidosis, and liver failure probably related to mitochondrial toxicity. Severe toxicity in 10% taking non-nucleoside reverse transcriptase inhibitor nevirapine.
- Tumours, including non-Hodgkin's lymphoma, Kaposi's sarcoma.
- Biliary disease. HIV-cholangiopathy associated with low CD4 count, with diffuse <u>biliary strictures</u> similar to <u>primary sclerosing cholangitis</u>, or distal biliary stricture/papillitis.

Clinical features Variable, dependent on type of liver injury. Hepatomegaly common.

Investigations

- In view of high frequency of LFT derangement, clinical balance needed between not missing important/reversible liver disease, and exposing otherwise well patient to invasive investigations.
- See <u>Approaches to recent-onset jaundice</u> and <u>well patient with abnormal liver tests</u>. Viral serology should be performed in all cases.
- <u>U/S</u> or <u>CT</u> may exclude biliary dilatation or liver masses.
- <u>ERCP</u> may be necessary to diagnose HIV cholangiopathy.
- Liver biopsy abnormalities in 90% (e.g. *hepatic granulomas*, steatosis), but 'new' diagnoses only made in 8% of biopsies in HIV patients (e.g. Kaposi's sarcoma, mycobacterium).

Management

- Depends on making a specific diagnosis.
- <u>Hepatitis B</u> coinfection usually treated with lamivudine, which is also active against HIV, as part of combination HAART.
- Standard treatment for <u>hepatitis C</u> appears to be less effective in patients with, than without, HIV, but sustained responses possible.
- LFTs should be regularly monitored during HAART (especially first 8 weeks and with reverse transcriptase inhibitors), and stopped if signs of significant hepatotoxocity (e.g. serum ALT > ×5 ULN).
- Mitochondrial toxicity and liver failure have been successfully treated with <u>liver transplantation</u>.

Common drug causes of liver derangement in HIV patients

Drug	Type/use
Indinavir	Anti-HIV protease inhibitor
Saquinovir	
Ritonovir	
Stavudine	Anti-HIV reverse transcriptase inhibitor
Didanosine	
Nevirapine	
Trimethoprim–sulfamethoxazole	*Pneumocystis* prophylaxis/treatment
Ketoconazole	Antifungal
Isoniazid	Anti-TB
Rifampicin	

Hookworms

See: <u>round worms</u>.

Hydatid disease (see Colour Plate 14)

Epidemiology + pathogenesis

Caused by tapeworm *Echinococcus*. Most commonly seen in farming or rural communities, where man is an accidental host for *E. granulosum*, whose life cycle usually involves the ingestion of eggs by a definite host (carnivore, e.g. dog), from an infected intermediate host (e.g. sheep).

Clinical features

Cystic echinococcosis affects the liver (63% of cases), lungs (25%), and more rarely bones, kidneys, brain.

Many cysts asymptomatic, but may cause symptoms due to mass effect (e.g. obstructive jaundice, abdominal pain) or cyst complications (rupture with anaphylaxis, secondary infection).

Investigations

- Echinococcus ELISA has 90% sensitivity for hepatic echinococcosis.
- Eosinophilia in 25%; LFTs may be elevated in patients with hepatic disease.
- CT is 98% accurate, and highly sensitive at demonstrating characteristic daughter cysts.

Management

- Surgery is optimal approach, as only 30% are cured with medical therapy alone. Surgery includes cystectomy alone, or partial affected organ resection. During surgery, sterilization of the cyst, and prevention of spillage, with risk of anaphylaxis, is essential. Chemotherapy with benzimidazoles (e.g. albendazole, mebendazole) is given for at least 1 month over perioperative period to prevent secondary infection.
- If surgery is not an option, 'PAIR' technique of aspiration of cyst contents and injection of a scolicidal agent, followed by isotonic saline, in conjunction with oral benimidazole treatment, may be effective.

Hydrogen breath test

See: <u>breath tests</u>.

Hypogammaglobulinaemia

See: <u>immunoglobulin deficiency</u>.

I

Ileal pouch–anal anastomosis (IPAA)

The procedure of choice for patients requiring proctocolectomy for <u>ulcerative colitis</u> or <u>familial adenomatous polyposis</u>. Advantages include:

- Removal of nearly all mucosal disease (in contrast to ileorectal anastomosis).
- Stoma not required.
- Anal sphincters not disturbed.
- Pelvic dissection should not affect sexual function.

A pouch needs to be constructed from ileum because direct anastomosis of ileum to anal verge results in excess stool frequency and anal seepage. There are several forms of pouch (see diagram): the J pouch is the easiest of these to construct and has functional outcomes identical to those of the more complex designs.

Clinical results. Average post-pouch stool frequency is 6 times a day and once at night. Incontinence more than twice per week occurs in 5% by day and 12% by night: minor nocturnal incontinence occurs in up to 30% at 1 year post op. 30% need to wear a pad to protect against see page.

Long-term results. Overall morbidity is 25–30%. Failure is rare provided the operation is not done in error in patients with <u>Crohn's disease</u>. The most important factor is probably an experienced surgeon.

Complications are shown in the table opposite.

<u>**Pouchitis:**</u> see separate entry.

Technical issues

Role of defunctioning ileostomy. Reported rates of pelvic sepsis vary from 0 to 25% but are higher in patients undergoing a one-stage procedure. Indications for defunctioning ileostomy include steroids at the time of surgery, nutritional compromise, emergency surgery, and any concerns at operation about blood supply or anastomotic tension.

Stapled vs hand-sewn anastomosis. A debate arising because of the opposing benefits of removing all colonic mucosa (implying a mucosal strip and technically demanding hand-sewn anastomosis) and preserving a cuff of colonic mucosa to improve functional outcome. A randomized trial at the Mayo clinic found no difference in complication rate, but less night-time incontinence and better anal pressures in the stapled group. Most surgeons use a stapled anastomosis.

Risk of cancer and dysplasia. There is a small risk of cancer in the retained rectal mucosa, estimated at less than 1% at 2 years post-op. This risk is higher if there was cancer or dysplasia in the original colectomy specimen.

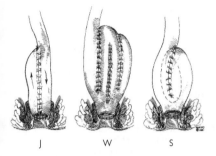

J   W   S

Fig. 2.16 Three types of ileal pouch. Reproduced from Feldman M, Friedman LS, and Sleisenger MH (2003). *Sleisenger and Fordtran's Gastrointestinal and Liver Disease*, with permission from Elsevier

Complications of ileal pouch–anal anastomosis (IPAA)

Complication	Rate
Pelvic infection	5%
Abdominal sepsis	6%
Small bowel obstruction	17%
Peritonitis on closing ileostomy	4%
Anastomotic stricture	Very high: usually easy to dilate digitally
Impotence and retrograde ejaculation	1.5% and 4% men
Dyspareunia	7%

Ileostomy

Operations that expose the ileal serosa to ileal effluent result in serositis. The **Brooke ileostomy** invented in the 1950s involves everting the mucosa and suturing it to the skin. This ileostomy is incontinent: a variation called a 'Koch pouch' features an ileal pouch, a nipple valve, and an ileal conduit leading to a cutaneous stoma that can be flush with the skin.

All ileostomies should discharge between 300 and 800 g material per day: 90% of this is water.

Sequelae of ileostomy. Urine is more concentrated. Incidence of urolithiasis is about 5%. Resection of terminal ileum may lead to <u>bile acid malabsorption</u> and <u>vitamin B12</u> deficiency.

Complications of ileostomy. Stomal obstruction causes pain, increased ileal discharge, and fluid and electrolyte depletion. Mechanical problems with poorly fitting stomal appliances can cause skin excoriation or even fistula formation.

Ileus

The failure of forward passage of intestinal contents in the absence of mechanical obstruction. There are several common causes in hospitalized patients—see box.

Intestinal motility is impaired after abdominal surgery or injury. Small bowel motility usually returns in 24 h, followed by gastric motility in 2 days and colonic motility in 3–5 days. The duration of operation and degree of manipulation do not appear to influence the length of ileus.

Clinical features. Poorly localized abdominal pain. Nausea, vomiting, reduced or absent bowel sounds. Differentiation from obstruction is usually possible based on gas in stomach, small intestine, and colon on plain X-ray. Passage of contrast, either on barium or CT imaging can assist in the diagnosis. CT can also show inflammatory processes like pancreatitis, abscesses, or retroperitoneal haemorrhage.

Management. Post-laparotomy, limit oral intake, maintain intravascular volume, correct electrolyte imbalances. Pass a nasogastric tube if there is distension or vomiting. Search for a cause (see box) if ileus lasts for more than 5 days. Giving a poorly absorbed opioid antagonist may shorten post-operative ileus: this approach is currently under evaluation.

Immunoglobulin deficiency

Congenital causes

X-linked (Bruton) defect of B-cell maturation resulting in absence of functional antibodies. Patients present with recurrent pyogenic infection in infancy or childhood: GI infections occur in 30%, usually with *Campylobacter* or less often *Giardia*. T-cell function is normal. There is an increased risk of <u>lymphoma</u> and leukaemia.

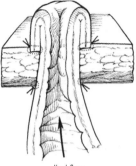

Ileal flow

Fig. 2.17 Ileostomy, showing evertal mucosa. Reproduced from Feldman M, Friedman LS, and Sleisenger MH (2003). *Sleisenger and Fordtran's Gastrointestinal and Liver Disease*, with permission from Elsevier

Causes of ileus

- **Laparotomy**
- **Electrolyte disturbance:** low K or Na, low or high Mg
- **Drugs:** narcotics, phenothiazines, anticholinergics
- **Intra-abdominal inflammation:** <u>appendicits</u>, <u>diverticulitis</u>, perforated DU
- **Retroperitoneal inflammation:** lumbar fracture, <u>pancreatitis</u>, pyelonephritis
- **Intestinal ischaemia:** arterial embolus or thrombosis, mesenteric venous thrombosis
- **Thoracic disease:** MI, lower lobe pneumonia
- **Systemic sepsis**

Selective IgA deficiency has a prevalence of 1/500 to 1/3000. Usually sporadic; reversible deficiency has been reported after salazopyrine, phenytoin, and penicillamine. There is little if any increased risk of GI infection: there is an association with coeliac disease and pernicious anaemia but the main risk is false negative tests for IgA anti-reticulin and anti-endomysial antibodies.

Acquired causes

Common variable hypogammaglobulinaemia usually involved defective terminal differentiation of B cells. Patients present in second or third decades with chest infections or diarrhoea. 2/3 of those with diarrhoea have malabsorption; *Giardia* is common. There is increased risk of bacterial overgrowth, parasitic and bacterial enteric infection. Atrophic gastritis and pernicious anaemia can develop.

Inflammatory bowel disease

See: microscopic colitis, ulcerative colitis, and Crohn's disease.

Intestinal ischaemia

Can be acute or chronic, due to arterial disease or venous disease, and can affect small bowel, colon, or both. The anatomy of splanchnic circulation is shown in the figure opposite.

Collateral circulation to stomach, duodenum, and rectum accounts for rarity of ischaemic episodes affecting these organs. The splenic flexure and sigmoid colon are most at risk.

Acute mesenteric ischaemia

Usually arterial, most commonly superior artery embolus, less commonly non-occlusible mesenteric ischaemia or thrombosis of SMA. Venous thrombosis accounts for only 5–10% of patients with acute mesenteric ischaemia. Most patients with arterial thrombosis have significant generalized arteriosclerosis.

Colonic ischaemia (ischaemic colitis). The commonest form of intestinal ischaemia.

Clinical features. Sudden onset cramping pain in left iliac fossa, with fresh or altered blood pr mixed with stool within 24 h, and mild to moderate tenderness over the bowel. Diagnosis is made by careful colonoscopy or (perhaps better) contrast-enhanced CT scanning. Barium studies are less sensitive than colonoscopy: the classical 'thumbprinting' disappears in days as submucosal haemorrhages are resorbed and overlying mucosa sloughs. Management is conservative (fluids IV, bowel rest, broad spectrum antibiotics) if there is no sign of perforation or gangrene. Increasing tenderness, fever, ileus suggest infarction and mandate operative intervention. More than 50% resolve on conservative management.

Intestinal angina (chronic mesenteric ischaemia)

Uncommon, causing pain due to small bowel ischaemia as gastric blood flow increases after a meal. Clinical features: classically pain within 30 minutes of eating, resolving over 1–3 h. The best test is angiography, with balloon angioplasty as the preferred therapy. Recurrence after angioplasty is common but may be reduced by stenting.

Vasculitis of splanchnic circulation

<u>Polyarteritis nodosa</u> and rheumatoid arthritis can affect large vessels and any cause of systemic vasculitis can cause small vessel occlusion and segmental ischaemia.

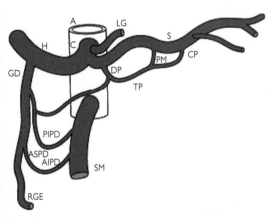

Fig. 2.18 Diagram of typical coeliac axis anatomy and branching pattern.
A, aorta; C, coeliac axis; H, hepatic artery; GD, gastroduodenal artery; LG, left gastric artery; S, splenic artery; DP, dorsal pancreatic artery; TP, transverse pancreatic artery; PM, pancreata magna; CP, caudal pancreatic artery; SM, superior mesenteric artery; PIPD, posterior inferior pancreaticoduodenal artery; ASPD, anterior superior pancreaticoduodenal artery; AIPD, anterior inferior pancreaticoduodenal artery; RGE, right gastroepiploic artery.
Reproduced from Feldman M, Friedman LS, and Sleisenger MH (2003).
Sleisenger and Fordtran's Gastrointestinal and Liver Disease, with permission from Elsevier

Intramural haematoma

Rare but can occur spontaneously, especially in patients using anticoagulants, anti-platelet drugs, and with clotting disorders. Commonest in the **oesophagus**, in patients with a history of retching.

Clinical features include sudden onset chest pain, dysphagia, and haematemesis. The suddenness of onset can mimic that of MI, dissecting aneurysm, or pulmonary embolus.

Diagnosis is best made by contrast radiology or by CT.

Endoscopy is not always necessary and should be pursued with caution as many intramural haematomas are contained perforations: there is no serosal layer in the oesophagus, so air inflation can convert a contained perforation into a free perforation. Most haematomas resolve over 7 to 10 days.

Intrinsic factor (IF)

- A 50 kDa glycoprotein secreted by human parietal cells, IF is one of two proteins that bind cobalamin (<u>vitamin B12</u>)—the other is called R binder protein. Most B12 initially binds to R binder in the stomach: the complex is cleaved by pancreatic trypsin, and the freed B12 then binds to IF. The IF–B12 complex binds to a specific ileal receptor called cubilin that mediate endocytosis of the IF–B12 complex (autosomal recessive mutation in this receptor causes juvenile megaloblastic anaemia, the Imerslund–Graesbeck syndrome). B12 is then transported to tissues bound to transcobalamin II.
- Diagnosis of vitamin B12 deficiency due to loss of functioning IF clarified by <u>Schilling test</u>.
- Secretion of IF usually in physiological excess: most patients with hypochlorhydria produce enough to prevent B12 deficiency and histamine receptor antagonists/PPIs do not induce IF deficiency.
- Circulating antibodies to IF are found in <u>pernicious anaemia</u>.

Intussusception

- The invagination of a proximal segment of bowel (the intussusceptum) into an adjacent distal segment (intussuscipiens). Important cause of small bowel obstruction in children, and is aetiology of 5% of cases in adults. The important point is that in adults intussusception always needs investigating since there is usually a pathological cause (tumours (e.g. ileocaecal <u>carcinoid</u>), inflammatory lesions, <u>Meckel's diverticulum</u>). This usually results in surgical resection of the affected segment.
- Clinical presentation is usually with partial small bowel obstruction. Occult or overt rectal bleeding may occur.
- Diagnosis is usually by ultrasound or CT.

Iron

Dietary iron comprises haem (meat, fish, poultry) and non-haem iron (vegetables, grains, and fruits). Poor intake alone rarely causes anaemia but may deplete stores and combines with any cause of malabsorption or blood loss to produce anaemia. Absorption and losses are about 1 mg/day in adults: menstrual loss in women is 5–50 mg per month

Absorption takes place in duodenum and upper small bowel. Absorption is increased by <u>vitamin C</u> because it maintains iron in the ferrous state which is more soluble. Increased in <u>haemochromatosis</u> and can also increase 2–3 fold to compensate for increased loss. Reduced in cases of reduced acid secretion (atrophic gastritis, gastric surgery, prolonged antacid treatment) and small bowel disease (e.g. <u>coeliac disease</u>).

Iron deficiency. Common (5–10% of pre-menopausal women, 1–5% men). In groups other than pre-menopausal women, the assumption is usually of chronic occult GI bleeding and this underlies the routine search for GI pathology. 12% pre-menopausal women with iron deficiency anaemia have significant GI abnormalities, so investigation in this group is also important.

Diagnosing iron deficiency is a crucial step. Key routine tests are a low serum ferritin and low transferrin saturation as assessed by ratio of serum iron to total iron binding capacity (TIBC). TIBC is usually elevated.

Finding the cause. Overall, upper GI lesions are twice as common as colonic lesions (40% compared with 20% respectively in several large series). Trivial lesions such as mild gastritis and small adenomas do not contribute to Iron deficiency: *Helicobacter pylori*-associated gastritis has been implicated in iron deficiency, as have large <u>hiatus hernias</u> and gastric achlorhydria and atrophy. Right-sided <u>colon cancers</u> are the classical occult colonic source of bleeding: <u>angiodysplasia</u> and adenomas are nearly as frequent.

Investigations

Symptoms are not a reliable guide. Investigation should include upper GI endoscopy and low duodenal biopsy (undiagnosed <u>coeliac disease</u> is an unusual, but important cause), and colonoscopy. There may be a role for <u>enteroscopy</u>, video capsule endoscopy, and occasionally angiography or labelled red cell studies in cases where iron deficiency persists, and initial endoscopies are negative.

Treatment of iron deficiency

Oral iron. If possible give oral iron 100–200 mg per day, with vitamin C which improves absorption. Ferrous sulphate 200 mg tablets contain 65 mg elemental iron. Continue treatment for 3 months to replenish stores. In general differences in tolerability are due to differences in concentration of iron. Prophylactic iron may be appropriate in malabsorption, pregnancy, post-gastrectomy.

Parenteral iron. Reserved for patients who cannot tolerate oral iron, where there is continued blood loss, or malabsorption. Anaphylactoid reactions can occur and patients should be given a small test dose first.

Irritable bowel syndrome (IBS)

A common, chronic recurrent illness (rather than a specific medical disease: there being no recognized pathology and no specific cause) characterized by abdominal pain or discomfort and a disturbed bowel habit (see box for diagnostic criteria).

Epidemiology

Found all over the world but different cultures have varying perceptions of disease and illness seeking behaviour. In the West, more common in women and more common in those under 50 years.

Pathophysiology

Motility

Intestinal contractile and electrical activity is increased in patients with IBS, but this is probably an exaggerated response to stimuli rather than physical pathology. There is increased senstivity to visceral stimulation, although there are wide variations in subgroups of IBS patients with diarrhoea or constipation.

Triggers for sensitization

There is currently much interest in the role of inflammatory cells or mediators in at least some types of IBS. Proliferation of intestinal mast cells, or sympathetic afferent excitation via increased neuropeptide release have been proposed as mechanisms by which food or stress may trigger symptoms.

There is an association between emotion and gut motility and this has been proposed as a further factor in IBS.

Post-infective sensitization

Culture positive gastroenteritis is a very strong risk factor for IBS, which does not seem linked to continuing infection. A change in microbial flora seems to be associated with changes in colonic transit and rectal sensitivity but the mechanisms are largely undefined.

Food intolerance

Studies of dietary restriction followed by reintroduction suggest food intolerance in 30–60% of IBS patients. Immunological or biochemical correlation has been lacking: despite a reported association with atopy, skin testing with food-derived allergens is of dubious relevance. A recent study reports positive results of food elimination based on serum IgG antibodies in IBS patients (Atkinson, W et al. (2004). Gut **53**: 1459).

Diagnosis

- IBS is not a diagnosis of exclusion. Diagnosis is based on criteria agreed at a conference in Rome (see box).
- The decision to investigate is based on the age of the patient, family history, and the presence of 'alarm' symptoms (see box).

Treatment

Successful management combines individualizing treatment of predominant symptoms and conferring insight on how symptoms may related to emotional stresses. Time spent in exploring association between symptoms and life events often pays dividends.

Rome II criteria for irritable bowel syndrome

At least 12 weeks in the preceding 12 months of abdominal discomfort or pain with 2 or more of the following features:
- Relief by defecation
- Onset associated with a change in stool frequency
- Onset associated with a change in stool appearance

Symptoms supporting a diagnosis of IBS:
- Abnormal stool frequency
- Abnormal stool form
- Difficulties in evacuation
- Passage of mucus
- Bloating or feelings of distension

Clinical features supporting the diagnosis of irritable bowel syndrome

- Rome II criteria
- Long history with relapsing and remitting course
- Exacerbations triggered by life events
- Coexistence of anxiety and depression
- Associated with symptoms in other organ systems
- Symptoms aggravated by eating

Clinical features suggesting organic disease other than IBS

- Onset in old age
- Progressive deterioration
- Fever
- Weight loss
- Rectal bleeding (not caused by fissures or haemorrhoids)
- Steatorrhoea
- Dehydration

Investigations in suspected IBS

- Routine haematology/biochemistry and sigmoidoscopy with rectal biopsy (if there is diarrhoea) are reasonable starting investigations
- If the diarrhoea is persistent, serum B12, folic acid, iron studies, thyroid function, coeliac antibodies, liver function tests, and stool microsopy should be done
- Consider colonoscopy to exclude <u>microscopic colitis</u>
- Faecal urgency or incontinence suggests a need for <u>anorectal manometry</u>

Evidence for efficacy of therapies is complicated by a high placebo effect with all modes of treatment. This may relate to the benefit observed with alternative or complementary remedies (see box).

Drugs useful in managing IBS are shown opposite. Sometimes drugs useful for one symptom can make another worse. In particular, dietary fibre or stimulant laxatives can make bloating and abdominal pain worse. We recommend the use of non-stimulant osmotic laxatives such as movicol for constipation. Antidepressants used in low doses have a visceral analgesic effect that should be explained to the patient as this often facilitates acceptability. Tricyclics can have a supplemental effect in relieving insomnia.

Newer drugs are aimed at modifying visceral sensitivity and reactivity by using ligands for intestinal serotonin receptors. The long-term benefit of this approach remains to be determined.

Diet and IBS

Patients often believe that <u>food intolerance</u> contributes to their symptoms and some sufferers benefit from eliminating certain foods from the diet. Detection of food intolerance is often difficult even with the help of food diaries and dieticians. Many studies rely on the use of exclusion diets that are labour-intensive and time-consuming. They depend on the principle of stabilizing the patient on a very bland diet for a few days and then gradually introducing favourite foods one or two per day. About 30% of patients can identify a precipitating food using this approach. Attempts to test for food intolerance have in the past focused on classic food allergy based on IgE-mediated antibody responses, although immediate type 1 hypersensitivity is rare in IBS. A recent study supports the role of IgG antibodies in IBS (see above).

Prognosis in IBS

There is a high probability of remaining free of severe symptoms in IBS patients but symptoms usually persist for a long time (5% free of symptoms at 5 years). Medical intervention relieves or improves symptoms and quality of life in about 2/3 patients with IBS. Outcome is best in males with a short history, predominant constipation, and a good initial response to treatment. Long-term response is best where psychosocial issues have been explored and patient education emphasized.

Islet cell tumours

See: <u>pancreatic endocrine tumours</u>.

Isospora

See: <u>coccidia</u>.

IBS: all in the mind?

- IBS is more common in those attending psychiatric clinics, and there is an association with psychological factors including anxiety and depression. The only prospective data comes from IBS triggered by an episode of gastroenteritis: psychological factors at onset of infection appear to predict development of chronic bowel symptoms
- IBS patients appear to show particular illness behaviour: they consult doctors more frequently about minor ailments and there is an overlap with illnesses such as chronic fatigue syndrome and fibromyalgia
- IBS patients report more stressful life events, ranging from loss to familial disruption, domestic or career dissatisfaction, or abuse (physical or sexual). Loss of self-esteem and autonomy is frequently manifest in somatic symptoms including those of IBS

Complementary and alternative therapies in IBS

Evidence is accumulating that a variety of therapies can modulate stress hormones and other physiologic functions. Different therapies are directed at different aspects of healing

- **Physical therapies** (massage, acupuncture, reflexology, shiatsu) may work on the release of tension
- **Meditation and hypnotherapy** produce focused relaxation that may facilitate cognitive behavioural change
- **Biofeedback** may help patients gain control over their symptoms

Drugs useful in managing IBS

- **Antispasmodics** for abdominal pain: mebeverine, buscopan, colpermin, alverine citrate
- **Antidiarrhoeal** agents: <u>LOPERAMIDE</u>, <u>CHOLESTYRAMINE</u>
- **Anticonstipating** agents: movicol
- **Antidepressants:** tricyclics, SSRIs

J

Jaundice

See: <u>Approach to recent-onset jaundice</u>.

Jejunal diverticulum

A common location for small bowel diverticula (also seen in the duodenum and <u>Meckel's diverticula</u>): found in 0.5% to 7% of small bowel series. Most are asymptomatic but they can cause pain, bleeding, diarrhoea, and fever. Malabsorption can arise from stasis and <u>bacterial overgrowth</u>.

Diagnosis is most efficient with a barium contrast radiograph. Treatment is surgical for significant bleeding or diverticulitis. Malabsorption can be treated with oral antibiotics to treat bacterial overgrowth.

Juvenile polyps and polyposis

Mucosal tumours consisting of excess lamina propria and dilated cystic glands rather than epithelial cells. They are hamartomas and appear to be acquired, being most common from ages 1–7. They usually regress spontaneously but can occur in adults. They are usually single, range in size from 3 mm to 2 cm, and are commonest in the rectum. They may prolapse during defecation.

They have no malignant potential when single but removal is suggested because of their blood supply and tendency to bleed. Association with proximal adenomas is rare.

The juvenile polyposis syndrome is defined by 10 or more juvenile polyps; juvenile polyps occurring throughout the GI tract; or any number of juvenile polyps with a family history of juvenile polyposis. Associated with germline mutations in PTEN and DPC4, which are tumour suppressor genes (DPC4 has a role in signalling through TGFβ). When juvenile polyps are multiple, there is an increased risk of cancer because of the adenomatous tissue present in some polyps rather than the juvenile polyps *per se*.

If colonoscopy reveals polyps, upper GI endoscopy should be done. The lifetime risk of cancer is 1 in 3. Screening is recommended in early teens and surveillance colonoscopy every 3 years.

K

Kayser–Fleischer rings

- Greenish-brown ring around edge of iris, best seen by ophthalmologist using slit lamp. Due to deposition of copper-containing pigment in Descemet's membrane at posterior surface of cornea. See Colour Plate 16.
- Found in 90% of people with <u>Wilson's disease</u>, but also rarely seen in other conditions of chronic cholestasis (e.g. <u>primary biliary cirrhosis</u>).

L

Lactose intolerance

- Deficiency of brush border lactase can lead to lactose intolerance. Symptoms are bloating, cramps, wind, and diarrhoea after milk or dairy ingestion (although milk protein allergy or fat intolerance are alternative causes).
- Commonest cause is acquired primary lactase deficiency. This is regulated at gene transcriptional level and varies in different populations. Even in populations where lactase activity persists, levels are lower than for other disaccharidases, making lactose digestion more susceptible to impairment by acute gastrointestinal infections where the brush border is lost.
- Diagnosis can be confirmed by a lactose hydrogen <u>breath test</u>. Treatment consists either of a lactose-free diet or dietary supplementation with lactase.

Laser therapy and the GI tract

Bleeding peptic ulcers

Argon and Nd:YAG lasers were the first endoscopic therapies for haemostasis to be assessed in large randomized controlled trials. These show that lasers stop bleeding and reduce the risk of re-bleeding, but they are expensive and cumbersome and have been replaced by more portable methods (see <u>heater probe</u>, <u>argon plasma coagulation</u>).

Oesophageal carcinoma

- Endoscopic laser is a non-contact method of thermally ablating tumours: it enables tissue vapourization and coagulation necrosis. Tissue effects vary with the wavelength used: Nd:YAG, KTP, and argon lasers have been used. Luminal patency and relief of dysphagia can be achieved in 70–85% patients, with 25% patients symptom-free at 3 months. Usually maximum patency is achieved in 2–3 sessions. Minor side effects include chest pain, odynophagia, low grade fever, and leucocytosis. Major side effects include perforation in 2%, fistula or bleeding in 1%, sepsis in 0.5–1%.
- Characteristics favouring successful lasering include an exophytic and straight short tumour (< 6 cm), rather than extensive angulated one.

Other applications of laser in the GI tract

Laser has been used to ablate <u>Barrett's oesophagus</u>: multiple treatments are required, perforation has been reported, and the technique is less widely used than <u>photodynamic therapy</u>. Laser has been used to treat non-surgically respectable colonic cancers and polyps but use has declined recently: for malignant growths, endoscopic stenting has increased in popularity, while for large benign sessile growths techniques of endoscopic mucosectomy have advanced rapidly.

Laxative abuse

Also see <u>LAXATIVES</u>.

Patients abusing laxatives fall into one of four categories (see table). Detection depends on a high level of suspicion. Hypokalaemia may complicate purgative abuse. Melanosis coli suggests ingestion of anthracene laxatives. A large faecal osmotic gap may suggest magnesium ingestion. Faecal osmolality less than 290 mOsm/kg suggests dilution of the stool with water. Mixing stool with hypertonic urine gives a very high faecal osmolality, with a negative faecal osmotic gap because of the high urinary concentrations of Na^+ and K^+.

Groups of patients abusing laxatives

Group	Characteristics
Patients with <u>bulimia</u>	Usually adolescent/young adult women concerned about weight
Secondary gain	May have disability claim pending, or abuse laxatives to induce concern in others
Munchausen's syndrome	Feigned illness to confound physicians
Munchausen's syndrome by proxy	Poisoning by caregivers

(Adapted from Feldman, M, Friedman, LS, Sleisenger, MH, and Scharschmidt, BF (1998). *Sleisenger and Fordtran's gastrointestinal and liver diseases*, 7th edn, W.B. Saunders, Philadelphia)

Leiomyomas

See: <u>GIST (gastrointestinal stromal tumours)</u>.

Leptin

A 16 kDa protein encoded by the obese (*ob*) gene and expressed mainly in adipocytes, providing a signal of fat mass and hence of nutritional status. It has a role in regulating body weight through effect on hypothalamic centres controlling feeding behaviour and hunger. Exogenous leptin decreases hunger and food consumption and increases energy expenditure. Leptin levels tend to be increased in obese people, suggesting reduced sensitivity rather than leptin deficiency. True leptin deficiency is a rare cause of human obesity and suggests that leptin therapy is unlikely as a significant therapy for obesity.

Leptospirosis

Background

- Weil's disease refers to the 10% of infections due to spirochaete *Leptospira* that result in clinical liver disease. Endemic human infection in the tropics (30% seropositivity for exposure), but in West *L. icterohaemorrhagiae* mainly carried by rats.
- Direct contact with infection in soil, water, or urine (organisms entering through skin abrasions/cuts) explains epidemiological link with sewage workers, farmhands.

Clinical features

- 7–14 day incubation period, followed by initial septicaemic phase, with influenza-like illness, including headache, myalgia, leg pain, dyspnoea. Lasts 4–7 days, and improvement associated with clearance of circulating leptospira. Second immune-mediated phase occurs after further 2 days, characterized by fever, meningeal irritation, iritis, skin lesions (bleeding, petechiae, purpura, ecchymosis), renal failure (acute tubular necrosis), jaundice, and hepatomegaly.
- Death (5–10%) due to renal/cardiorespiratory disease, and rarely liver failure.

Investigations

Diagnosis never made unless thought about! Careful history of possible exposure essential (e.g. caving, 'outward bound' course). See <u>Approach to recent-onset jaundice</u>.

- FBC: ↓Hb, ↑WCC, ↓platelets.
- LFTs: ↑Bn, ↑AST, ALP normal. Deranged clotting in severe disease.
- Creatine kinase elevated in > 50% with liver disease.
- Blood/CSF culture: high yield in first phase.
- Urine (dark field) microscopy positive in second phase (and for several weeks).
- ELISA for *Leptospira* IgM highly sensitive and specific, and is most widely used diagnostic test.

Management
• Effective supportive care essential (may need renal dialysis).
Doxycycline (100 mg bd PO) highly effective if given early, or IV penicillin.

Lichen planus

A chronic inflammatory disease affecting oral mucosa and skin, commoner in women. Increased risk of squamous cell cancer. Topical steroids are effective. Oesophageal involvement may occur rarely.

Listeria

Gram-positive bacteria. Can cause outbreaks of disease. Sources include raw or unpasteurized milk or cheese and prepackaged meats. Immuno-competent people can develop gastroenteritis with fever, headache, pain, nausea, and diarrhoea. This is usually not accompanied by bacteraemia, whereas listeriosis is a systemic disease that can attack immunocompromised patients and pregnant women—it is often associated with bacteraemia that can seed heart valves, meninges, or other organs.

Lithotripsy

See: extracorporeal shock wave lithotripsy.

Liver abscess

Epidemiology/aetiology

- In pre-antibiotic era most pyogenic liver abscesses occurred following appendicitis. Abscess formation may occur in pre-existing liver lesions, including hepatocellular carcinoma, especially in those with prior instrumentation, or in setting of significant tumour necrosis (e.g. following chemoembolization/radiofrequency ablation). May also arise from biliary tract, in association with cholangitis, choledocholithiasis, and *Clonorchis* infection, and following ERCP. Intraabdominal disease (e.g. colon cancer, diverticular disease) may give rise to portal bacteraemia and liver abscess.
- Infections usually polymicrobial, involving gut-derived Gram-negative (e.g. *E. coli*, *Klebsiella*), Gram-positive (e.g. *Enterococci*, *Streptococcus milleri*), and anaerobic organisms (e.g. *Bacteroides* spp). Rarer causes include hydatid disease, TB, and *Candida albicans*. *Entamoeba histolytica* is an important cause in developing countries (see amoebiasis). Portal vein thrombosis (PVT) is associated with local/systemic infection, and portal pyaemia. In patients who present with cholangitis, but who remain septic despite relief of biliary obstruction, it is vital to exclude liver abscess.

Clinical features

- Significant variability in severity and duration of symptoms. May present acutely with right upper quadrant pain, high fever, and septic shock, or more indolently (> 1 month) with pyrexia of unknown origin (PUO), malaise, anorexia, weight loss, and dull abdominal discomfort.
- Examination may reveal tender hepatomegaly, and occasionally jaundice.

Investigation

- Bloods show mildly abnormal LFTs (often ↑ALP/GGT, even in absence of large duct obstruction), ↑ WCC (neutrophilia), ↑ ESR/CRP.
- Blood cultures positive in 50–80%.
- Imaging. Abscesses may be single or multiple. <u>Ultrasound</u> is usually first modality, and is highly specific. <u>CT scanning</u> is nearly 100% sensitive for liver abscess, often showing hypodense lesion with 'rim enhancement' with contrast. Vital to exclude biliary obstruction.
- Differential diagnoses of liver abscess on imaging include amoebic liver abscess (<u>amoebiasis</u>), <u>hydatid disease</u>, simple cysts, necrotic tumour.
- Abscess aspiration needed if blood cultures negative, and failure to respond to initial treatment (but organism isolated in 90% of cases if abscess aspirated prior to antibiotics).
- Look hard for a reason for liver abscess (e.g. colonoscopy to exclude <u>colon cancer</u> in *Streptococcus milleri* abscess).

Management

- If abscess associated with biliary obstruction, biliary drainage (preferably endoscopically by <u>ERCP</u>) is essential.
- Antibiotics tailored to culture sensitivities but, until available, broad-spectrum empirical cover (e.g. 3rd generation <u>CEPHALOSPORIN</u> and <u>METRONIDAZOLE</u>, or <u>PIPERICILIN/TAZOBACTAM</u>). Be guided by microbiologists. Antibiotics usually given for 2 weeks IV, then further 6 weeks orally. May take weeks/months for resolution of abscess—be guided primarily by clinical progress, not radiological change.
- Percutaneous aspiration/drainage of large abscesses used in combination with antibiotics (important to give metronidazole prior to aspiration if amoebiasis suspected).
- Surgery for abscess drainage rarely required.

Liver biopsy (LBx)

No investigation in medicine should be performed unless the result might change management (especially if it carries risk), and LBx demonstrates this point *par excellence*. Studies show that the results of LBx affect subsequent management in only 30% of cases.

Indications

- LBx has a central role in diagnosis of wide range of diffuse parenchymal and focal liver disease.
- Chronic viral <u>hepatitis B and C</u> (histological grade (inflammation) and stage (fibrosis) may determine need/timing of treatment); genetic <u>haemochromatosis</u> (enables cirrhosis to be excluded, but improvements in genetic, biochemical, and imaging assessment are reducing need for LBx); unexplained hepatitis/abnormal liver function tests (where non-invasive tests, such as serology, are non-diagnostic); <u>autoimmune hepatitis</u> (role during initial work-up, and probably in assessing treatment response); <u>nonalcoholic fatty liver disease (NAFLD)</u> (allows identification of steatohepatitis, which may show histological progression); <u>alcoholic liver disease</u> (especially exclusion of <u>alcoholic hepatitis</u>, as clinical diagnosis wrong in >20% of cases); focal liver masses (e.g. liver metastases, <u>focal nodular hyperplasia</u>, <u>hepatocellular carcinoma</u> (but see comments below *re* seeding)).
- Routine use of LBx, where diagnosis has been established by other modalities, remains unclear for <u>primary biliary cirrhosis</u>, <u>primary sclerosing cholangitis</u>, <u>Wilson's disease</u>.
- Rarely needed in proven acute viral hepatitis.

Contraindications to percutaneous LBx

- Uncooperative patient (sudden movement may lead to liver laceration).
- Biliary obstruction ± <u>cholangitis</u>.
- Deranged clotting. Usual advice is to avoid percutaneous LBx if INR > 1.3 (i.e. prothrombin time (PT) prolonged >3 s), but little clear data, and 90% of biopsy-related bleeds occur in patients with INR < 1.3. If INR 1.4–1.6, may give fresh frozen plasma (FFP), and perform LBx if INR reduces to <1.4. Percutaneous 'plugged' LBx, in which gelatin is injected down biopsy track after removing needle, may be considered if 'moderate' coagulopathy persists (e.g. INR 1.4–1.6, platelets 40–60 × 10^9/l). However, technique is 'fiddly', and this author feels that necessity to keep metal sheath within liver for extended period (e.g. 5–10 seconds) whilst gelatin is injected increases risk of movement/breathing, and capsular laceration. If coagulopathy present, and cannot be corrected sufficient to allow safe percutaneous LBx, consider transjugular LBx.

- Low/dysfunctional platelets. Minimum safe lower limit of platelets 60 x 109/l for percutaneous LBx (but recommendations vary). If platelets 40–60 x 109/l, LBx may be performed immediately after platelet transfusion, if count increased to 'safe' level. Bleeding time should be considered in patients with suspected impaired platelet function (e.g. renal failure, recent anti-platelet drugs), as bleeding time >10 minutes associated with increased risk of bleeding.
- Significant ascites. Drain ascites first (see paracentesis), but transjugular LBx is alternative.
- Amyloidosis. Historical data suggests an increased risk of intraperitoneal bleeding.
- Cystic liver lesions. If communicate with biliary tree biopsy may precipitate biliary leak. Risks of anaphylaxis if inadvertently biopsy hydatid cyst.
- Confirmatory LBx generally avoided in presumed resectable hepatocellular carcinoma, in view of risk of needle track seeding (but reported incidence from diagnostic LBx <2%).

Pre-procedure care

- Informed written consent.
- Stop anti-platelet medication at least a week prior to procedure, if clinically possible. Anticoagulation must be stopped prior to percutaneous LBx.
- Pre-procedure blood tests, as discussed above (within last 2 weeks if stable chronic disease, more recent if change likely (e.g. recent onset jaundice).
- Imaging. U/S or CT scanning of liver is essential prior to LBx, in part to exclude unexpected pathology that may increase risks (e.g. intrahepatic gall bladder, liver cyst). Debate continues as to whether 'untargeted' LBx should be performed under U/S guidance in all cases (as argued by most radiologists).
- Prophylactic antibiotics should be given for patients at risk of endocarditis, or if there is a risk of biliary sepsis.

Complications/risks

Mortality 0.1–0.3%, morbidity 5.9% following liver biopsy. Complications and death most commonly related to intraperitoneal bleeding or peritonitis following gallbladder perforation. Risk factors for bleeding include increasing patient age, intrahepatic malignancy, and > 2 needle passes. Puncture of lung (pneumothorax), colon, and kidney are all recognized. Small subcapsular haematomas are seen on U/S in > 20%, but are rarely symptomatic.

Procedure

- Patient lies supine, with right hand behind head.
- Liver identified by percussion or (ideally) U/S. Usual approach in mid-axillary line, between the lower ribs.
- Aseptic technique, with skin cleaned with iodine-based solution, and skin infiltrated down to the liver capsule using 22G needle and ligno-caine 1–2% 4–6 ml. Line of infiltration just above edge of lower rib (to avoid neurovascular bundle running on underside of upper rib). 5 mm scalpel cut into skin to allow advancement of biopsy needle.
- Biopsy performed with patient having been instructed to stop breathing after full expiration (this raises diaphragm, so reducing risk of pneumothorax).
- 2 types of biopsy needle used: cutting needle (e.g. Trucut) provides good cores of tissue, but may carry slightly higher complication rate than suction needle (e.g. Menghini). It is important that those under-taking LBx gain confidence and experience using one needle type.
- After biopsy patient lies in right lateral position for 1 hour (helps 'tamponade' liver capsule against chest?), then supine for 2 hours, and stays in hospital for 6 hours. Vital signs monitored quarter hourly for 2 hours, then half hourly for 2 hours, then hourly (> 80% of complications occur within first 10 hours, and > 60% within 2 hours).

Liver function tests (LFTs)

Conventional 'liver function' tests (AST, ALT, ALP, GGT) provide little information as to synthetic function of the liver. This is best indicated by serum albumin, clotting (prothrombin time) and bilirubin.

Bilirubin (normal serum range 3–17µmol/l)

↑ levels may reflect ↑ production (e.g. haemolysis), ↓ hepatic uptake/ conjugation (e.g. Gilbert's syndrome), ↓ biliary excretion (e.g. choledo-cholithiasis). See bilirubin metabolism and Approach to recent-onset jaundice.

Prothrombin time (PT; normal range 12–15 s)

In absence of vitamin K deficiency (excluded by giving vitamin K 10 mg PO/IV/day for 3 days), PT provides good indicator of liver synthetic function. Strong prognostic indicator of poor outcome and need for liver transplantation in acute liver failure and after paracetamol overdose (and so do not correct PT in this setting (e.g. with fresh frozen plasma), unless bleeding.

Albumin (normal serum range 35–50 g/l)

Reasonable indicator of liver synthetic function. In chronic liver disease, serum albumin reflects disease severity and prognosis (see Child–Pugh score). Always consider other causes of low albumin (malnutrition, se-vere intercurrent illness, renal losses (e.g. nephrotic syndrome), and gut losses (protein-losing enteropathy).

Aspartate aminotransferase (AST; normal range 5–45 IU/l)

Intracellular enzyme present in a number of tissues other than hepatocytes (e.g. striated muscle). As with ALT, ↑ levels in many types of liver disease, but levels > 1000 IU/l suggest acute hepatocyte injury due to drugs (e.g. paraceta-mol overdose), viruses (e.g. hepatitis A, hepatitis B), or ischaemia (e.g. hypotensive episode). AST > x2 higher than ALT characteristic of alcoholic liver disease.

Alanine aminotransferase (ALT; normal range 5–50 IU/l)

Also intracellular enzyme, but more specific than AST for hepatocyte injury. ALT > AST often found in viral hepatitis and non-alcoholic fatty liver disease.

Alkaline phosphatase (ALP; normal range 40–165 IU/l)

Present in biliary epithelial cells, bone, and intestine. Isoenzyme may identify source, but associated ↑ GGT in setting of ↑ ALP rarely makes measuring this necessary. ↑ ALP seen in intrahepatic cholestasis (e.g. primary biliary cirrhosis) or extrahepatic biliary obstruction (e.g. pancreatic cancer).

Gammaglutamyl transpeptidase (GGT; normal range 10–60 IU/l)

Marker of cholestasis, but may be ↑ due to alcohol and other drugs through enzyme induction. Extensive investigation of ↑ GGT, in absence of other LFT derangement, rarely identifies significant pathology.

Liver support devices

- <u>Liver transplantation</u> as the only therapeutic option for the patient with end-stage acute or chronic liver failure is unsatisfactory for many reasons (e.g. lack of donors; life long immunosuppression; ethical issues).
- Artificial liver support systems remain a 'holy grail' in hepatology, and could have particular role as a 'bridge' to transplant in those with <u>acute liver failure</u> awaiting a donor liver, and to allow time for spontaneous recovery of native liver (e.g. post <u>paracetamol overdose</u>).
- 2 broad types of devices:
  - **Non-biological.** These devices use non-cellular technologies to mimic some aspects of liver function. Molecular absorbance recirculation system (MARS) is an extracorporeal device attached to a conventional haemodialysis machine. Patient's blood circulates through a special hollow-fibre filter with a membrane, and protein (albumin)-bound toxins pass through membrane and attach to albumin in the dialysate compartment. The dialysate albumin is cleaned of toxins by continuously passing over charcoal and anion exchange resin columns, and then recirculates. MARS reduces hyperbilirubinaemia and may improve <u>hepatic encephalopathy</u> and intractable pruritis, but definite effect on outcome in liver failure not yet established.
  - **Biological.** These devices employ isolated liver cells to mimic liver function, often in conjunction with charcoal and resin columns. Advantage of providing some synthetic activity and toxin clearance that is comparable to native liver function. In trial of commercial system, overall 30 day survival not improved, but survival benefit shown in small subgroups. Devices appear to be safe, but more expensive than non-biological systems.
- Other methods of liver support under development include hepatocyte transplantation, stem cell transplantation, and transgenic xenografts.

Liver transplantation

Background

- Management of chronic liver disease has been transformed by orthotopic liver transplantation (OLT) over the last 20 years.
- Alternatives to human livers for transplantation (e.g. xenotransplantation from other mammals such as pigs, or large-scale production of functioning hepatocytes) remain an elusive goal (also see <u>liver support devices</u>).
- End-stage liver disease due to cirrhosis accounts for 60% of OLT, malignancy 10% (see <u>hepatocellular carcinoma</u>), <u>acute liver failure</u> 5–10%, cholestasis 10–15%. In UK, OLT for <u>paracetamol overdose</u> is falling (probably due to introduction of blister packs), but proportion of transplants for <u>hepatitis C</u> continues to rise (> 20%).
- Overall patient survival post-OLT at 1 and 3 years are 86% and 76%.

When to refer for OLT consideration?

This is not an exact science, but simple answer is 'sooner rather than later'. Liver units don't want to first hear of the patient with acute liver failure when in grade III <u>hepatic encephalopathy</u>, or of the decompensated cirrhotic when they have become cachectic and malnourished. Broadly, consider OLT when anticipated survival < 2 years.

Acute liver failure (see emergencies and table opposite). Note that progression of liver synthetic dysfunction determines timing/need for OLT. Prothrombin time (PT) is an ideal marker of this (and so do not correct elevated PT (e.g. with fresh frozen plasma) unless actively bleeding).

Chronic liver disease

Indications

- Refractory ascites (see <u>Approach to ascites</u>), <u>hepatic encephalopathy</u>, and variceal bleeding (not effectively controlled with medical/endoscopic therapy—see <u>portal hypertension</u>).
- After 1st episode of <u>spontaneous bacterial peritonitis</u> (SBP), as predicts 50% 2 year mortality.
- Poor quality of life (e.g. pruritis, severe fatigue) in cholestatic liver disease (e.g. <u>primary biliary cirrhosis</u>).
- <u>Child–Pugh score</u> >7, and more recently MELD score (see box) have been used as indicators of need for referral.

Contraindications

- HIV positivity (although some transplant programmes are reviewing this in view of efficacy of highly active antiretroviral therapy (HAART)).
- Active sepsis.
- Advanced cardiopulmonary disease.
- Extrahepatic/extensive intrahepatic malignancy (also see <u>hepatocellular carcinoma</u> and <u>cholangiocarcinoma</u>).
- Active <u>alcohol dependency</u> or substance abuse (most programmes require 6 months abstinence prior to transplantation for alcoholic cirrhosis).
- Psychosocial factors that may impair ability to comply with immunosuppression.

Technique

Pre-transplant assessment, surgical approach, and post-operative care, are outside remit of this text.

Types of transplant

- Whole cadaveric graft—represents great majority of transplants. Totally reliant on limited supply of organs.
- Split-liver graft—also cadaveric, but splitting liver may allow 2 recipients to be transplanted.
- Auxiliary liver transplantation—donor liver is implanted next to part, or whole, of recipient liver. May be used for acute liver failure (when regeneration of native liver might occur) or metabolic liver disease.
- Live-related transplantation—hemi-hepatectomy and liver lobe donation from family member. Likely good immunological match, but huge ethical considerations (e.g. small but definite risk of donor mortality).

Post-transplant complications

Myriad complications, related to immunological rejection, technical problems, drug effects, infection, and recurrence of underlying disease. All may contribute to early or late graft dysfunction.

- **Rejection.** Three types:
  - **Hyperacute**—antibody and complement-mediated reaction, with massive hepatic necrosis < 10 days after OLT. Only treatment is urgent retransplantation.
  - **Acute**—occurs in 30–70% of patients, often clinically silent, diagnosed on liver biopsy, usually day 7–9 post-OLT. Often rapid response to high dose immunosuppression (e.g. methylprednisolone 1 g IV od for 3/7).
  - **Chronic**—progressive bile duct loss, with fibrosis and cholestasis. Associated with previous recurrent acute rejection, cytomegalovirus (CMV), and hepatitis C infection. Adjustment of immunosuppression may help but graft failure is usual.
- **Technical problems.** Hepatic artery, portal vein, vena cava thrombosis (may necessitate urgent retransplantation if occurs acutely), or anastomotic leak and haemorrhage. Biliary anastomotic leaks in 10%, with anastomotic strictures in 3–20% (treatment with endoscopic stenting ± surgical revision).
- **Drug effects.** As well as predisposing to infective complications, immunosuppressives may have hepatotoxic, and extrahepatic, effects (see CORTICOSTEROIDS, AZATHIOPRINE, CYCLOSPORINE, TACROLIMUS).
- **Infection** may relate to immunosuppression. Bacterial infection accounts for most infective episodes (35–70% of patients), but viral infection may be linked to early or late graft dysfunction (e.g. herpes simplex virus (HSV), CMV). See table. Epstein–Barr virus (EBV) reactivation occurs 2–6 months post-OLT, and is linked with post-transplant lymphoproliferative disorder (PTLD).
- **Disease recurrence**. Reinfection of graft with hepatitis C is universal, and may lead to accelerated cirrhosis and graft loss. Hepatitis B reinfection may be prevented/limited with hepatitis B immunoglobulin (HBIg) and LAMIVUDINE ± ADEFOVIR DEPIXOL. 20–30% of patients transplanted for alcoholic liver disease return to drinking. Recurrence of autoimmune hepatitis, primary biliary cirrhoisis, and primary sclerosing cholangitis post-transplantation has been reported.

Selection criteria for liver transplantation in acute liver failure:
King's College criteria (Adapted with permission from O'Grady J.R.
(1997) *Acute liver failure. J Coll. Physicians Lond.* **31**: 603)

Paracetamol	Non-paracetamol
Arterial pH < 7.3 (should be interpreted with caution—may improve with N-Acetylcysteine and aggressive rehydration)	PT >100 s, INR > 6.7
Or all 3 of:	Or any 3 of:
• PT >100 s	• Aetiology: halothane hepatitis, drug reaction, seronegative hepatitis
• Creat >300 µmol/l	• Age <10, > 40 years
• Grade III or IV encephalopathy	• PT > 50, INR > 4.0
	• Serum bilirubin > 300 µmol/l

MELD score

Model for end-stage liver disease (MELD) score based on retrospective study of prognosis with chronic liver disease in absence of OLT.

$$3.8 \times \log(e) \text{ (bilirubin mg/dl)} + 11.2 \times \log(e) \text{ (INR)} + 9.6 \log(e) \text{ (creatinine mg/dl)}$$

- MELD scores range from 6 to 40. (< 9 = 4% 3 month mortality, > 30 = 83% 3 month mortality.)
- Advantage of MELD over <u>Child–Pugh score</u> in having no subjective components (e.g. clinical ascites).
- In 2002, MELD adopted in USA as means of determining OLT candidate's priority for organ allocation.

Infectious agents post-liver transplantation	
Bacterial	Gram-positive, Gram-negative, anaerobes
Viral	Epstein–Barr virus, *cytomegalovirus*, *herpes simplex virus*, *varicella zoster virus*
Mycobacteria	*M. tuberculosis*, *M. avium intracellulare*
Fungal	*Aspergillus* spp, *Pneumocystis carinii*, *Candida* spp, *Cryptococcus*

Los Angeles grading

See: <u>oesophagitis.</u>

Lymphangiectasia

Obstruction of lymphatic drainage from the small intestine, resulting in dilatation of small lymphatic channels in serosa and mesentery. Consequences are reduced absorption of chylomicrons and fat soluble vitamins, and excess loss of lymph into the lumen, with hypogammaglobulinaemia and lymphocytopenia (especially of T cells): there is a loss of cell-mediated immunity. Blockage of lymphatics can result in chylous ascites or a chylous pleural effusion. GI symptoms are not prominent, although there can be diarrhoea, pain, and vomiting. Causes are outlined in the box.

Diagnosis. Suspect in any patient with unexplained hypoalbuminaemia: especially if there is lymphopenia and/or steatorrhoea. Small bowel biopsy can demonstrate dilated lacteals. Radiology may reveal oedematous bowel folds. Faecal concentrations of α_1-antitrypsin can be used to measure intestinal protein loss (not gastric protein loss, as α_1-antitrypsin is degraded at pH less than 3). The optimal test is to measure clearance during a 72 hour stool collection, with plasma clearance expressed as ml/day.

Treatment. Acquired lymphangiectasia should be treated by correction of the primary disease. Congenital lymphangiectasia can be partially controlled with dietary restriction of long-chain fatty acids with enrichment by medium chain triglycerides (which do not require lymphatic transport).

Causes of lymphangiectasia

Primary (congenital): asymmetric lymphoedema dating from infancy or early childhood.

Secondary (acquired): abdominal or retroperitoneal carcinoma, chronic pancreatitis, mesenteric TB or sarcoid, Crohn's, Whipple's, scleroderma, constrictive pericarditis, congestive heart failure, and systemic lupus erythematosus.

Lymphoma in GI tract

Solid malignancies of lymphoid tissue. The GI tract is very rarely affected by Hodgkin's lymphoma, but accounts for 30–40% of extranodal cases of non-Hodgkin's lymphoma.

Gastric lymphomas

- Lymphoma accounts for 5% of gastric neoplasms (see also gastric cancer and gastrointestinal stromal tumours (GIST)). Great majority are B-cell lymphomas, either non-Hodgkin's or low-grade mucosa-associated lymphoid tissue (MALT) lymphomas (or MALTomas). The latter account for 40% of primary gastric lymphomas.
- The term MALT lymphoma has come to be used interchangeably with marginal zone B cell lymphoma, which in the stomach is associated with *Helicobacter pylori* infection. *Helicobacter pylori* found in up to 98% of cases of MALT lymphoma, with CagA-positivity particularly linked. Incidence is about 1:50 000 *H. pylori*-infected people. MALT lymphomas usually found in antrum, but may be multifocal, and tend to metastasize late.
- About 50% of gastric lymphomas are diffuse large cell B lymphomas. Relationship to *H. pylori* infection is uncertain but these tumours are of high grade and do not respond to antibiotics alone. Treatment of this condition now involves combined chemotherapy and radiotherapy, since surgery is no longer needed for diagnosis or staging.
- Early gastric lymphoma may be asymptomatic, but later clinical presentation is similar to gastric cancer, but night sweats and fever may be prominent. Polypoid, fungating mass may be seen, and be difficult to distinguish endoscopically from adenocarcinoma. Endoscopy and biopsy provides 95% sensitivity, and endoscopic ultrasound allows assessment of stage of disease. CT used to assess distant spread.
- Eradication of *H. pylori* may lead to complete remission of MALT lymphoma in > 80% of cases, but for *H. pylori*-negative MALT lymphomas, or where eradication has not induced remission, newer agents including monoclonal antibodies against B-cell antigen CD20 (e.g. rituximab) show promise.

Small bowel lymphomas

- B-cell lymphomas encompass immunoproliferative small intestinal disease (IPSID) and non-IPSID subtypes including marginal zone B-cell lymphoma (MALT type, but not associated with *H. pylori*), large B-cell lymphoma, mantle cell lymphoma, follicular lymphoma, and Burkitt's lymphoma. T-cell lymphomas are usually associated with coeliac disease.
- Of the B-cell small bowel lymphomas, marginal zone and follicular lymphomas are regarded as indolent processes, incurable but controllable by chemotherapy. Diffuse large cell lymphomas and mantle cell lymphomas are more aggressive and require chemotherapy.

Enteropathy-associated T-cell lymphoma occurs as a complication of <u>coeliac disease</u>. Intraepithelial T cells in coeliac are $CD3^+CD8^+$ and are polyclonal. Monoclonal proliferation of T cells in coeliac can result in a spectrum of processes from refractory sprue, where response to gluten-free diet is lost, through ulcerative jejunitis to enteropathy-associated intestinal T-cell lymphoma. Clinical features include diarrhoea, abdominal pain, weight loss, and vomiting. A minority present with intestinal perforation or obstruction. Anaemia is common, albumin usually low, LDH is elevated in 25%. Treatment is usually combined surgery and chemotherapy, but prognosis is poor (response rate 60%, remission rate 40%, but relapse in 6 months 80% with 1 and 5 year survival rates of 30–40% and 10–20% respectively.

Immunodeficiency-related lymphoma

- Post-transplant immunoproliferative disorders (PTLD) occur in 1–20% of solid organ transplants (e.g. <u>liver transplantation</u>) and bone marrow transplants and usually result from proliferation of Epstein–Barr virus transformed cells. Treatments include antiviral agents, B cell antibodies (rituximab), and donor leucocyte infusions.
- B-cell NHl can develop in HIV positive patients. EBV is implicated in about 50%.

M

Mallory–Weiss syndrome

First described by Quincke in 1879, Mallory and Weiss described 15 cases of this syndrome in 1929.

Lacerations in the region of the gastro-oesophageal junction though to be caused by retching. They account for 5–10% cases of <u>upper GI bleeding</u>. Bleeding stops spontaneously in 80–90% and rebleeding is rare. Endoscopic therapy to stop bleeding may be necessary but surgical intervention is very rare.

Magnetic resonance imaging

See: <u>MRI</u>.

MALT lymphoma

See: <u>lymphomas in GI tract</u>.

Manometry

- Measuring intraluminal pressure in the gastrointestinal tract is one way of studying motility, abnormalities in which cause a number of common clinical problems. See separate entries under <u>oesophageal manometry</u>, <u>anorectal manometry</u>, and <u>sphincter of Oddi dysfunction</u>.
- Gastroduodenal manometry is established as a research tool but is not widely used, partly because mild to moderate symptoms correlate poorly with manometric findings and partly because the techniques are somewhat invasive and prolonged.

Meckel's diverticulum

- Arises from persistence of the omphalo-mesenteric or vitelline duct which connects the embryonic gut tube with the yolk sac but normally disappears early in fetal life. It occurs in 2% of people and is the commonest congenital GI tract abnormality. Can be as proximal as ligament of Treitz but most are within 100 cm of ileocaecal valve. Associated with other congenital anomalies (cleft palate, annular pancreas).
- **Clinical features.** Painless <u>lower GI bleeding</u> in the young (mean age 5 years); obstruction (commonest presentation in adults). Diverticulitis, perforation, and carcinoma are much less common.
- **Diagnosis** is with technetium pertechnate scan('Meckel's scan'): this assumes uptake by heterotopic gastric mucosa, but nearly all bleeding diverticula contain gastric mucosa. False positives may occur with <u>intussusception</u> and <u>Crohn's disease</u>.
- **Surgical resection** is the treatment of choice.

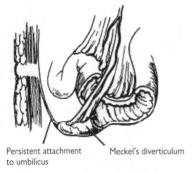

Persistent attachment
to umbilicus   Meckel's diverticulum

Fig. 2.19 Meckel's diverticulum. (Reproduced with permission from Feldman, M, Friedman, LS, Sleisenger, MH, and Scharschmidt, BF (1998). *Sleisenger and Fordtran's gastrointestinal disease*, 7th edn, W.B. Saunders, Philadelphia.)

Megacolon

Defined as a radiological diameter of the rectosigmoid or descending colon of >6.5 cm, ascending colon of >8 cm, or caecal diameter >12 cm. Can be **congenital** (Hirschsprung's, and may be subtle congenital abnormalities resulting in autonomic denervation) or **acquired** (can be associated with any cause of constipation, and rarely with infection by trypanosomiasis in Chagas' disease). See also toxic megacolon.

- Acquired megacolon is assumed if there is no congenital lesion or when symptoms did not appear in infancy. Look for an underlying cause (see box).
- Idiopathic megarectum and megacolon relate to dilatation of the rectum and/or colon in the absence of demonstrable organic disease. Patients with megarectum tend to present with faecal soiling and impaction and are young.

Diagnosis. Water soluble contrast media are useful in defining colonic anatomy. Anorectal manometry is useful in differentiating congenital from acquired causes: an intact recto-inhibitory reflex depends on intact ganglia and if present the patient does not have Hirschsprung's disease. Colonic transit is usually delayed in those with megacolon but may be normal in those with isolated megarectum.

Management. Optimal treatment is to empty the bowel completely (phosphate enemas) and then titrate an osmotic laxative. Disimpaction may be required: stimulant laxatives should be avoided. Usually lifelong laxatives are needed and follow up is important. Behavioural treatment and surgery may be helpful.

Acute or toxic megacolon is covered separately.

Melanosis coli

Brown discoloration of colonic epithelium, caused by accumulation of lipofuscin pigment in lamina propria macrophages resulting from laxative-induced apoptosis. Found in 70% of people who use anthroquinone laxatives (cascara, aloe, senna, rhubarb). It does disappear within 12 months of stopping laxatives. Colonic tumours lack pigment-containing macrophages and are thus very easily seen (see Colour Plate 17).

MELD score

See: liver transplantation.

Causes of acquired megacolon

Neurologic: Chagas' disease, Parkinson's disease, myotonic dystrophy, diabetic neuropathy
Smooth muscle: scleroderma, <u>amyloidosis</u>
Metabolic: hypothyroidism, hypokalaemia, <u>porphyria</u>, phaeochromocytoma
Drugs
Mechanical obstruction

Ménétrier's disease

- Characterized by giant hypertrophic gastric folds, mainly involving gastric fundus (enlarged gastric folds also seen in other conditions, e.g. gastrinoma (Zollinger–Ellison syndrome)). Associated hypochlorhydria, hypergastrinaemia, excess mucus production, and hypoalbuminaemia due to protein-losing gastropathy. Cause uncertain, but increased expression of the epidermal growth factor (EGF) reported. High prevalence of *H. pylori*.
- Symptoms include epigastric pain (may mimic peptic ulcer), nausea, peripheral oedema, anorexia, and weight loss. Premalignant condition, with gastric cancer reported in 10–15%.
- Diagnosis often made on endoscopy, but full thickness biopsy (e.g. with endoscopic ultrasound) required to adequately assess histology.
- Histological changes of marked foveolar hyperplasia, glandular atrophy, and increased mucosal thickness. Little controlled data on treatment, but response to *H. pylori* eradication, acid suppression (PROTON PUMP INHIBITORS, H2-ANTAGONISTS), CORTICOSTEROIDS, OCTREOTIDE, and monoclonal antibodies against the EGF receptor reported. Partial/total gastrectomy reserved for refractory/recurrent bleeding, severe hypoproteinemia, or gastric cancer.

Mesenteric venous thrombosis

Accounts for perhaps 10% of cases of acute mesenteric ischaemia: intestinal infarction is rare unless the branches of peripheral arcades and vasa recta are involved. Causes are similar to those for portal vein thrombosis.

Clinical features. **Acute mesenteric venous thrombosis** presents with pain in 90%: lower GI bleeding or hamatemesis occurs in 15% and suggests bowel infarction. Most patients are febrile and 25% show signs of septic shock. Patients with **chronic mesenteric venous thrombosis** are usually asymptomatic at time of diagnosis but may develop GI bleeding from varices secondary to portal vein thrombosis.

Diagnosis. Selective angiography can establish a definite diagnosis and can differentiate arterial from venous ischaemia but is not always available in an emergency. CT angiography is very useful and probably the investigation of choice.

Treatment. Most patients with acute mesenteric venous thrombosis are treated as for intestinal ischaemia. If surgery is required, postoperative heparinization reduces recurrence and progression. Treatment of chronic mesenteric venous thrombosis centres on controlling bleeding from varices.

Microscopic colitis

Comprises two distinct diseases, <u>**collagenous colitis**</u> and **lymphocytic colitis**, united by their clinical presentation of watery diarrhoea with macroscopically normal colonic mucosa on endoscopy but evidence of histological inflammation.

Epidemiology

Initially thought commoner in women age 50–70, but recognized in both sexes. Prevalence as high as 10–15 per 100 000. Historically probably underreported because of failure to biopsy normal appearing mucosa in patients with watery diarrhoea. Association with <u>coeliac</u> and autoimmune disease.

Pathology

Increased CD8 T cells, plasma cells, macrophages. In collagenous colitis, there is a thickened subepithelial collegan layer, greater than 10 μm thick. It tends to be collagen type I and III rather than the normal type IV, and is commoner on the right side of the colon than the left (see Colour Plate 18).

Aetiology and pathogenesis

Thought broadly to involve epithelial immune responses to antigens derived from luminal contents. Faecal diversion produces improvement but the condition relapses once intestinal continuity is re-established. Dietary factors, intestinal pathogens, drugs (particularly NSAIDs), and toxins have all been proposed as important causative factors. The collagen band may be partly a result of reduced collagenases rather than increased deposition, and its thickness does not relate to clinical severity; it may be a secondary phenomenon rather than causative for the diarrhoea.

Clinical features

Usually chronic watery diarrhoea, sometimes associated with crampy pains and weight loss. Examination normal, routine blood tests normal, stool microscopy negative for blood but 50% positive for leucocytes. Colonoscopy is normal or only mildly and variably abnormal endoscopically.

Treatment

The range of therapies tried (<u>METRONIDAZOLE</u>, <u>BISMUTH</u>, <u>5-ASA</u>, bile acid resins, <u>CORTICOSTEROIDS</u> or other immunosuppressants, as well as simple anti-diarrhoeal agents such as loperamide) reveals that the diseases are poorly understood. Long-term steroid therapy is not desirable: there are however reports of successful treatment with <u>BUDESONIDE</u>.

Microsporidia

Obligate intracellular protozoan parasites that can cause disease in the immunocompromised patient. Commonest is *Enterocytozoon bieneusi* which infects small intestine and causes severe diarrhoea. Diagnosis is best made by PCR from faeces or biopsies.

Mirizzi's syndrome

Refers to the impaction of a gallstone in the cystic duct, with obstruction of common bile duct/common hepatic duct, and gallbladder. Patients present with jaundice, right upper quadrant pain, and fever, and may mimic <u>choledocholithiasis</u> or <u>cholangitis</u>. Distended gallbladder may be palpable and tender (see <u>cholecystitis</u>), and gallbladder empyema may develop. Ultrasound or CT scan reveals biliary dilatation above the cystic duct. ERCP may demonstrate the obstructing stone, and a <u>biliary stricture</u> in region of common hepatic duct with obstructed cystic duct (features may mimic <u>cholangiocarcinoma</u>).

Endoscopic stone removal is often not possible, and definitive treatment is usually surgical, with open <u>cholecystectomy</u> and surgical repair of bile duct if necessary.

MRI (magnetic resonance imaging)

Technique. Patient is placed within a strong magnet, which causes hydrogen nuclei (protons) to align with magnet field. Radiofrequency pulse displaces the protons, and on switching off pulse protons relax back to alignment, and release absorbed radiofrequency energy, which is detected. 'T1 and T2 weighted' refer to relaxation constants related to timing of proton realignment. Different tissues display different T1/T2-weighted characteristics. MRI does not use radiation.

Indications for MRI in GI disease include staging of <u>pancreatic cancer</u> and defining other solid lesions (usually as second line to <u>CT scan</u>), and in investigation of fistulating perianal disease (see <u>Crohn's disease</u>). MR cholangiopancreatopathy (MRCP) increasingly used in delineation of biliary and pancreatic ductal anatomy, allowing higher-risk <u>ERCP</u> to be reserved for therapy.

Contraindications include claustrophobia, morbid obesity (e.g. > 60 cm abdominal diameter), displaceable metal *in-situ* (e.g. cochlear implants, pacemaker). MRI more expensive and longer procedure than CT scanning.

Multiple endocrine neoplasia (MEN)

MEN should be considered in all patients with <u>pancreatic endocrine tumours</u>. 3 main syndromes:

- **MEN-1** (Wermer syndrome). Autosomal dominant. Hyperparathyroidism in >90%, pancreatic neuroendocrine tumours (NET) in 80% (mainly <u>gastrinoma</u> and insulinoma), and pituitary adenomas (usually prolactin secreting). Gene defect on chromosome 11. Pancreas demonstrates diffuse microadenomatosis, but in those with Zollinger–Ellison syndrome 80% of gastrinomas are in duodenum, not pancreas.
- **MEN-2a** (Sipple syndrome). Phaeochromocytoma (20–40%) and bilateral medullary thyroid carcinoma are characteristic.
- **MEN-2b:** similar to MEN-2a, but thyroid carcinoma at younger age and more aggressive, and additional Marfanoid features and mucosal neuromas.

N

Nasogastric tubes

Indications for passing a nasogastric tube include:
- Decompression of the stomach with aspiration of gastric contents in the case of gastric outlet or small bowel obstruction.
- Reduction of risk of aspiration pneumonia in at risk patients, e.g. prolonged vomiting, reduced conscious level.
- Occasionally in the patient with upper GI bleeding.
- To provide temporary (usually less than 2 weeks) nutritional support in patients with a functioning GI tract but who cannot or will not eat. Longer periods of enteral nutrition can be provided by percutaneous endoscopic gastrostomy (PEG) tube placement.

  Most tubes for feeding are thin (about 5 F) made of silicone or polyurethane and contain weighted tips with a stylet for easy placement. Tubes for gastric decompression or drainage are larger (about 12 F).

Complications of tube placement:
- Intubation of the bronchial tree is not uncommon.
- Intracranial placement is a risk in patients with skull fractures.
- Erosive tissue damage can produce nasopharyngeal trauma, pharyngitis, sinusitis, otitis media, pneumothorax, GI tract perforation, and oesophageal ulceration.
- Tube occlusion can occur through inspissated feedings or pulverized medications.

Nematodes

See: roundworm (nematode) infection.

Neuroendocrine tumours (NET)

Background
NETs within the GI tract classified into two main groups: carcinoid tumours and pancreatic endocrine tumours. These are discussed separately, although both types arise from neuroendocrine cells, and may be histologically indistinguishable. Particular systemic syndromes are caused by hormones and biogenic amines released from cytoplasmic membrane-bound neurosecretory granules.

Investigation
- Aimed at identifying functional activity, and site of primary/metastatic tumour.
- Histology of tumours shows small cells with regular, round nuclei, which stain positive for neuroendocrine markers, including neuron-specific enolase, synaptophysin, and chromogranin.
- 'Gut hormone profile' usually includes serum gastrin, vasoactive intestinal polypeptide (VIP), glucagons, somatostatin.
- CT scan/MRI cross-sectional imaging required in all cases, but may fail to identify small (<3 cm) NETs. Endoscopic ultrasound (± FNA) increasingly used to define small pancreatic lesions.

- Scintigraphic scanning with radiolabelled meta-iodobenzylguanidine (MIBG) or octreotide (Octreoscan) may identify primary or metastatic NETs (particularly carcinoid, which has higher somatostatin receptor expression than most other NETs). <u>Positron emission tomography (PET)</u> scanning has low yield in NET, in view of low metabolic turnover of tumours.

Clinical features

May be asymptomatic (e.g. incidental lesion seen on abdominal U/S), or present with syndromes related to hormone release, or mass effect of primary/metastatic disease.

Management

- Referral to specialist unit important, for multidisciplinary approach.
- Surgical cure attempted for localized disease (see <u>carcinoid</u> and <u>pancreatic endocrine tumours</u>).
- Palliative approaches to metastatic NET include systemic chemotherapy, somatostatin analogues (e.g. octreotide, lanreotide), and ^{131}I-MIBG if diagnostic scintigraphy positive.
- Options for liver lesions (commonest site for NET metastases) include surgical resection, embolization, radiofrequency ablation, and rarely <u>liver transplantation</u>.

Nodular regenerative hyperplasia (NRH)

- Most common cause of non-cirrhotic <u>portal hypertension</u> in the West. May be associated with other multisystem diseases (e.g. rheumatoid, <u>polyarteritis nodosum</u>). May present with malaise, fever, abdominal discomfort, ascites, or variceal bleeding. Liver function is usually well preserved.
- **Diagnosis** may be difficult. Histology shows nodule formation, but without fibrous septae (in contrast to cirrhosis). These nodules are usually 0.2–2 cm, and may be seen on imaging. Finding on vascular studies of pre-sinusoidal portal hypertension in presence of patent portal vein supports diagnosis of NRH.
- **Treatment** is based on the management of <u>portal hypertension</u>.

Non-alcoholic fatty liver disease (NAFLD)

Background and aetiology

- NAFLD is gaining acceptance as the term for a chronic liver disease with histological features similar to those of alcohol-related liver disease, but without significant alcohol intake. Non-alcoholic steatohepatitis (NASH) constitutes 20% of NAFLD, and is part of spectrum of disease.
- Increasing prevalence of NAFLD closely parallels rate of obesity in population, and 25% of patients have fatty liver on U/S in study from USA.
- Mechanism of steatosis and liver injury uncertain, but may involve hyperinsulinaemia, endotoxaemia, oxidative stress. Wide range of conditions is associated with NAFLD (see box opposite).

Risk factors for NAFLD

- Middle age female
- Obesity
- Diabetes mellitus/glucose intolerance
- Hyperlipidaemia
- Total parenteral nutrition
- Jejuno-ileal bypass
- Starvation
- Drugs (e.g. amiodarone, methotrexate, tetracycline)
- Metabolic disease (e.g. abetalipoproteinaemia, glycogen storage disease, Wilson's disease)

Clinical features

- Many patients asymptomatic, with diagnostic suspicion raised by incidentally raised serum aminotransferases (e.g. ALT) or 'fatty liver' on U/S. Fatigue, malaise, right upper quadrant discomfort may be reported.
- Hepatomegaly common.
- Can progress to end-stage liver disease and portal hypertension, but natural history remains poorly defined, and many patients run indolent course.
- As with other aetiologies of chronic liver disease, patients with cirrhosis related to NAFLD are at risk of hepatocellular carcinoma (HCC).

Investigation

- Important to exclude other causes of chronic liver disease (see Approach to well patient with abnormal liver tests), including careful alcohol history.
- Characteristic pattern of LFTs showing ↑ALT/AST, ↑GGT (ALP usually normal) with ↑fasting cholesterol, lipids, glucose. Elevated serum ferritin may be seen, and role of heterozygosity for HFE haemochromatosis gene in accelerated fibrosis in NAFLD remains controversial.
- U/S, CT, and MRI are all accurate at showing fatty liver.
- Liver biopsy is the only definitive way to define liver injury, as LFT derangement poorly predicts fibrosis, and approximately 20% of patients with persistent ↑ALT have advanced fibrosis/cirrhosis. Histology may show steatosis (fatty liver), steatohepatitis (fatty liver plus inflammation, which may progress to fibrosis/cirrhosis), or established fibrosis. Role of liver biopsy remains controversial, as carries definite risk, and many hepatologists advise initial identification and treatment of risk factors prior to biopsy in otherwise uncomplicated case.

Management

- Cornerstone is control of risk factors (weight loss, treatment of hyperlipidaemia and hyperglycaemia, and discontinuation of possible drug causes). However, these measures effective in only minority.

- Control of hyperinsulinaemia shows promise, even in non-diabetics, with preliminary trials of metformin, and also rosiglitazone (a ligand for the peroxisome proliferator-activated receptor-γ which promotes insulin responsiveness), showing improved liver biochemistry and histology in NASH. However, NASH returns on stopping rosiglitazone, and there are concerns about liver toxicity. Routine use of these agents awaits clarification, but evidence supports consideration of metformin in diabetic patients with NASH.

Nonsteroidal anti-inflammatory drugs (NSAIDs) and the GI tract

NSAIDs, even as low dose aspirin for cardiovascular protection, cause bleeding and ulceration in the GI tract (2–4% users per year: relative risk compared to matched controls of 4 for gastric ulcers and 2 for duodenal ulcers).

Site of damage: as well as gastric and duodenal injury, NSAIDs cause small bowel ulcers and are associated with web like small intestinal strictures. In the colon they can cause acute colitis and precipitate relapses of IBD. They may potentiate bleeding from diverticulosis or established vascular malformations.

Mechanism of injury

Topical damage is largely prevented by enteric-coated preparations. It is very common (erosions seen in 30–50% patients on NSAIDs and, although associated with increased blood loss, probably not associated with serious ulcers or perforations).

Systemic damage. Reduced mucosal prostaglandins caused by NSAIDs inhibiting COX-1 result in lowered mucosal defence and reduced mucosal blood flow (this is nitric oxide (NO) dependent and can be reduced by NO donors).

Risk factors for NSAID-associated complications are shown in the box. There is current uncertainty about the role of *Helicobacter* as a risk factor for NSAID-induced GI damage, but current consensus favours the two being independent risk factors.

Relative frequency of injury with different NSAIDs

Generally this correlates with COX-1 inhibitory efficiency. Ibuprofen and naproxen have the lowest relative risk, and indomethacin and piroxicam have the highest.

Clinical studies with COXIBs

Celecoxib was released in 1999. Rofecoxib was released in the same year but withdrawn in September 2004 because of increased risk of cardiovascular toxicity. Celecoxib produces comparable effects on pain and inflammation to diclofenac in rheumatoid arthritis, with less GI ulceration and withdrawal due to GI side-effects and less admission to hospital in elderly patients due to GI complications. The incidence of endoscopically assessed GI ulceration is comparable to that with placebo. However, COX-2 inhibitors are not cardioprotective and the reduction in GI side-effects is not seen in patients co-prescribed aspirin at cardioprotective doses.

Risk factors for NSAID-induced <u>peptic ulceration</u> and complications

- Age over 60
- Previous ulcer disease
- Concomitant corticosteroids
- High dose NSAIDs
- Chronic major organ impairment
- Concomitant anticoagulant use

Methods of limiting GI toxicity of NSAIDs

- Enteric-coated preparations, antacid buffers, histamine receptor antagonists, PPIs, and natural prostanoids all attenuate mucosal injury caused by NSAIDs
- Agents that include nitric oxide (NO) or induce release of NO exert a protective effect against mucosal injury by vasodilatation and reducing cell-endothelial adhesion. Such agents show reduced GI toxicity but good anti-inflammatory actions
- Selective COX inhibition: cyclo-oxygenase 1 (COX-1) is involved in control of mucosal blood flow, platelet aggregation, renal tubular function, and regulation of gastric acid. COX-2 is inducible and is the main source of pro-inflammatory prostanoids. This has led to development of COX-2 selective inhibitors

Non-ulcer dyspepsia

See: <u>Approach to dyspepsia and gastro-oesophageal reflex</u>.

Norwalk virus

See: <u>Approach to acute diarrhoea</u>.

Nutrition

See: <u>Approach to nutritional support</u>.

O

Obesity surgery

Anti-obesity ('bariatric') surgery is now an enormous growth industry in USA (so to speak). Of 9 million morbidly obese adults, approximately 140 000 undergo weight-loss surgery each year, with the number increasing. Surgical approaches vary, with commonest operation involving division of the stomach at the fundus, with a loop of small bowel, following Roux-en-Y anastomosis, brought up to the small remnant of stomach (which accommodates <30 g of food). Following surgery 30% develop gallstones, and 30% metabolic bone disease, including osteoporosis. Gastric banding procedures are also widely used. Also see Approach to obesity.

Obstetric cholestasis

Background
- Form of intrahepatic cholestasis that is responsible for 20% of cases of jaundice in pregnancy.
- Prevalence reported as 0.5–1% of pregnancies. In those women who developed cholestasis on high oestrogen oral contraceptive pill, 50% developed obstetric cholestasis in subsequent pregnancies.

Clinical features
- Usual onset in 3rd trimester, but may develop earlier.
- Itch predominates, but jaundice in 20–60% develops 2–3 weeks later.
- Right upper quadrant pain unusual.

Investigation
- Vital to exclude other causes of symptomatic cholestasis (e.g. choledocholithiasis; and see Approach to liver problems in pregnancy.
- ↑ Bilirubin (largely conjugated), but usually <100 μmol/l, ↑ ALP (usually <1000 U/l), ↑ AST/ALT (sometimes >1000 U/l). Curiously, GGT often normal. ↑ PT may be due to deficiency of vitamin K-dependent clotting factors, rather than liver failure.
- Imaging with ultrasound essential to exclude biliary obstruction.
- Liver biopsy rarely necessary, but shows intrahepatic cholestasis, bile plugging, and minimal inflammation.

Management
- Symptoms most reliably controlled by delivery.
- URSODEOXYCHOLIC ACID 15–20 mg/kg/day usually very effective at controlling itch. CHOLESTYRAMINE is alternative, but may exacerbate vitamin K-deficiency, necessitating parenteral vitamin K in latter stages of pregnancy.
- Antihistamines, phenobarbitone, S-adenosylmethionine (SAMe), and steroids have also been tried.
- Pregnancy should not continue beyond term, and condition carries significant risks, with perinatal mortality up to 35%. Recurrence of cholestasis in future pregnancies in 60% of mothers.

Occult blood

See: <u>faecal occult blood testing</u>.

Octreotide

See: <u>OCTREOTIDE</u> in index of drugs.

Oesophageal manometry and motility studies

Commonly used techniques to investigate <u>oesophageal motility disorders</u> include:
- Intraluminal manometry.
- Radiological studies using barium swallows or video fluoroscopy.

Radionuclide imaging to quantify bolus transit through the oesophagus is largely a research tool and will not be further described . Standard endoscopy is a poor method for assessing oesophageal function, although there is some interest in using small calibre endoscopes passed transorally or transnasally to diagnose tracheobronchial aspiration and test sensory thresholds.

Radiological assessment (barium swallow with videofluoroscopy) is essential to study the oropharyngeal phase of swallowing and the upper oesophageal sphincter and offers a less invasive alternative to manometry in some patients. It can be used by speech therapists working with radiologists to develop compensatory strategies to minimize tracheobronchial aspiration in patients with oropharyngeal swallowing disorders. Limitations of radiological examination of motility include subjective evaluation, study of only a small number of swallows, a lack of standardization of details of swallowing technique such as bolus size, and time delays between swallows.

Manometry is the gold standard for assessing oesophageal body motility, because of its quantitative approach. Equipment includes transnasally passed catheters with multiple water-perfused small calibre lumens or more high tech solid state devices using pressure transducers embedded into the probe at various levels. Developments in telemetry allow temporary fixation of pressure transducers at the level of the lower oesophageal sphincter and recording of data on a belt device.

Reading a manometry report. 4 aspects of function need to be characterized to enable most disorders to be diagnosed:
1 Peristaltic performance: percentage of swallows with progressive contraction sequences.
2 Contraction wave configuration (amplitude and duration).
3 Lower oesophageal sphincter basal and peak pressures.
4 Lower oesophageal sphincter relaxation with swallowing.

Limitations of manometry
- Poor toleration of probe by some patients.
- Longitudinal muscle contraction can result in axial displacement.
- Manometry cannot distinguish muscular from neural problems.

Oesophageal motility disorders

Hypermotility disorders

Non-<u>achalasia</u> disorders of hypermotility include:

- Diffuse oesophageal spasm.
- Nutcracker oesophagus.
- Hypertensive lower oesophageal sphincter.
- Non-specific oesophageal motor disorder.

Considerable overlap between these terms exists. All are diagnosed by <u>oesophageal manometry</u>: although (in 2005) stationary manometry remains the gold standard, full agreement between this and 24 hour ambulatory manometry is seen only in about 50% of cases.

Pathology is poorly defined but may involve increased oesophageal sensitivity to cholinergic stimulation.

Clinical presentation Chest pain occurs in 90%, can be severe, is usually retrosternal, and may radiate to the back. There may be some persisting discomfort after the acute episodes, which may help to differentiate it from angina. Dysphagia occurs in 30–60%, and heartburn is seen in up to 20%.

Diagnosis. Upper GI endoscopy is usually normal, but may show alternative reasons for symptoms such as oesophagitis or stricture. Barium studies, especially fluoroscopic studies swallowing soft solids, can be very helpful because they can link faulty transit with symptoms and also show up features such as non-propulsive contractions (so-called 'corkscrew oesophagus').

Manometric abnormalities can include:

- **Non-peristaltic contractions after wet swallows.** Diffuse oesophageal spasm is (somewhat arbitrarily) diagnosed if abnormal swallows occur more than 30% or the time. The term nutcracker oesophagus is reserved for a subgroup with very high contraction amplitude.
- **Abnormal wave of contraction.** This can be variable and is best labelled as a non-specific spastic disorder: there is no agreed classification.
- **Hypertension or poor relaxation** of the lower oesophageal sphincter. This often accompanies spastic abnormalities of the oesophageal body.

Treatment. These disorders are not progressive and not associated with more serious underlying pathology, so symptom reduction is the goal.

- If symptoms suggest abnormal transit (e.g. regurgitation or dysphagia) then treatment similar to that for <u>achalasia</u> may help, especially if manometry shows abnormalities of the lower oesophageal sphincter. Botox injections into the LOS or balloon dilatation have been used effectively in this context.
- Treating reflux can be dramatically beneficial, even in the absence of a classical history.
- Therapeutic trial of nitrates, calcium antagonists, and anticholinergics (see index of drugs) can help and have all been shown experimentally to produce at least short-term improvement in manometry. Remember that nitrates and calcium antagonists will worsen any coexistent oesophageal reflux.

- The tricyclic antidepressant trazodone is the only agent found to improve symptoms in a prospective controlled study (although improvement did not depend on any change in manometry).

Hypomotility disorders

This is usually secondary to systemic disease (see box). The clinical manifestations include:

- Dysphagia, secondary to impaired peristalsis or associated sicca syndrome in scleroderma or associated connective tissue disorders.
- Oesophageal reflux due to the low pressure LOS. Complications of reflux such as <u>oesophagitis</u>, strictures, and <u>Barrett's oesophagus</u> are all more common.

Management of symptoms of impaired GI motility in scleroderma is described elsewhere (see <u>Oesophageal obstruction</u>).

Oesophageal pH monitoring

Ambulatory 24 h pH monitoring is the most widely used test to investigate gastro-oesophageal reflux and to correlate symptoms with reflux. The test involves positioning a transnasal pH probe 5 cm above the lower oeso-phageal sphincter (determined manometrically). The patient then conducts life as normally as possible while recording symptoms, meals, and sleep in a diary. Oesophageal acid exposure is defined as pH less than 4: this should occur for less than 3.5% of total recording time (this is an arbitrary threshold: there is no value that reliably identifies GORD patients).

It is not necessary in most patients with typical reflux symptoms but can be useful in patients with refractory or atypical symptoms not re-sponding to empirical treatment.

Recent technology allows measurement of alkaline reflux from the duodenum into the oesophagus, using a different probe positioned in exactly the same way. This can allow rational prescribing with prokinetics such as <u>DOMPERIDONE</u> or mucosal protective agents such as <u>SUCRALFATE</u> in patients with symptomatic reflux not responding to empirical acid suppressant treatment (see index of drugs).

Oesophageal rings

The mucosal ring, located at the gastro-oesophageal junction, was first described by Schatski in 1953.

Found in approximately 6–14% of adult population on barium swallow, but causes symptoms in minority. Usually considered a congenital struc-tural variant, although chronic reflux may contribute.

Clinical presentation is classically with intermittent non-progressive dysphagia to hurriedly eaten solids (classically bread or meat bolus— 'steakhouse syndrome').

Diagnosis can be by barium swallow or endoscopy: if using barium, the oesophagus must be well distended by getting the patient to perform a valsalva manouevre and including a solid bolus during the exam to iden-tify the lesion. See Colour Plate 19.

Management. In symptomatic patients <u>endoscopic dilatation</u> per-formed, with intention of splitting ring, using bougies or pneumatic balloons. Repeat treatments may be required.

Causes of impaired oesophageal motility

- Usually secondary to multisystem disease
- 80% of <u>scleroderma</u> patients have altered oesophageal motility (second commonest affected organ)
  - Vascular obliteration, secondary fibrosis
  - Reflux, oesophagitis, and Barrett's all seen
- Also seen in mixed connective tissue disease, rheumatoid arthritis, and systemic lupus erythematosus
- Amyloid, alcohol, myxoedema, MS
- Diabetes: 60% of patients with peripheral or autonomic neuropathy have disordered motility, but symptoms are only seen in a minority
- Pseudo-obstruction

Oesophageal stricture

Can be a feature of oesophageal malignancies or due to extrinsic compression of oesophagus. Commonest benign cause is acid reflux but also seen after caustic injury, after variceal sclerotherapy or band ligation, and after mediastinal chemo/radiotherapy. Prevalence of peptic strictures in patients with reflux oesophagitis is 8–20% but may be decreasing with widespread use of proton pump inhibitors. Strictures can develop weeks to months after sclerotherapy; incidence is 2–13% and the major risk factor is large persistent oesophageal ulcers.

Treatment centres on endoscopic dilatation, healing oesophagitis, and minimising recurrence. Dilatation can be done with Celestin or Savary–Gillard graded dilators over a guide wire or using a through the scope balloon. Results are equally effective although the balloon exerts a lower radial force than the rigid dilators. Dilatation to 15 mm generally relieves dysphagia. The schedule varies but repeating the procedure every 1–2 weeks with no more than three step dilatations at any one occasion is advised. More than 50% patients need repeat dilatation: risk factors are number of previous dilatations and persistent oesophagitis. Maintenance proton pump inhibitors are advised.

Risks of dilatation

- Perforation (less than 0.5% for benign structures, but higher for malignant structures (2–6%)).
- Bleeding (less than 0.5%).
- Bacteraemia (give antibiotic prophylaxis to at-risk patients).

Oesophageal tumours

Classified into epithelial or non-epithelial, benign or malignant: see table.

Malignant epithelial tumours

- Mostly primary oesophageal cancers: squamous cell carcinoma (SCC), adenocarcinoma of oesophagus, and adenocarcinoma of oesophago-gastric junction.
- Worldwide, 5th commonest lethal cancer, with SCC commonest subtype, but in Western countries adenocarcinoma has increased 5-fold in last 30 years so that this is now commoner than SCC: the rise is particularly marked for cancers of the oesophago-gastric junction.

Epidemiology and risks for oesophageal cancer are shown in table.

Clinical features

- SCC occurs in the upper two-thirds of the oesophagus; adenocarcinoma occurs in the lower third and at the oesophago-gastric junction.
- Symptoms include dysphagia and odynophagia (pain on swallowing), often accompanied by anorexia and weight loss. Both cancer types can infiltrate submucosally but SCC is more locally aggressive, and can cause vocal cord paralysis due to recurrent laryngeal nerve invasion and <u>tracheo-oesophageal fistula</u> in 5%. Pulmonary, hepatic, brain, and bone metastasis occurs. Adenocarcinoma is less locally invasive, but haematogenous and lymphangitic spread occurs to regional and distant lymph nodes and to liver. Most patients present with advanced disease because the oesophagus has a rich lymphatic supply and lacks a serosa, so that local spread occurs before luminal stenosis causes symptoms.
- Hepatomegaly may be present if there are liver metastases.

Diagnosis

- **Screening** of high risk groups includes surveillance of patients with <u>Barrett's oesophagus</u> (e.g. see <u>Barrett's surveillance</u>). Non-endoscopic balloon cytology involves a latex balloon covered with nylon mesh that is advanced into the cardia and withdrawn through the oesophagus. It is much cheaper than endoscopic surveillance and has been used with some success in China where the risk of SCC is high, but has not yet been shown effective in other populations.
- **Laboratory** tests may reveal low albumin, anaemia (bleeding or chronic disease), and hypercalcaemia due to PTH-related peptide, especially in SCC (seen in 15–30% patients).
- **Radiology.** Chest X-rays can be helpful in diagnosing pulmonary metastases of lung infiltrates suggestive of oesophago-bronchial fistula. Contrast radiology with barium can confirm fistulation or obstruction. Cross-sectional imaging is needed for staging (see below).
- **Endoscopy.** This allows histological diagnosis but also characterization of length and configuration and an opportunity for therapeutic dilatation. 6 biopsies are needed for an accuracy of nearly 100%.

Classification of oesophageal tumours

Epithelial	Non-epithelial
Malignant	
Squamous cell carcinoma	Lymphoma
Adenocarcinoma	Sarcoma
Adenocarcinoma of the oesophago-gastric junction	Metastases
Other rare malignancies e.g. small cell carcinoma (1–5% of oesophageal cancers)	
Benign	
Papilloma	Leiomyoma
Adenoma	Granular cell tumours
	Others (lipoma, haemangioma)

Epidemiology and biology of oesophageal cancer

Squamous cell cancer	Adenocarcinoma
Incidence	
Incidence varies by region: commonest in China, Iran, Turkey, N. Africa. Commoner in (black) men in 6th and 7th decades	Commoner in white men
Environmental risk factors	
Nitrosamines in the diet, exposure to hydrocarbons from cooking in confined spaces, and chewing of betel nuts have been implicated. Alcohol and tobacco are both linked to SCC	An apparent inverse relation with *Helicobacter pylori* has been claimed
High risk diseases	
Achalasia (possible due to prolonged stasis of oesophageal contents) Caustic strictures	Gastro-oesophageal reflux and Barrett's oesophagus are associated factors, with most cancers arising from areas of intestinal metaplasia. Annual incidence of cancer in Barrett's quoted as 0.5–1% per annum
Plummer–Vinsen/Patterson–Kelly syndrome	
Tylosis	
Concurrent head or neck SCC	
Human papilloma virus	
Biology	
Associated oncogenes include cyclin D1	P53 and E cadherin are both important tumour suppressor genes.

Staging

Staging is largely based on retrospective Japanese data (most patients had SCC rather than increasingly common adenocarcinoma). Treatment and outcome are stage-dependent (see tumour staging TNM classification) Patients with T1 or T2 lesions who are N0, M0 have significant surgical cure rates. T3N1 patients are potentially curable but do poorly with surgery alone. Patients with local spread into aorta, airway, pleura, and spine and those with haematogenous spread should be treated palliatively, although there is some evidence that patients with positive abdominal lymph nodes can undergo curative resection.

- **Cross-sectional imaging.** CT is accurate at identifying solid organ metastases but less good at identifying lymph node metastases, especially in the chest. MRI has no significant advantage over CT. PET scanning has high sensitivity and specificity for distant metastases but is not widely used at present in staging.
- **Endoscopic ultrasound** is probably the most accurate tool for staging; overall accuracy for T stage is 75–85% and N stage is 65–75%. EUS for the guiding fine needle aspiration (FNA) improves diagnosis of malignant lymphadenopathy. EUS has been shown to have high sensitivity and negative predictive value for submucosal invasion of cancer in patients with Barrett's and highgrade dysplasia (HGD) or intramucosal carcinoma.

Treatment

Primary treatment

- Options include surgery alone, chemoradiotherapy, endoscopic mucosal resection, and photodynamic therapy. Combined modality therapy with e.g. surgery plus chemoradiotherapy is under evaluation.
- Surgery is indicated for superficial tumours. Operative mortality is 3–10%. Surgical approach is either trans-hiatal or involves thoracotomy.
- Squamous cell tumours are more sensitive to radiotherapy than adenocarcinomas, but even in SCC, combined chemo- and radiotherapy is more effective than radiation therapy alone. Results suggest a 75% local control rate, with 18% survival at 5 years for stage I/II patients.

Endoscopic mucosal resection. Accurate staging and histological diagnosis of HGD or carcinoma limited to mucosa allows endosopic resection using submucosal saline injection and electrocautery techniques. Complete resection appears possible in over 75% but long-term follow up data are limited at present. Photodynamic therapy (PDT) is being evaluated as a curative modality.

Palliative treatment includes radio- and chemotherapy, intraluminal brachytherapy, endoscopic dilatation or stent placement, contact thermal therapy, endoscopic laser therapy, and PDT. Argon plasma coagulation does not penetrate deeply enough to give relief of dysphagia, and injection of cytotoxic drugs, although theoretically attractive, has not been standardized or compared with other ablative techniques.

Prognosis in oesophageal cancer is related to TNM classification

Stage	5 year survival	Comments
T1	46%	Surgically resectable. 5 year survial is 40% for N0 but 17% for N1
T2	30%	
T3	22%	
T4	7%	

- **Chemotherapy.** Objective response rates of 30–50% are seen with platinum based regimes with 5FU, a taxane, or topoisomerase inhibitor.
- **Endoscopic therapy** aims at palliating dysphagia, although bleeding and oesophago-respiratory fistulae can also be treated endoscopically. Endoscopic dilatation can be done using bougies or through-the-scope (TTS) balloons. Advantages include simplicity, low cost, and relative safety. Disadvantages include short duration of efficacy and the frequent need for repeated procedures. It is not adequate palliation for most patients. The best results using thermal ablation are with endoscopic laser, Nd:YAG being the commonest wavelength (see lasers in the GI tract).
- **Endoscopic stents** offers good palliation of malignant strictures and tracheo-oesophageal fistulae. Self-expanding metallic stents have replaced rigid plastic stents because they are easier to place, give better palliation, and are associated with fewer complications (see Colour Plate 20).
- **Photodynamic therapy**. This is discussed in detail elsewhere.

Other oesophageal tumours

- **Malignant non-epithelial tumours.** The oesophagus is a rare site of primary lymphoma and sarcoma: leiomyosarcoma are the most common. Diagnosis can be difficult with conventional biopsy—EUS-guided FNA is the best way of getting a diagnosis.
- **Benign tumours.** Leiomyomas arise from smooth muscle cells; they have been subsumed into the category gastrointestinal stromal tumours (GIST). There is a risk of malignant transformation into sarcomas that appears to increase with size over 5 cm diameter. EUS is the most accurate diagnostic modality (see Colour Plate 21). Surgery should be considered if there are symptoms, uncertainty about the diagnosis, or a suspicion of malignant transformation. Other benign tumours include granular cell tumours, fibrovascular polyps or hamartomas, and lipomas.

Oesophagitis

- Most commonly due to gastro-oesophageal reflux (see <u>Approach to dyspepsia and gastro-oesophageal reflux</u>) but remember other causes (see box).
- Diagnostic evaluation of oesophagitis is usually by endoscopy, although only 30–40% patients with GORD have endoscopically obvious inflammation. Endoscopic evaluation can be confusing: the commonest classification is the Los Angeles grading system (see box).

Ogilvie's syndrome (acute pseudo-obstruction)

Acute pseudo-obstruction localized to the colon, precipitated by trauma, orthopaedic surgery, obstetric procedures, pelvic surgery, or electrolyte disturbances such as hypokalaemia. The precise cause is not known, but the condition results from a dilatation of the colon in response to non-mechanical factors.

Diagnosis is by abdominal X-ray, which shows gaseous distension of the colon, with no bowel sounds on examination.

Treatment

- Nil by mouth, <u>nasogastric tube</u>, IV fluids. Water soluble contrast exam to exclude mechanical obstruction: hyperosmolarity often helps to evacuate colon.
- Try and decompress the colon with a rectal decompresson tube. Neostigmine (2.5 mg IV over 1–3 minutes) can be very helpful in management of acute colonic pseudo-obstruction. Patients should be on an ECG monitor: have IV atropine available in case of bradycardia. Response is usually within 20 minutes: treatment can be repeated up to three times until successful.
- **Surgery** is advisable for patients with caecal diameter over 11 cm and refractory to medical or endoscopic management. Tube caecostomy can be helpful: for patients with fever, leucocytosis, or peritoneal signs, right hemicolectomy may be required.

Old age

See: <u>elderly and the GI tract</u>.

<u>Opiates</u>

See: index of drugs and <u>pain control</u>.

Causes of oesophagitis

- Infections: fungal (*Candida*, *Aspergillus*), bacterial (staphylococcus, stretococcus), and viral
- Systemic diseases: pemphigus, Behçet's syndrome
- Graft versus host disease
- IBD: the oesophagus is rarely affected in Crohn's disease
- Pill-induced oesophagitis
- Chemoradiation: mucositis can affect oesophagel mucosa. Radiation above 30 Gy is associated with oesophagitis. Chemotherapy potentiates radiation-induced oesophagitis

Los Angeles grading system for oesophagitis

Grade A: one or more mucosal breaks no longer than 5 mm that do not extend between the tops of two mucosal folds

Grade B: one or more mucosal breaks more than 5 mm long that do not extend between the tops of two mucosal folds

Grade C: One or more mucosal breaks that are continuous between the tops of two or more mucosal folds but involve less than 75% of the circumference

Grade D: One or more mucosal breaks that involve at least 75% of the oesophageal circumference

Note that the Los Angeles system does not describe strictures, hiatus herniae, or Barrett's: these have to be described separately.

Oral contraceptive pill (OCP)

OCPs, particularly those containing higher doses of oestrogens are associated with range of gastrointestinal conditions:

- Hepatic adenomas are benign tumours of liver, clearly associated with OCPs (risk of 3–4 per 100 000 exposed women). Complications include pain due to size, and rupture. May disappear after stopping OCP.
- Cholestasis due to OCPs is similar to intrahepatic cholestasis of pregnancy (and occurs on taking OCPs in 50% of women who have suffered condition in pregnancy). May be dose-dependent oestrogen effect on bile secretion. Appears <6/12 after starting OCPs.
- Focal nodular hyperplasia probably not caused by OCPs, but drug may promote growth and risk of rupture.
- Hepatocellular carcinoma very rare in patients on OCPs, but risk may be increased in those using for >8 years.
- Relative risk of Budd–Chiari syndrome in patients on OCPs >2.
- Intestinal ischaemia reported in patients with blood group A taking OCPs. Portal vein thrombosis reported in patients on OCPs, usually in conjunction with other prothrombotic tendencies.

In contrast to the detrimental effects of OCPs, they have also been used as medical therapy to treat recurrent blood loss due to angiodysplasia.

Oral rehydration solutions (ORS)

- Can be life-saving in treating children with diarrhoeal illnesses; in Western countries it can be helpful in treating patients with high output ostomies, short-bowel syndrome, and HIV infection.
- The principle is to stimulate sodium and water absorption by the sodium glucose co-transporter in the intestinal epithelial brush border. Glucose enhances sodium absorption by an active carrier process: water absorption follows passively. For treating severe diarrhoea, rehydration solutions should contain an alkalinizing agent to counter acidosis and be slightly hypo-osmolar (about 250 mM/l) to prevent osmotic diarrhoea.
- The precise composition is controversial; there is debate about the type of carbohydrate that should be used and the best concentrations of sodium, potassium, chloride, and base.

Components of feed

- Glucose is the most commonly used substrate and should be provided at 70–150 mM: higher concentrations can cause osmotic diarrhoea. Replacing glucose with polymeric carbohydrate such as rice syrup solids provides a hypotonic solution that is better in decreasing stool output.
- In developed countries oral rehydration solutions contain lower concentrations of sodium (Na^+ 50–60 mM) than the WHO formulation (75 mM) since patients tend to suffer less severe sodium loss. Stool sodium concentration in cholera is about 90 mM; maximal absorption of sodium occurs at a concentration of 120 mM and this higher concentration may be optimal in patients with short-bowel syndrome and high stoma output.

- The concentration of potassium in ORS is about 20 mM although stool potassium concentrations are often higher and 30–35 mM may be more appropriate.

Composition of oral rehydration solutions

Solution	Na (mM)	K (mM)	Cl (mM)	Citrate (mM)	Glucose (mM)	Osmolarity
WHO	75	20	65	10	75	245 mOsm/l
UK formulations	60	20	50	10	90	Approx 300

Osler–Weber–Rendu syndrome

See: hereditary haemorrhagic telangiectasia.

Osteoporosis and metabolic bone disease

See also: bone densitometry.

Definitions

- Osteoporosis refers to defective bone formation, defined by WHO as T-score > –2.5 standard deviations below the average (T-score compares bone mineral density (BMD) to controls with peak BMD (i.e. young fit adults), whereas Z-score matches for age and sex).
- Osteopenia refers to less severe reduction in BMD (see table), but affects >15% of young women, and 40% >50 years.
- Osteomalacia refers to defective bone mineralization, due to vitamin D deficiency.

At risk groups in gastroenterology/hepatology

- Chronic cholestatic liver disease (e.g. primary biliary cirrhosis (PBC) and primary sclerosing cholangitis (PSC)). 20% of patients with PBC have osteoporosis at time of referral, and 50% have severe bone loss at time of liver transplantation. All patients with cirrhosis appear at risk.
- Coeliac disease. Osteoporosis in 5–10%, and osteomalacia in association with vitamin D deficiency.
- Inflammatory bowel disease (Crohn's disease and ulcerative colitis). Malnutrition and bowel resection may predispose to osteoporosis, but long-term steroid therapy appears main reason for ↓BMD, with 40% increase in fracture risk over controls.
- Post-gastrectomy status (e.g. Billroth I/Billroth II partial gastrectomy). Calcium and vitamin D malabsorption may both contribute to osteomalacia in 10–20%, osteoporosis in > 30% > 10 years post-surgery.
- Chronic pancreatitis. Malabsorption of fat soluble vitamins.
- Malnutrition, low BMI, eating disorders.
- Long-standing steroid use (e.g. autoimmune hepatitis and see drugs).
- Any cause of body mass index (BMI) < 19, or physical inactivity.

Investigation

- Bloods
  - Serum calcium. Usually normal in osteoporosis.
  - Parathyroid hormone (PTH). ↑ PTH, with ↓ serum phosphate, and normal/↓ calcium suggests secondary hyperparathyroidism, vitamin D deficiency, and osteomalacia.
  - 25-(OH) vitamin D. Deficiency usually dietary, contributing to osteomalacia.
  - LFTs. ↑ ALP in presence of normal GGT suggests ALP of bone origin (e.g. in osteomalacia). ALP isoenzymes can be performed to differentiate bone from liver.
  - Thyroid function tests.
- Plain X-rays: osteopenia may be visible on plain X-rays, but only after 30–40% bone loss has occurred.
- <u>Bone densitometry</u>. Bone mineral density (BMD) most accurately assessed by bone densitometry using dual energy X-ray absorptiometry (DEXA), usually of femoral neck and lumbar spine. If steroid use planned (e.g. prednisolone 7.5 mg/day for > 3 months) baseline DEXA and follow-up DEXA in 6–12 months should be performed. Spine measurements unreliable in elderly due to presence of osteophytes, extraskeletal calcification, and spinal deformity.

Management

- Give oral calcium supplements (e.g. calcium carbonate 1–1.5 g/day) and vitamin D 800 IU (e.g. Calcichew® D3) if in at risk group. If T score <–2.5 repeat DEXA in 2 years; if T score >–2.5 consider additional therapy:
  - Hormone replacement therapy (HRT) in postmenopausal women.
  - Bisphosphonates (e.g. alendronate 70 mg/week). May be used in conjunction with calcium, vitamin D, and HRT.
  - Parathyroid hormone supplementation reserved for severe osteoporosis and fractures, if patient is unresponsive to bisphosphonates, and in absence of secondary hyperparathyroidism.
- Avoid smoking and excess alcohol.
- In patients with chronic liver disease, <u>liver transplantation</u> is associated with further reduction in BMD over first year, then improvement.

WHO diagnostic criteria for osteoporosis	
Normal	BMD value within 1 standard deviation (SD) of young-adult mean (T-score at or above –1)
Osteopenia	BMD value between –1 S.D. and –2.5 SD below young-adult mean (T-score between –1 and –2.5)
Osteoporosis	BMD value at least –2.5 SD below young adult mean (T-score at or below –2.5)
Severe osteoporosis	BMD value at least –2.5 SD below young adult mean and presence of fracture

Overlap syndromes

Refers to clinical scenario in which 2 chronic liver diseases are simultaneously present. Found in 10% of patients with autoimmune liver disease.

- <u>Autoimmune hepatitis</u> (AIH)/<u>primary biliary cirrhosis</u> (PBC) overlap occurs as 2 variants: one with predominant cholestatic LFTs, anti-mitochondrial Ab (AMA) positive, but histological evidence of AIH; the other (also known as autoimmune cholangitis or AMA-negative PBC) with histological criteria for PBC, but AMA-negative, but often anti-nuclear Ab (ANA) and anti-smooth muscle Ab (SMA) positive. <u>URSODEOXYCHOLIC ACID</u> (UDCA) is usually given (12–15mg/kg/day) in addition to steroids ± <u>AZATHIOPRINE</u> in those with prominent AIH features.
- AIH/<u>primary sclerosing cholangitis</u> (PSC) overlap mainly reported in children/young adults, with cholangiogram (MRCP/ERCP) and histological features consistent with PSC, but biochemical and serological markers of AIH. UDCA ± immunosuppressants used, but response unpredictable.
- AIH/<u>hepatitis C</u> characterized by chronic HCV infection with anti-LKM-1, ANA, SMA Abs, and ↑serum IgG. Treatment difficult, as <u>INTERFERON</u> may worsen liver disease if AIH predominant (e.g. Ab titres > 1:320), yet immunosuppression for AIH may increase HCV replication.

Oxalate stones

- Dietary oxalate (found in tea, chocolate, cola, vegetables) is usually precipitated out as calcium oxalate in the bowel and lost in stool.
- In conditions associated with <u>bile acid malabsorption</u>, and thus fat <u>malabsorption</u> (e.g. <u>short bowel syndrome</u>, terminal ileal <u>Crohn's disease</u>), unabsorbed long-chain fatty acids compete with oxalate for available calcium. As a result, larger amounts of free oxalate reach the colon, are absorbed, and ultimately excreted in the kidney. Hyperoxaluria then predisposes to calcium oxalate kidney stones (> 20% of patients with short bowel syndrome).
- Urinary oxalate should be measured in at risk patients (no risk if colon removed).
- Management involves restricting high oxalate foods and maintaining adequate fluid intake. If hyperoxaluria continues, oral calcium citrate may be used to enhance oxalate precipitation.

P

Paget's disease

See: <u>anal cancer</u>.

Pain control

> 'It is easier to find men who will volunteer to die, than to find those who are willing to endure pain with patience'. Julius Caesar

- Pain associated with GI disease may be due to range of mechanisms—inflammation (e.g. <u>familial Mediterranean fever</u>), colic (e.g. biliary colic), tumour invasion (e.g. <u>pancreatic cancer</u>).
- Pain control is rarely effective (and potentially dangerous) in the absence of a clear diagnosis as to the cause.
- WHO recently proposed a 3 step 'pain ladder' for cancer pain relief:
    - **Step 1**: prompt oral administration of non-opioids (e.g. aspirin 600 mg 4 hourly PO and paracetamol 1 g 4 hourly PO) ± adjuvants (to treat anxiety, depression, e.g. tricyclic antidepressants).
    - **Step 2**: mild opioids (e.g. codeine 30–60 mg 4 hourly PO, dihydrocodeine 30 mg 4 hourly PO, tramadol 50–100mg qds PO) ± non-opioids ± adjuvants.
    - **Step 3**: strong opioids (e.g. morphine 5–10 mg 4 hourly PO/IM/IV, slow release fentanyl 25–100 µg transdermal patch every 72 hours) ± non-opioids ± adjuvants.
- Step-wise increase in opioids advised until patient pain free. Normal release opioids given 'by the clock' (e.g. 4 hourly), rather than 'on demand'. Same dose of morphine used for 'breakthrough' pain as frequently as 1–2 hourly, and total daily intake used to calculate 4 hourly requirement for next day. Once maintenance dose achieved, can swap to 12 or 24 hourly slow-release preparation. Diamorphine preferred to morphine if IV drug required (but third of total 24 hour morphine dose required).
- Prevent opioid-induced constipation using stool softener and stimulant laxative (e.g. co-danthramer 25/200 in 5 ml od PO or senna 2 tabs at night PO + sodium docusate 200 mg bd PO). <u>ANTI-EMETICS</u>, particularly for first week of opioids, may be needed (cyclizine 50 mg tds PO/IM/IV, <u>METOCLOPRAMIDE</u> 10 mg tds PO/IM/IV).
- Involve the experts (e.g. palliative care service, pain team).
- Type of GI disease will influence approach to pain control, e.g:
    - **Functional bowel disorders** (e.g. <u>irritable bowel syndrome</u>, simple constipation) may benefit from behavioural therapies (<u>biofeedback</u>, cognitive therapy, hypnotherapy). Antispasmodics may help with colicky pain (e.g. mebeverine 135 mg tds PO).
    - **Pancreatic disease.** Opioids often required for cancer and <u>chronic pancreatitis</u>. Percutaneous/<u>endoscopic ultrasound</u> guided coeliac plexus block (with bupivacaine + triamcinolone) useful, but usually short term. Radiotherapy may reduce <u>pancreatic cancer</u> pain.
    - **Decompensated liver disease**. NSAIDs may worsen liver + renal dysfunction, and risk GI bleeding. Opioids may cause <u>hepatic encephalopathy</u>, particularly if precipitate constipation. Ironically, paracetamol probably safest analgesic, but at dose < 3 g/day.

Pancreas divisum

- In embryonic development, dorsal and ventral pancreatic buds join, so that body and tail of pancreas drain predominantly through major papilla, with common bile duct, via ventral pancreas. In 4% of population ventral duct not linked to dorsal duct, which then drains through smaller accessory duct (duct of Santorini). See figure on previous page.
- May be a cause of recurrent <u>acute</u> or <u>chronic pancreatitis</u>, and accessory sphincterotomy/sphincteroplasty may improve symptoms. However, aetiological link controversial, as minimal increase in prevalence of pancreatitis in patients with pancreas divisum.

Pancreatic cancer

Epidemiology

- 4th leading cause of cancer death in USA and Europe (incidence approximately 10 cases per 100 000). Median age at diagnosis 65 years, slightly more common in males (and blacks, in USA).
- No clear cause in most cases, but risk factors include <u>chronic pancreatitis</u> and cigarettes. 8% of patients with pancreatic cancer have 1st degree relative with disease, related to both underlying <u>hereditary pancreatitis</u> (40% risk by age 70 years) and familial pancreatic cancer.
- Onset of diabetes within previous 2 years in patients without family history of diabetes is linked.

Pathogenesis

- Pancreatic cancer usually refers to ductal adenocarcinoma, which accounts for 90% of pancreatic tumours (others include <u>pancreatic cystic tumours</u> and <u>pancreatic endocrine tumours</u>).
- Genetic mutations within *KRAS2* and *CDKN2* genes in > 80% of cancers.
- 75% of cancers in pancreatic head, 10–15% in body, 5–10% in tail.
- Metastases to regional lymph nodes, liver, and occasionally lung.

Clinical features

- Jaundice (at presentation in 50%), weight loss, anorexia, and upper abdominal pain radiating to back are classical symptoms. Symptoms of <u>chronic pancreatitis</u> (e.g. <u>pancreatic insufficiency</u>) occasionally present.
- Nausea and vomiting may relate to duodenal obstruction.
- Palpable gallbladder in 30% (Courvoisier's sign—see opposite).
- Migratory thrombophlebitis (i.e. Trousseau sign) and venous thrombosis (including <u>portal vein thrombosis</u>) occur at increased frequency.
- Differential diagnosis includes distal <u>cholangiocarcinoma</u>, <u>ampullary cancer</u>, focal pancreatitis in head of pancreas, and rarely <u>autoimmune pancreatitis</u>.

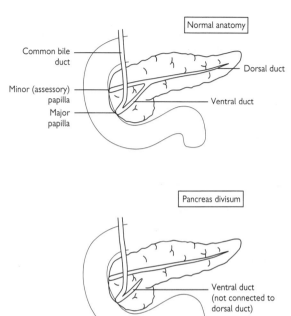

Fig. 2.20 Anatomic arrangement of pancreatic ducts. (a) The most common arrangement, where most pancreatic secretions empty with the bile through the major duodenal papilla. In about 70% adults, the proximal portion of the dorsal duct remains patent and some pancreatic secreations empty through the accessory papilla. (b) Pancreas divisum: the embryonic dorsal and ventral ducts fail to fuse, with 80–95% of pancreatic secretions emptying from the dorsal duct through the accessory papilla.

Courvoisier's law

Ludwig Georg Courvoisier, Swiss surgeon 1843–1918

'Jaundice in the presence of a palpable gallbladder is not explained by gallstone obstruction of bile duct'.

Probably explained by slow onset of biliary dilatation with distal bile duct tumours (e.g. pancreatic cancer, ampullary cancer), and fact that chronically inflamed, thick-walled gallbladders less likely to dilate. Exceptions to this rule include gallbladder empyema with cystic duct stone obstruction, and Mirizzi's syndrome.

Investigation
- Aimed at making diagnosis, and <u>tumour staging</u>.
- LFTs may show cholestatic picture—↑Bn, ↑ALP/GGT (see <u>Approach to recent-onset jaundice</u>).
- ↑ serum CA19–9 elevated in 75–85% of patients, but value > 100 U/ml only highly specific for malignancy in absence of biliary obstruction. <u>Carcinoembryonic antigen</u> (CEA) ↑ in 40% of patients, but of little diagnostic use.
- Transabdominal <u>ultrasound</u>: accurately shows biliary dilatation, but views of pancreas often incomplete. Pancreatic-protocol <u>CT</u>: defines tumour and size, demonstrates local vascular involvement (portal vein, superior mesenteric artery/vein), retroperitoneal invasion, and liver metastases. Only imaging modality needed to make diagnosis in > 90 % of cases. Very accurately demonstrates irresectability, but falsely suggests resectability in 25–50% of cases.
- <u>MRI</u> rarely used instead of CT, but has comparable accuracy.
- <u>ERCP</u>: allows endoscopic stenting (with plastic stent until histological confirmation of inoperable cancer), and cytological brushings. '<u>Double duct sign</u>' strongly suggests head of pancreas cancer.
- <u>Endoscopic ultrasound</u> playing increasing role in staging (as good as <u>CT</u> for defining vascular involvement), allows FNA cytology, and useful for 'trouble-shooting' small pancreatic lesions/unexplained strictures.

Management
- Curative resection in <15% of patients (very rare for cancers in body/tail, as present late), and overall survival at 1 year and 5 years 20% and 4%. In those undergoing curative resection (<u>Whipple's procedure</u>), 5 year survival 10–25%. Histological diagnosis not usually needed or sought prior to attempted curative surgery.
- Palliative chemotherapy with gemcitabine provides some survival benefit, but newer combination regimes are awaited. Role of chemo-radiotherapy, including as neoadjuvant therapy (to 'downstaging' inoperable tumours to operable), remains uncertain.
- <u>Pain control</u> may be a particular problem, necessitating regular opiates. Radiotherapy and coeliac plexus block may help.
- ERCP and biliary stenting dependent on presentation (i.e. obstructive jaundice). Metal stents should not be inserted unless histology and clinical assessment/imaging confirm inoperable malignancy. In patients with unresectable tumour and biliary and duodenal obstruction (5% of patients), surgical <u>biliary bypass</u> or enteral and biliary mesh-metal stents (see Colour Plate 22) are options.

Differential diagnosis of pancreatic mass

- <u>Pancreatic cancer</u> (ductal adenocarcinoma)
- Distal <u>cholangiocarcinoma</u>
- <u>Ampullary cancer</u>
- <u>Lymphoma</u>
- TB
- <u>Pancreatic endocrine tumour</u>
- <u>Autoimmune pancreatitis</u>
- <u>Acute</u> and acute-on-<u>chronic pancreatitis</u>
- Von Hippel–Lindau disease
- <u>Pancreatic cystic tumour</u> .
- <u>Pancreatic pseudocyst</u>

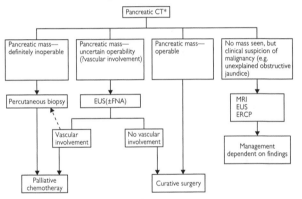

* Includes CT cuts through abdomen and chest, to exclude metastases.

Fig. 2.21 Staging and management of suspected pancreatic cancer.

Pancreatic cystic tumours

Background

- Cystic neoplasms of pancreas account for 10–15% of cystic lesions (<u>pancreatic pseudocysts</u> (80–90%), true cysts, and acute fluid collections after acute pancreatitis account for rest), and represent only 1% of pancreatic neoplasms.
- Mucinous cystic neoplasm (MCN), serous cystadenoma, and intraductal papillary mucinous tumour (IPMT see Fig. 2.22) account for > 90% of pancreatic cystic neoplasms (see table).

Clinical features

- Increasingly diagnosed incidentally on abdominal imaging.
- IPMT may be misdiagnosed as idiopathic recurrent or <u>chronic pancreatitis</u>, with pancreatic duct abnormalities, and <u>pancreatic insufficiency</u> caused by mucus obstruction of pancreatic duct.
- May occasionally present as for <u>pancreatic cancer</u> (i.e. weight loss, jaundice, pain).

Investigation

- <u>CT</u> and <u>MRI/MRCP</u> may define cyst architecture and relationship with pancreatic duct.
- <u>Endoscopic ultrasound</u> (EUS) has increasing role, and allows cyst fluid aspiration, but may not be necessary where surgery is planned and cross-sectional imaging unequivocal.
- Fluid analysis allows differentiation from <u>pancreatic pseudocyst</u>. Elevated cyst CEA levels suggest malignancy, but CA19–9 not of use.
- <u>ERCP</u> may demonstrate mucus, either emanating from wide-open papilla (pathognomonic of IPMT), or within dilated pancreatic duct.

Management

No standardized policy. Management in specialist centres. Need to balance potential cure from surgery, against requirement for radical resection (<u>Whipple's procedure</u> or distal pancreatectomy, dependent on site) in asymptomatic patients with cystic tumours of low malignant potential.

Pancreatic endocrine tumours (PET)

- <u>Neuroendocrine tumours</u> of the GI tract classified into 2 groups—<u>carcinoid</u> tumours and PETs. Latter arise from pancreatic islet cells.
- Primary insulinomas and glucagonomas occur exclusively in pancreas, but 50–70% of <u>gastrinomas</u> arise from extra-pancreatic sites. May be associated with other conditions, including <u>multiple endocrine neoplasia (MEN)-1</u>, Von Hippel–Lindau disease, neurofibromatosis type 1 (NF1), and tuberous sclerosis (e.g. >10% NF1 patients develop <u>carcinoid</u> tumour, often duodenal).
- PETs may be functional (associated with clinical syndrome related to hormone release (see table and p.489)) or non-functional.

Pancreatic cystic tumours

	Mucinous cystic neoplasm (MCN)	Serous cyst—adenoma	Intraductal papillary mucinous tumour (IPMT)
Sex	> 80% female	> 80% female	> 50% male
Peak age	50 years	70 years	60–70 years
Presentation	Mass/pain	Mass/pain	Recurrent pancreatitis
Pancreatic site	Body/tail	Head/body	Head
CT findings	Septae, Ca^{2+}	Septae, Ca^{2+}	No septae
ERCP findings			
Pancreatic duct dilatation	No	No	Yes
Duct–cyst communication	No	No	Yes
Malignant potential	Yes (8–33% of cases)	Very rare	Yes (15–40% of cases)

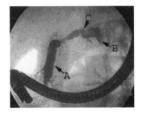

Fig 2.22 IPMT in tail of pancreas. ERCP shows dilated main pancreatic duct (A), abnormal ducts in tail (B), and filling defects due to mucus (C).

Insulinoma

- Located throughout pancreas (1/3rd head, 1/3rd body, 1/3rd tail), usually < 5 cm, with multiple lesions in approx 10%. Clinical features relate to symptomatic hypoglycaemia, and patients may become morbidly obese due to overeating to stave off hypoglycaemia.
- As with other functional PETs, diagnosis depends on localizing tumour, and demonstrating excess hormone. In > 90%, 48 hour fast with 3–6 hourly blood glucose, plasma insulin, and C-peptide levels induces hypoglycaemia and demonstrates disproportionately elevated insulin. CT/ MRI localize lesion in < 40% if 1–3 cm, and <u>endoscopic ultrasound</u>, angiography, and selective venous sampling may be required.
- Management includes advice to take small regular meals and diazoxide, a nondiuretic benzothiazide analogue, that inhibits insulin release (this drug and <u>OCTREOTIDE</u> may control symptoms in 60% of cases). Surgery provides complete cure in 70–95%.

Glucagonoma

- Glucagon stimulates glycogenolysis and insulin secretion, and inhibits pancreatic and gastric secretion and gut motility. Association with <u>MEN-1</u> in 20%. Metastases/local invasion in 50–80%.
- Usually > 5cm, secrete excess glucagons, causing dermatitis (migratory necrolytic erythema), weight loss, glucose intolerance, and anaemia. Hyperglycaemia in 40–90%.
- Diagnosis made on demonstrating elevated plasma glucagons >1000 pg/ml (normal < 200 pg/ml). Treatment includes control of diabetes and use of octreotide (may improve weight loss, diarrhoea, and rash).
- Surgery performed for local disease, but cure in only 20%.

VIPoma

- Usually solitary tumours in tail of pancreas.
- Characterized by profound watery diarrhoea, dehydration, hypokalaemia and hypochlorydia.
- Diagnosis made on basis of large volume diarrhoea (> 3 l/day in > 75% of patients), and raised serum VIP levels.
- Medical management includes careful fluid and electrolyte replacement. May need > 5 l fluid, and 350 MEq of potassium/day). <u>OCTREOTIDE</u> controls symptoms, but effect may be short-lived. Surgery completely relieves symptoms in approximately 30%.

Non-functional PETs (1/3rd of PETs) usually occur in pancreatic head, are generally larger than functional ones, and 60–90% malignant.

Pancreatic endocrine tumours (PET)

Syndrome	Hormone released	Clinical features	Rate of malignancy %	Incidence per million
Gastrinoma (Zollinger–Ellison syndrome)	Gastrin	Recurrent upper GI tract ulceration	60–70	1
Insulinoma	Insulin	Hypoglycaemic episodes Obesity	< 10	1–2
Glucagonoma	Glucagon	Weight loss Diarrhoea Dermatitis (migratory necrolytic erythema)	60	0.1
VIPoma	Vasoactive intestinal polypeptide	Watery diarrhoea ↓K, ↓Mg^{2+} Flushing	> 60	0.5
Somato-statinoma	Somatostatin	Diarrhoea	> 70	< 0.1

For details on practical aspects of measuring gut hormones, see gut hormone profile.

Pancreatic function tests

- Pancreatic **endocrine** function usually assessed with glucose tolerance test. Malabsorption and steatorrhoea only occur when > 90% of **exocrine** pancreas function lost. Exocrine function tests used to assess chronic pancreatitis and other causes of exocrine pancreatic insufficiency, and variety of direct and indirect tests available.
- **Direct tests** involve sampling of pancreatic secretions after administration of secretagogue (e.g. secretin, cholecystokinin). Duodenal aspiration and measurement of volume, bicarbonate, and enzyme concentration (e.g. amylase, trypsin, lipase). Direct tests remain 'gold standard', but invasive to perform, and rarely used in clinical practice.
- **Indirect tests** involve measurement of pancreatic enzymes in stool, or of metabolites of pancreatic enzyme breakdown in urine/plasma/stool.
  - **3 day faecal fat.** Normally < 7% of ingested fat appears in stool, but steatorrhoea only develops if pancreatic lipase output falls to < 10% of normal, so test poorly sensitive for mild to moderate pancreatic insufficiency. Unpleasant test for patients and laboratory staff, and rarely performed. Qualitative microscopic examination of single stool for oil nearly as sensitive.
  - **Faecal elastase 1 (FE1).** Increasingly used, as is simple, non-invasive, and accurate (sensitivity/specificity > 90% for significant exocrine insufficiency). Uses monoclonal antibody and ELISA to detect elastase in single spot stool sample. Falsely low FE1 levels (< 200 µg elastase/g of stool) may occur in watery diarrhoea, but level < 50 µg elastase/g of stool highly specific for significant exocrine pancreatic insufficiency. Measurement not affected by concomitant use of PANCREATIC SUPPLEMENTS.
  - **Pancreolauryl test.** Fluorescein dilaurate is split by pancreatic enzymes into lauric acid and fluorescein. Fluorescein absorbed in the intestine, partly conjugated in the liver, and excreted in the urine. On day one of test, tablet of fluorescein dilaurate taken and urine collected for 10 hours. On day two, same procedure, but tablet contains free fluorescein (allows for correction of individual variations in intestinal, hepatic, and renal function). Results expressed as the ratio of fluorescein excreted after fluorescein dilaurate (T) and after free fluorescein (K) (T/K ratio < 20% abnormal). Para-aminobenzoic acid (PABA) test employs similar technique, but, as with pancreolauryl test, only accurate at diagnosing significant exocrine insufficiency. Test unreliable in patients with previous gastric surgery, small bowel disease, liver disease, and renal dysfunction, and when using range of drugs (e.g. paracetamol, chloramphenicol, sulfonylurea). In clinical practice these tests largely being replaced by FE1 measurement.

Pancreatic insufficiency

- Clinical exocrine insufficiency only occurs when > 90% of exocrine pancreas function lost.
- Causes include chronic pancreatitis, pancreatic resection (see Whipple's procedure), and cystic fibrosis.
- Clinical features relate to malabsorption and include steatorrhoea (pale, loose/bulky stools, which may contain visible droplets of oil, float, and be difficult to flush away), weight loss, abdominal bloating and discomfort. Malabsorption of fat soluble vitamins (see vitamins A, D, E, K) may give rise to a range of clinical problems, including metabolic bone disease (see osteoporosis). In patients with chronic pancreatitis and significant exocrine insufficiency, pain is often absent, reflecting loss of functioning pancreas.
- Diagnosis confirmed using pancreatic function tests, but significant exocrine insufficiency unusual in absence of structural abnormality of pancreas (e.g. pancreatic atrophy, calcification, pancreatic duct abnormalities). Anatomy usually accurately assessed with pancreatic protocol CT scan, but other complementary modalities include endoscopic ultrasound, ERCP, and MRCP. The latter may be performed before and after secretin injection, providing some indication of volume of pancreatic juice output, and functional hold up at pancreatic sphincter.
- Management includes treating underlying cause, PANCREATIC ENZYME SUPPLEMENTS, treatment/prevention of osteoporosis, and replacement of fat soluble vitamins. Also see Approach to malabsorption and steatorrhoea

Pancreatic pseudocyst

Background

- Localized fluid collection (2–30 cm) with non-epithelialized wall, usually sited within lesser sac. Accounts for 80–90% of pancreatic cystic lesions.
- Arises due to pancreatic duct disruption. Complicates 16–50% of cases of acute pancreatitis, 20–40% of chronic pancreatitis, and rarely associated with pancreatic cancer or trauma. By convention, cyst needs to be present for > 4/52 after acute pancreatitis to make diagnosis ('acute fluid collection' < 4/52).

Clinical features/complications

May be asymptomatic, or cause symptoms related to:
- Local compression: biliary obstruction; gastric outlet obstruction.
- Vascular involvement: portal vein thrombosis (PVT); pseudoaneurysm: involvement of gastroduodenal/splenic artery. May present with rapidly increasing pain, ↓Hb, or hypovolaemic shock due to rupture.
- Infection: occurs in 10%, usually following instrumentation (e.g. drainage).
- Rupture: may be associated with development of largely asymptomatic pancreatic ascites, or generalized peritonitis.

Investigations

- Diagnosis usually made with transabdominal <u>U/S</u> or contrast <u>CT scan</u>.
- Diagnostic cyst aspiration occasionally needed (via <u>endoscopic ultrasound</u> (EUS)), as high cystic <u>amylase</u> differentiates pseudocyst from <u>pancreatic cystic tumours</u>.
- <u>ERCP</u> avoided unless transpapillary drainage considered, or diagnosis unclear, as may introduce infection.

Management

- Pancreatic rest (e.g. with nasojejunal feeding) may hasten resolution of <u>acute pancreatitis</u> and associated pseudocyst.
- Asymptomatic pseudocysts < 6 cm can be managed conservatively, as most will resolve spontaneously (but may take months).
- Drainage considered (without clear scientific basis) for symptomatic, > 6 cm pseudocysts, present for > 6 weeks. Approaches include:
  - **Percutaneous**. Effective, but may develop cutaneo-pancreatic fistula if pancreatic duct leak continues, so percutaneous, transgastric puncture ideal (allowing drainage into stomach after drain removal, or endoscopic internalization of drain).
  - **Linear EUS**. Favoured approach by specialist units, as linear EUS allows cyst drainage into stomach/duodenum, delineation and avoidance of pericystic varices (common in view of PVT). Less than 1 cm between gastric and pseudocyst wall necessary.
  - **Transpapillary** drainage via <u>pancreatic stent</u> insertion at ERCP depends on cyst–duct communication.
  - **Surgery** with internal cyst drainage may provide resolution, but 24% complication rate. Persistent or recurrent pseudocysts may ultimately require pancreatic resection if duct rupture does not resolve (<u>Whipple's procedure</u> for cysts in head, distal pancreatectomy if in tail).
- Pseudoaneurysm treated with angiographic embolization, rarely surgery.
- ERCP and plastic stent insertion for biliary obstruction.

Pancreatic stents

- Insertion of small 3–5F polyethylene stents into main pancreatic duct at ERCP increasingly used to prevent post-ERCP pancreatitis, particularly in high risk patients (e.g. suspected <u>sphincter of Oddi dysfunction</u>, previous post-ERCP pancreatitis—also see <u>endoscopic complications</u>). In series from specialist centres, pancreatic stent insertion does seem to reduce risk, but unsuccessful attempts at insertion may worsen outcome further, with risk of pancreatic trauma. 80% of stents fall out within 3 weeks, but checking X-ray at this time is essential, with endoscopic stent removal if stent still *in situ*.
- Long-term pancreatic duct stenting for relapsing or <u>chronic pancreatitis</u> not of proven benefit, and may cause further duct stricturing.
- In patients with <u>pancreatic pseudocyst</u> or fistulae, pancreatic stent insertion, particularly across the point of duct disruption, may acceler-ate resolution. Should only be undertaken by endoscopists with spe-cialist experience of pancreatic endotherapy.

Pancreatitis

See: <u>acute pancreatitis</u>, <u>autoimmune pancreatitis</u>, <u>chronic pancreatitis</u>, and <u>hereditary pancreatitis</u>.

Paracentesis

Refers to the drainage of fluid in the peritoneal cavity (i.e. ascites; see Approach to ascites).

Most common indication is for diuretic-resistant ascites related to portal hypertension, but other causes include malignant ascites. TIPSS (transjugular intrahepatic portosystemic shunt) may occasionally be alternative to recurrent paracentesis for diurectic-resistant ascites.

Technique

- As with most procedures in medicine, best way to perform safely and effectively is to watch and learn from experienced colleague.
- Ensure clotting optimized prior to drainage (e.g. INR < 1.4, platelets > 60 ×10^9/l), although normalization of clotting parameters may be impossible to achieve in end-stage liver disease, even with FFP and platelet infusions.
- Patient supine or with head of bed elevated approximately 30°. Examine abdomen, particularly noting lower margin of liver and spleen. Moving laterally from umbilicus, percuss into flanks, until reach area of stony dullness (usually anterior axillary line). On rolling patient, confirm that area of dullness related to fluid (see Approach to GI examination). Use hub end of needle to mark site of planned needle insertion. If in doubt, ask radiologists to perform ultrasound, and mark skin at point of safest and most effective insertion.
- Perform under sterile conditions (i.e. wear sterile gloves + gowns, sterile drapes around 'surgical field'). Clean around insertion point with betadine/iodine solution (> 8 cm radius). Using 22G needle and 5 ml syringe, raise a subcutaneous bleb with lidocaine 2%, then inject further anaesthetic through skin, until reach peritoneal cavity. Using 20 ml syringe, send fluid for analysis (see Approach to ascites and spontaneous bacterial peritonitis). Using pointed-tip scalpel, make 5 mm incision through skin. Drainage catheter (e.g. Bonanno suprapubic catheter) inserted over trocar, at 90° to skin. Depending on patient adiposity, peritoneal cavity entered approximately 4 cm from skin, often indicated by ascitic fluid seeping back along catheter. At this point, advance further 1 cm, then withdraw trocar whilst advancing catheter (should occur without resistance or discomfort). Tape catheter securely to skin (no need to stitch), and attach bladder drainage bag to catheter. Keep bag below level of patient, and leave on free drainage.
- Reduced circulating blood volume, with secondary hyperaldosteronism and sympathetic drive may occur 12–24 hours post large (e.g. 4–6 litre) paracentesis. To prevent this, most hepatologists advise use of albumin as plasma expander (e.g. give 100 ml 20% human albumin solution (HAS) after every 3 litres drained). Alternatives to HAS are being sought (see albumin (use in liver disease)), but trials of dextran 70 and hemaccel show that they are less effective in this setting. No logic in giving albumin infusion in malignant ascites (as low serum–ascites albumin gradient).

- Drain should be removed within 12 hours.
- Rare complications include intraperitoneal bleeding, bowel perforation (particularly if history of abdominal surgery i.e. possible adhesions), and infection.

Paracetamol (acetaminophen) overdose

Background
- UK has dubious reputation for having the highest incidence of acute liver failure related to paracetamol in the world (although rate is falling, following introduction of 'blister packs').
- Drug very safe at therapeutic levels (< 4 g/day), but in overdose (particularly > 10 g), depletion of hepatic glutathione leads to accumulation of toxic metabolites (para-amino benzo quinonamaine), and liver injury.
- Increased toxicity associated with chronic alcohol excess, fasting, late presentation (> 16 hours since ingestion), and concomitant use of certain drugs (phenobarbitone, phenytoin, isoniazid, zidovudine) that promote paracetamol metabolism to toxic metabolites.

Clinical features
- Patients may be well, or have nausea/vomiting for first 24 hours.
- Liver failure, with progressive jaundice, hypoglycaemia, <u>hepatic encephalopathy</u> (often associated with cerebral oedema), and multiorgan failure develops from approximately 48 hours post-overdose.
- Acute renal failure may occur independent of liver failure.

Investigation
- Plasma paracetamol levels (see nomogram) taken > 4 hours post-ingestion predict toxicity (and need for treatment).
- Baseline U&Es, LFTs, Glu, FBC, PT/INR. Abnormalities at presentation suggest overdose > 18 hours previously, or pre-existing liver disease.

Specific management
- <u>N-ACETYLCYSTEINE</u> (NAc) replenishes hepatic glutathione stores, virtually abolishes severe hepatotoxocity if given < 12 hours post-ingestion, and may provide benefit even if started up to 36 hours after overdose.
- Indications for Nac include:
  - Serum paracetamol levels above cut off > 4 hours post-ingestion.
  - Patients presenting > 12 hours post-overdose.
  - History of staggered overdose, or history unreliable.
  - Serum paracetamol levels below treatment line, but risk of increased toxicity (as above).

General management
- See <u>acute liver failure</u>.
- Daily bloods: U&Es, LFTs, Glu, FBC, PT/INR.
- AST/ALT may rise massively (10 000 U/l not uncommon) at day 2–3, but patient's clotting (INR/PT), and overall clinical state (e.g. <u>hepatic encephalopathy</u>) much more important prognostic markers. If INR normal at 48 hours significant liver damage will not occur.
- Contact specialist liver unit early, especially if any of following: arterial pH < 7.3; INR > 3; creatinine > 200 µmol/l, hypoglycaemia, or any degree of encephalopathy, 48 hours after ingestion.
- Paracetamol overdose remains important indication for urgent <u>liver transplantation</u>.

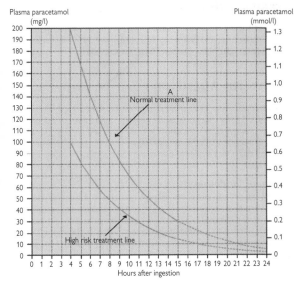

Fig 2.23 Nomogram of paracetamol toxicity.

Parasitic infection

Parasites of the GI tract are classified into worms or helminths (<u>round-worms</u>, <u>tapeworms</u>, and <u>flukes or flatworms</u>) and protozoal infections (see <u>amoebiasis</u>, <u>giardiasis</u>, <u>coccidia</u> and <u>trypanosomiasis</u>).

Parenteral nutrition

Indications

Prevention or correction of specific nutrient deficiencies or to prevent malnutrition when GI tract cannot be used (also see <u>nasogastric tubes</u>). It is usually recommended if enteral intake is inadequate for more than 7 days, but this is not evidence-based and the duration of tolerable starvation varies.

Techniques for delivery

Parenteral feeds can be given through peripheral catheters (including standard venous cannulae or mid-length fine bore catheters), peripherally inserted central catheters (PICC), or skin-tunnelled central venous catheters.

The major limitation to using peripheral catheters is the high incidence of thrombophlebitis. This relates to several factors:
- Osmolality, pH, lipid content of nutrition solution.
- Catheter characteristics (diameter, composition).
- Infusion protocol.
- Diameter and position of vein and insertion technique.

The incidence of thrombophlebitis can be minimized by following the principles outlined in the box opposite.

Peripherally inserted central lines can be used for TPN and under optimal circumstances (i.e. if inserted by a dedicated member of a nutrition team) show similar incidences of catheter-related complications to those of subclavian lines. See box for practical points on placing lines.

Tunnelled central venous catheters use a subcutaneous skin tunnel from a point of the anterior chest wall distant from the point of entry of the catheter into the vein. They are indicated when feeding is likely to be for longer than 2 weeks, when peripheral access is poor, and when the osmolality is higher than 1000 mOsm/L. The tip of the catheter needs placing as for a PICC.

Calculating requirements and choosing the feed

In most hospitals this will be done by dieticians or members of the nutrition team. The following principles apply.
1. **Calculate the energy requirements**. This can be done by calculating the basal metabolic rate (available from charts developed by Schofield, WN (1985). *Hum. Nutr. Clin. Nutr.* **39** (suppl. 1): 5).
   - Add 10% for each degree C rise in temperature.
   - Adjust for mobility (add 10% if bed-bound: 20% if sitting in chair; 30% if mobile on ward).
   - Add up to 600 kCal if weight gain is required.

Pa 505

Practical principles in peripheral TPN

- Use as large a vein as possible: avoid standard venflons, and use a fine bore (22 or 23 g) polyurethane catheter
- Put a GTN patch over the infusion site
- Add 500–1000 IU heparin/l of TPN solution
- Add 5 mg/l of hydrocortisone
- Buffer the solution to pH 7.4
- Keep daily infused volume below 3.5 l; use an infusion pump
- Use an inline 1.2 micron filter
- Provide at least 50% of total energy as lipid: this serves to keep the osmolality low

Placing a PICC (peripherally inserted central catheter)

- Use the basilic (medial) vein at the antecubital fossa (avoid lateral (cephalic vein because it joins the axillary vein at a right angle, which can make further advancement beyond this point very difficult)
- Thrombosis rates are much lower if the catheter tip is in the SVC rather than the axillary or subclavian vein. Therefore, check on a PA chest X-ray that the catheter tip is no more than 2 cm below a line joining the lower borders of the medial ends of the clavicles

2. **Calculate the protein requirements**. Most hospitalized patients need 0.8 to 1.5 g protein/kg/day. Any catabolic illness, protein-losing enteropathy, or nephropathy (or dialysis) increases protein requirements. Protein balance can be checked in most patients if necessary by calculating urinary nitrogen loss from urinary urea excretion and comparing this with content of the prescribed feed.

3. **Consider the amount of fat infused**. The optimal percentage of calories that should be infused as fat is not known, but most complications occur at rates over 1 kCal/kg/h, so a max of 0.7 kCal/kg/h is usually observed: this translates to 500–1500 ml of a 10% lipid solution.

4. **Consider infused carbohydrate**. Intravenous carbohydrate, usually dextrose, is a vital source of calories that stimulates insulin secretion and reduces muscle breakdown (reduces hepatic gluconeogenesis, which needs amino acid precursors from skeletal muscle).

5. **Consider parenteral electrolytes, vitamins, and trace elements**. Sodium: Provide patients weight in kg as basline, and add calculated losses remembering that bile and small intestinal/ileostomy fluid is near isotonic at 150 mM). Monitor potassium but also calcium (5–10 mM required per day) and phosphate (10–30 mM needed per day).

Clinical management of the patient on TPN

1. Daily weight. This contributes to assessing fluid balance.
2. Blood glucose may be raised if there is insulin resistance.
3. Watch for pyrexia. Any spike may indicate line sepsis: take blood from the feeding catheter and peripheral vein; stop TPN until culture results are known.
4. Beware overenthusiastic feeding of critically malnourished: there is a danger of <u>refeeding syndrome</u>, which can cause death.

Complications of parenteral nutrition

- **Mechanical damage** to veins or local structures (pneumothorax, brachial plexus injury, thoraci duct injury, haemothorax).
- **Vascular complications**: air embolism, catheter thrombosis, embolic complications including pulmonary emboli.
- **Metabolic**. Fluid overload, hyperglycaemia, metabolic bone disease, hyperlipidaemia.
- **Infectious complications**: line sepsis rates should be below 3–5%.
- **GI complications**. Abnormal liver function is common (most commonly cholestatic pattern, but steatohepatitis is seen on histology. Acalculous <u>cholecystitis</u> (5%), <u>acute pancreatitis</u>, <u>gallstones</u> (30%), and gallbladder sludge (approaching 100%) also occur and presumably relate to bile stasis in the absence of enteral feeding.

Clinical applications of parenteral nutrition

See sections on nutrition in entries under <u>Crohn's disease</u>, <u>ulcerative colitis</u>, <u>short bowel syndrome</u>, and <u>hepatic encephalopathy</u>. Parenteral nutrition also has a role in management of gastrointestinal fistulae, and in <u>acute pancreatitis</u>.

Parkinson's disease and the GI tract

Parkinson's disease can be associated with **swallowing problems** and **constipation**. See also elderly and the GI tract.

- **Drooling** is a result of reduced swallowing, correlates with the severity of the Parkinsonism and can be severe. Anticholinergics can dry the mouth but may lead to confusion. Irradiation of the salivary glands is effective, as is botox injection.
- **Dysphagia** occurs in 50% of patients.
  - Oropharyngeal problems arise because of poor tongue control, difficulty in bolus formation, and delayed transit to the pharynx. Food retention in the pharnx and consequent aspiration is common.
  - Oesophageal dysmotility is common in manometric studies and there may be incomplete relaxation of the lower oesophageal sphincter. L-dopa may help the oropharyngeal phase of swallowing but does not always lead to improved swallowing.
- **Heartburn** and documented oesophageal reflux are more common in Parkinson's disease.
- **Constipation** in Parkinson's is common and results from slow intestinal transit and sometimes from outflow obstruction due to pelvic floor problems. It can be masked by overflow incontinence. It may result from degeneration of the myenteric plexus and be aggravated by anticholinergic drugs as well as by inadequate intake of fibre and fluids.

Pellagra

Due to poor intake of niacin (vitamin B3) or reduced conversion of tryptophan to niacin. This latter reaction requires riboflavin, thiamine, and pyridoxine and is inhibited by excess intake of leucine. Pellagra is a wasting disease with dermatitis of exposed areas due to photosensitivity. Fatigue, insomnia, and apathy can lead on to hallucinations and psychosis. Widespread mucosal inflammation causes glossitis, stomatitis, vaginitis, and diarrhoea. Can be associated with drugs (isoniazid) or carcinoid.

Peptic ulceration

Note. Pathophysiology and epidemiology, treatment, and complications are discussed here. For approach to investigation and specific management recommendations, see gastric ulcers, duodenal ulcers, and also Approach to dyspepsia and gastro-oesophageal reflux).

- Includes all acid-related ulceration: gastric ulcers, duodenal ulcers but also oesophageal ulcers relating to gastro-oesophageal reflux and ulcers in Meckel's diverticulum. Textbooks and pathologists differentiate **ulcers** and **erosions** according to whether they erode through muscularis mucosae but this is not useful to clinicians or endoscopists because ulcers are diagnosed by morphological or radiological features.
- Before 1980s peptic ulcer was considered a chronic relapsing disease. Since the 1980s most peptic ulcers were shown to be related either to infection with *Helicobacter pylori* or to nonsteroidal anti-inflammatory drugs (NSAIDs), with hypersecretory states such as gastrinoma (Zollinger—Ellison syndrome) accounting for some others.
- Physiological stress (burns, sepsis, multi-organ failure) can cause multiple superficial erosions. Ulcers arising in burns patients are called Curling's ulcers. Ulcers in head injury patients are called Cushing's ulcers. Unlike other stress–related peptic injuries, Cushing's ulcers are associated with hypergastrinaemia.
- Pathogenesis appears related to impaired mucosal resistance due to reduced mucosal blood flow. Stress ulcer prophylaxis should be considered in multi-organ failure or if there is a history of peptic ulceration, cirrhosis, or renal failure. Sucralfate can be used via the enteral route: PPIs are reasonable if parenteral administration is essential.

Pathophysiology

Disordered epithelial defences. These include factors protecting the epithelial cells against acid, such as mucus and bicarbonate in the unstirred water layer covering cells as well as tight junctions between epithelial cells and also effective mucosal blood flow.

Abnormal acid and motility. Patients with duodenal ulcers are hypersecretors; some of this may relate to increased gastrin stimulated by HP or by an HP-mediated fall in somatostatin secretion. There may be high levels of pepsinogen (again related to HP) and possibly abnormal vagal control or disordered motility with a resulting increased delivery of acid to the duodenum.

Gastric ulcers in the body or fundus are associated with gastric atrophy, chronic gastritis, and low acid, while antral gastric ulcers and gastric ulcers associated with concomitant duodenal ulcers are associated with high acid output.

Risk factors for peptic ulceration

- **True**: _Helicobacter pylori_; NSAIDs; <u>gastrinoma</u>; cigarette smoking; associated diseases such as COPD and cirrhosis; probably some genetic factors (e.g. Lewis blood group antigens mediate HP attaching to musosa)
- **False**: alcohol in absence of cirrhosis, dietary factors
- **Uncertain**: emotional stress

Helicobacter pylori (HP). There is a strong association with both <u>duodenal ulcer</u> (DU) and <u>gastric ulcer</u> (GU), but although experimental HP infection produces a gastritis that if untreated can progress to gastric atrophy and cancer, still only 20% of infected people get peptic ulcers, so ill-understood host factors and virulence factors must be important. The paradox about HP is why infection in some produces high acid and duodenal ulceration, while in others it leads to chronic gastritis, gastric atrophy, and <u>gastric cancer</u>. Although this may relate to different patterns of infection (antral or body), more investigation is needed for proof of this hypothesis.

Nonsteroidal anti-inflammatory drugs (NSAIDS). These damage the GI mucosa by direct and systemic effects. Direct damage occurs within minutes of ingestion and can be reduced by enteric coating or rectal administration. Systemic affects are mediated by reduced mucosal prostaglandin synthesis with consequent effects on secretion of mucus and mucosal blood flow. Ulcers can be shown on endoscopy in 15–30% patients on chronic NSAID therapy. The risk is multiplied with concomitant corticosteroid ingestion. Risk is also increased by previous peptic ulceration, old age, and comorbidity. There is some evidence that risk of ulceration is also increased by concomitant HP infection: this is controversial.

Other drugs. Peptic ulcers are associated with some chemotherapeutic drugs (intra-arterial 5FU), potassium chloride tablets, crack cocaine, and bisphosphanates, especially alendronate.

Hypersecretory conditions. Suspect in the absence of HP or NSAID use, especially if there is diarrhoea, complications (perforation or haemorrhage), or if ulceration extends beyond the duodenal bulb. Relevant conditions include:
- <u>Gastrinoma</u>.
- <u>Systemic mastocytosis</u> and myeloproliferative disorders with increased basophils: both of these produce increased amounts of histamine, which can cause acid hypersecretion—DU is found in 40%.
- Antral G cell hyperplasia—although this is usually a consequence of HP infection.

Epidemiology
Rare before the 19th century, it became more common in the early 20th century, but incidence been declining since the 1960s. Hospitalization rates have not changed, probably because older people consume more NSAIDs. For risk factors, see box.

Clinical features. See box.

Investigations
See <u>Approach to dyspepsia and gastro-oesophageal reflux</u>. Remember that endoscopic examination alone is a poor predictor of malignancy and gastric ulcers should always be biopsied (take 6 biopsies, which gives 98% sensitivity of diagnosis: adding gastric brushing improves accuracy even more). Duodenal ulcers are very rarely malignant. Follow up endoscopy to confirm ulcer healing is traditional but dates from the radiological era when diagnosis of malignancy was inaccurate. Repeat endoscopy may not be necessary if the ulcer is benign on extensive brushing and biopsy sampling.

Clinical features of peptic ulcers

Do not attempt to diagnose peptic ulceration by the history alone despite the classic descriptions of abdominal pain in peptic ulcers:

- **Gastric ulcer**. Pain soon after meals, often not relieved by eating, associated with anorexia and weight loss in 50%
- **Duodenal ulcer**. Pain 2–3 h after meals, often wakes patient in middle of night, relieved by eating so most patients maintain or increase weight
- The pain of peptic ulceration can be mimicked by cancer, pancreatitis, cholecystitis, reflux, and mesenteric angina

Treatments

Test for HP; eradicate if present. Ask about NSAID ingestion.

Histamine receptor antagonists. Used by themselves, healing rate for DU is 70–80% and for GU is 55–65%. They are especially useful at decreasing basal acid output at night, although tolerance can develop rapidly. See H2 RECEPTOR ANTAGONISTS.

Proton pump inhibitors are the most effective inhibitors of gastric acid, but their efficacy is markedly limited in the fasting state when only 5% of the stomach's proton pumps are active. Even patients taking twice daily PPI often experience nocturnal acid breakthrough, which can be helped by nocturnal H2RA. Once daily PPI gives DU healing rate of 80–100%, and GU healing rate of 70–85%. Elevation of gastric pH impairs absorption of ketoconazole and facilitates absorption of digoxin. PPIs can affect levels of other drugs metabolized by cytochrome p450: omeprazole delays clearance of warfarin, diazepam, and phenytoin. For discussion of possible adverse effect of PPIs, see PROTON PUMP INHIBITORS.

Antacids. Although antacids can heal ulcers in high doses, they are poorly tolerated and often cause unacceptable GI side effects. See ANTACIDS.

Other drugs. SUCRALFATE and BISMUTH preparations both can heal ulcers but are infrequently used. The prostaglandin analogue MISOPROSTIL has similar efficacy to omeprazole for healing NSAID-induced ulcers.

Surgery (see gastrectomy and Approach to surgically revised anatomy and stomas). The need for surgery to treat uncomplicated peptic ulcers has almost disappeared because of effective drug treatment. Current indications for surgery include bleeding from ulcers not responding to endoscopic therapy, perforated ulcers, and gastric outlet obstruction that cannot be relieved by endoscopic dilatation. Operations for duodenal ulceration include patching a perforation with a tongue of omentum or removing the acid-producing tissue either with antrectomy or by vagotomy (usually highly selective vagotomy). Simple division of the vagus results in pyloric spasm so vagotomy needs to be combined with a drainage procedure such as pyloroplasty or gastro-jejunostomy. Operations for benign gastric ulcers depend partially on the site of the ulcer: an ulcer near the oesophageal junction refractory to medical treatment may need a subtotal gastrectomy and Roux-en-Y anastomosis.

Refractory peptic ulcers. See box.

Complications

Haemorrhage. Use of aggressive antisecretory therapy is reasonable. There is no benefit in using H2 receptor antagonists in controlling bleeding or preventing rebleeding. An important study from Hong Kong (Lau, J W et al. (2000). *N. Engl. J. Med.* **343**: 310) showed that, in patients who had received endoscopic treatment to control acute haemorrhage, a bolus of 80 mg IV omeprazole followed by 8 mg/h infusion for 72 h reduced rebleeding rates and shortened hospital stay. Also see: Acute upper GI bleeding.

What to do if a peptic ulcer is not healed by 8 weeks of a PPI (12 weeks for ulcers over 2 cm)

- Check compliance with drug treatment
- Is there HP infection?
- Is there ongoing and possibly surreptitious NSAID use?
- Smoking? Cigarette smoking delays healing
- Is there evidence for a hypersecretory condition?
- Is the ulcer peptic? Consider <u>gastric cancer</u> (very rarely duodenal cancer), infection, cocaine use, and IBD, e.g. <u>Crohn's disease</u>

Perforation. Can be life-threatening. Strong association with NSAIDs, smoking (especially in younger patients), crack cocaine. Diagnose by erect chest X-ray and possibly CT scanning. Avoid endoscopy, which will exacerbate any leak. Sometimes careful radiological exam with water soluble contrast will reveal site of perforation. Usual treatment is broad spectrum antibiotics, surgery to close perforation, and irrigation of peritoneum. Non-operative therapy rarely appropriate in highly selected patients where patient is well and perforation has sealed. **Watch these patients very carefully**—operation is indicated at first sign of clinical deterioration.

Penetration. Posterior DUs can invade the pancreas and GUs can penetrate the left lobe of liver. Choledochoduodenal fistulae and gastrocolic fistulae can occur.

Obstruction. Pain , bloating, early satiety, vomiting after a meal are suggestive. Weight loss can be dramatic. Examine for a succussion splash. A gastric aspirate of over 200 ml after overnight fasting is evidence of delayed gastric emptying. Management is medical and endoscopic using dilatation in 70% of cases, with only 30% needing surgical bypass of the gastric outlet obstruction.

Percutaneous endoscopic gastrostomy (PEG)

- PEG insertion increasingly widely performed when enteral feeding required for > 4 weeks (10% of nursing home residents in USA have had PEG sited).
- Main indications include neuromuscular disease (e.g. stroke, motor neurone disease, dementia), and oropharyngeal cancer.
- Ongoing debate surrounds maintenance of enteral feeding in patients with end-stage progressive disease, but PEG tubes are certainly better tolerated than long-term nasogastric feeding.

Technique

'Pull technique' entails:

1. Endoscopy to exclude any lesions within upper GI tract.
2. Endoscopic localization of anterior gastric wall, with corresponding point on anterior abdominal wall identified by transillumination.
3. Sterilization of skin, local anaesthetic infiltration (e.g. lignocaine 2% 4 ml), and 5 mm incision into skin at site of planned insertion.
4. Insertion of trocar, followed by looped string, percutaneously into stomach, under endoscopic vision.
5. String grabbed endoscopically with endoscopic snare, and drawn retrogradely out of mouth on removal of endoscope. 9–16F feeding tube attached to string, and drawn into position by traction at skin (see Fig. 2.24).
6. Button of PEG tube keeps it lightly impacted against gastric wall.

- Pre-procedure antibiotics (e.g. Cefuroxime 750 mg IV) reduce risk of peristomal infection.
- PEG can be modified with jejunal feeding tube, which may reduce risk of reflux and gastric aspiration.
- Alternatives to endoscopic gastrostomy insertion include percutaneous radiological approach or surgical. These may be considered for patients undergoing planned curative surgery for oropharyngeal cancer, as gastric stoma metastases due to endoscopic insertion rarely reported.

Contraindications to PEG include:

- Inability to bring the anterior gastric wall in apposition to the anterior abdominal wall (e.g. subtotal gastrectomy, ascites, hepatomegaly, severe obesity).
- Gastrointestinal tract obstruction.
- Malignant gastric/peritoneal infiltration.
- Gastric varices.
- Uncorrectable coagulopathy.

Complications

- Major complications in 3%, minor in 20%: infection (peritoneal, abdominal wall abscess, necrotizing fasciitis), local peritonitis, bowel perforation, tube displacement, haemorrhage, 'buried bumper'.
- Procedure-related mortality 0.5–2%, overall 30 day mortality 10–15% (largely reflecting underlying disease, but emphasizes need to be sure that patient not put through futile, unnecessary intervention in last few days of life).
- Pneumoperitoneum in 20%, but rarely of significance.

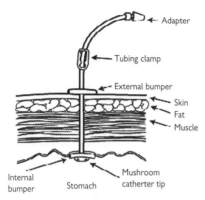

Fig 2.24 Percutaneous endoscopic gastrostomy tube placements. © The Cleveland Clinic (2004).

Perianal Crohn's disease

Incidence. Reported rates vary from 4 to 60%. More common with distal disease, occurring in about 90% patients with rectal <u>Crohn's disease</u>. Usually, perianal disease presents concurrently or after intestinal disease but in 25% perianal disease can precede intestinal manifestation by several years.

Spectrum of disease

- **Skin lesions** include skin tags (possibly arising from lymphoedema secondary to lymphatic obstruction) and abscesses that are usually linked to a fistula.
- **Anal canal lesions** include fissures, ulcers, and stenosis. Fissures tend to be eccentric rather than midline. Stricture can relate to smooth muscle spasm or to extramucosal fibrosis.
- **Perianal fistulae**. Often accompany perianal abscesses. Classified by Parkes in 1976: see <u>anorectal fistulae</u>. Rectovaginal fistulation occurs in about 5–10% with perianal disease.

Assessment of severity

- Conventional scoring systems like the <u>Crohn's disease activity index</u> correlate poorly with severity. A perianal disease activity index (PDAI) has been developed and validated by a Canadian group (Irvine, E J. et al. (1995). J. Clin. Gastroenterol.; **20**: 27).
- If examination is painful, examination under anaesthetic is appropriate.
- Imaging includes endoanal ultrasound (see <u>endoscopic ultrasound</u>) and <u>MRI</u>. Ultrasound is very useful at characterizing sphincter defects while MRI is useful for assessing sphincter integrity as well as defining fistula tract anatomy.

Treatment

Medical (also see index of drugs)

- **Steroids** can prevent fistula healing and may lead to abscess formation.
- Fissures are increasingly treated with pharmacological therapy including nitrates (GTN), botulinum toxin, and diltiazem.
- **Topical aminosalicylates** can be effective in rectal disease.
- **Antibiotics** are useful but metronidazole should not be used for longer than 3 months because of a risk of neuropathy. Ciprofloxacin has little effect against anaerobes but is of proven use in perianal Crohn's.
- **Immunomodulators**. Azathioprine/6MP will heal about 30% of fistulae, and methotrexate probably has similar efficacy.
- **Anti-TNF treatment** has been evaluated in perianal Crohn's. <u>INFLIXIMAB</u> has been shown to be highly effective in treating fistulae, and combination of infliximab and azathioprine/6MP seems to prolong effect.

Surgical

Surgical options range from drainage of fistulae to major interventions such as proctocolectomy with stoma formation.

- Emergency treatment of sepsis may involve incision of an abscess, with antibiotics. Fistulae after drainage often treated by placing a <u>seton suture</u>, aimed at preventing further abscess formation. An alternative bridging procedure prior to attempts at definitive treatment is the formation of a stoma as diversion of the faecal stream is of definite benefit in Crohn's disease.
- Operations for fistulae are complex and out of our scope here. An obvious concern and principle of surgery is the maintenance of faecal continence.

Pernicious anaemia (PA)

Called pernicious because it was fatal before treatment became available. Classic pernicious anaemia is caused by failure of gastric parietal cells to produce sufficient intrinsic factor (IF) to permit absorption of adequate amount of dietary vitamin B12 (cobalamin); this produces a megaloblastic anaemia. For other disorders that can cause cobalamin deficiency, see vitamin B12.

Aetiology

In adults PA is probably an autoimmune disorder (familial association, association with other autoimmune diseases and HLA A2, A3, B8, DR3, blood group A) .Anti-parietal cell antibodies occur in 90% of patients (5% of healthy controls); also both binding and blocking antibodies to IF are found. In adults PA is associated with atrophic gastritis and achlorhydria. In children the aetiology is different: there is usually a hereditary problem of cobalamin metabolism or of intrinsic factor production. Coexistent iron deficiency is common.

Epidemiology

Most cases occur after age 40, although there is a recognized incidence in children (juvenile pernicious anaemia): women outnumber men approx 2:1; prevalence is about 1 per 1000. 20–30% cases have a positive family history. There is an association with other autoimmune disorders—type 1 diabetes, Addison's, thyroid disease.

Diagnosis

Macrocytic anaemia, low B12, abnormal Schilling test. Elevated bilirubin due to haemolysis occasionally reported.

Therapy centres on B12 replacement.

- The standard regimen is to give hydroxocobalamin IM 1 mg three times a week for 2 weeks then 1 mg every 3 months. There is some evidence that giving larger doses orally (1–2 mg daily) may be effective.
- After initial parenteral replacement, most people can be maintained on oral supplementation of 250–1000 μg of B12.

Complications

There is a 2–3 fold increased risk of gastric adenocarcinoma.
Screening is not recommended because of a high cost–benefit ratio. The hypergastrinaemia resulting from achlorhydria causes enterochromaffin cell hyperplasia—there is an increased incidence of carcinoid tumours, which respond to antrectomy and are of relatively low grade malignancy.

Peutz–Jeghers syndrome

Peutz 1921; Jeghers 1949.
- Hamartomas represent a type of <u>polyp</u> characterized by glandular epithelium supported by a framework of smooth muscle continuous with muscularis mucosae. Usually multiple.
- The syndrome is autosomal dominant and involves germline mutation of a serine–threonine kinase gene of chromosome 19.
- There is characteristic mucocutaneous pigmentation that resembles freckles (see Colour Plate 23). Polyps can be anywhere in the GI tract but are commonly small intestinal.
- There is a high overall risk of cancer (90% by age 65). Risk of colon cancer is 40%, with similar rates for gastric and pancreatic cancers. There is an increased risk of breast cancer, uterine cancer, and testicular cancer.
- Guidelines for screening include colonoscopy from late teens every 3 years; upper GI endoscopy every 2 years; annual Hb and surveillance of small bowel; annual breast exam or mammogram; and annual pelvic examination.

Pharyngeal pouch ('Zenker's diverticulum')

- Present in 1% of people > 70 years. Diverticulum develops in area of weakness where fibres of cricopharyngeal sphincter meet oblique fibres of the inferior pharyngeal constrictor muscle. Incomplete relaxation of upper oesophageal sphincter may lead to ↑ pharyngeal pressure proximal to this during swallowing, with subsequent herniation.
- Symptoms: dysphagia, regurgitation, cough, aspiration, and halitosis.
- Diagnosis usually made by barium swallow. Oesophageal rupture is an important complication, often related to endoscope tip penetrating the base of the diverticulum.
- Traditionally, treatment was surgical, with > 90% subsequently symptom-free. Recently, new endoscopic stapling techniques have been shown to be effective.

Photodynamic therapy (PDT)

PDT involves the intravenous administration of a photosensitizing drug (e.g. porfimer sodium (Photofrin®), meso-tetrahydroxyphenyl chlorine (Foscan®)) , which is taken up by all dividing cells. Drug activated on exposure to low-power red light (630–675 nm) from a laser, leading to non-thermal local tissue destruction (usually to depth of 1–5 mm). Oxygenated tissue particularly affected, and connective tissue largely spared.

- PDT has been used for range of GI diseases, with laser inserted either percutaneously or endoscopically, including:
  - Barrett's oesophagus.
  - Oesophageal cancer.
  - Palliation of cholangiocarcinoma, and maintenance of biliary patency (with prolonged survival reported in a large single-centre study).
  - Palliation of pancreatic cancer reported with PDT.
  - Ablation of endoscopically accessible, small, inoperable tumours.
- Severe cutaneous photosensitivity may occur (patient kept in darkened room for 5 days after drug given, and direct sunlight avoided for >3 weeks, dependent on photosensitizer used). Viscus perforation and haemorrhage are rare.

Plummer–Vinson/Patterson–Kelly syndrome

A syndrome characterized by an iron-deficiency anaemia, atrophic changes in the buccal, glossopharyngeal, and oesophageal mucous membranes, koilonychia, and dysphagia. The dysphagia is due to an oesophageal ring/web formed in the post-cricoid region. Squamous carcinoma of the tongue and post-cricoid region are complications. It is most common in middle-aged women, rarely in the male. Aetiology unknown.

Pneumatosis coli

Multiple gas-filled cysts in the submucosa and subserosa. The name is misleading: most cases involve the small intestine and only 6% of cases affect the colon. There are several theories of pathogenesis, with most evidence supporting a bacterial aetiology; pneumatosis can be induced in laboratory animals by injecting gas-forming bacteria into the gut wall and successful treatment with antibiotics has been reported.

Clinical features: commonest in the 60s, no sex difference, usually asymptomatic but can cause diarrhoea, mucous discharge, rectal bleeding, constipation. Symptomatic patients can be treated by breathing high flow oxygen for several days (minimum 48 h). METRONIDAZOLE can also be effective.

Polyarteritis nodosa (PAN) and the GI tract

PAN is a necrotizing vasculitis affecting small and medium-sized arteries with aneurysmal dilatations up to 1 cm seen on angiography. Abdominal symptoms, usually pain, occur in about 50% of cases. Mesenteric vessels are abnormal in 80% cases; GI bleeding from ischaemia is seen in about 6% and perforation in 5%. Acalculous cholecystitis can occur in about 15%; acute pancreatitis, appendicitis, biliary strictures have all been reported. Polyarteritis is a recognized association of hepatitis B infection.

Polypectomy follow up

About 30% of people undergoing colonoscopic polypectomy will develop recurrent adenomas (although any lesions missed at index examination will be considered a recurrence).

Predicting recurrence

The main risk factor for recurrence is the presence of multiple adenomas at index examination. Lesser factors include polyp size over 10 mm, advanced age, and villous histology.

Frequency of surveillance colonoscopy

This is fertile ground for issuing of guidelines (see Bond, JH. *Am. J. Gastroenterol.* 2000; **95**: 3053). It is sensible to base frequency of surveillance on risk of recurrent polyps—see box. For high-risk patients, repeat colonoscopy at 3 years. For low-risk patients, repeat colonoscopy at 5 years. After one negative colonoscopy, increase the interval to 5 years.

Polyposis syndromes

See: colonic polyps and hereditary polyposis.

Porphyrias

- Rate-limiting step in haem production is conversion of porphyrins (comprising 4 pyrole rings) to δ amino-laevulinic acid (ALA), and haem provides negative feedback on δ ALA synthase.
- Deficiency of specific enzymes (including δ ALA synthase) leads to porphyrin accumulation. Porphyrias classified according to site of porphyrin accumulation (see table on facing page) and pattern of symptoms (i.e. acute (neurovisceral) and cutaneous (photosensitive)).
- **Acute intermittent porphyria and porphyria cutanea** tarda most common in GI practice.

Acute intermittent porphyria (AIP)

Autosomal dominant, incidence highest in Scandinavia (1:1000). Symptoms, even in heterozygotes, triggered by alcohol, surgery, fasting, drugs (e.g. sulphonamides, barbiturates, and many others).

Clinical features

- Abdominal pain. Severe, usually lasts several days, poorly localized, but no signs of peritonitis (see Acute abdominal pain). Nausea, constipation. Symptom-free between episodes.
- Tachycardia, sweating, hypertension during acute episode.
- Polyneuropathy (peripheral neuropathy, mononeuritis multiplex, cranial nerve palsy), epilepsy, agitation, anxiety, paranoia.

Risk for developing further adenoma or cancer after colonoscopic polypectomy

Low risk
- 1–2 adenomas less than 10 mm diameter

High risk
- Multiple (3 or more) adenomas
- Large adenoma over 10 mm
- Adenomas with villous component
- Adenoma with high grade dysplasia
- First-degree relative with colon cancer

Classification of porphyrias

Hepatic	Erythropoitic
Acute intermittent porphyria	X-linked sideroblastic anaemia
Porphyria cutanea tarda	Congenital erythropoietic porphyria
Hereditary coproporphyria	Erythropoietic protoporphyria
Variegate porphyria	

Diagnosis

Never made unless thought about (but, as with <u>familial Mediterranean fever</u>, immediate promotion for those who make the link in the patient with unexplained recurrent abdominal pain!).

- FBC: ↑ WCC during acute attack.
- U&Es: ↓ serum Na^+ may relate to syndrome of inappropriate ADH.
- Urine prophyrins: porphobilinogen (PBG) > × 4 ULN, and uroporphyrin and coproporphyrin moderately elevated during acute attack. Check that lab routinely does PBG on urine porphyrin screen (some don't!) PBG levels usually stay ↑ between attacks.

Management

- High-carbohydrate intake (oral, NG feed, or IV glucose infusion) inhibits haem synthesis. Total parenteral nutrition rarely required.
- Opiate analgesia often required (see <u>pain control</u>).
- Infusion of haem (e.g. Hematin) in severe attack is effective, as provides negative feedback to haem synthesis, and so ↓ production of porphyrins.
- 60–80% of patients never have another attack, provided precipitants sought and avoided (e.g. check BNF before prescribing any drug).

Porphyria cutanea tarda (PCT)

- Most common type of porphyria. Most cases either familial (25%) or sporadic (75%), but also linked with other conditions (e.g. alcohol, <u>hepatitis C</u>, <u>haemochromatosis</u>). Presents as scarring blisters in sun-exposed areas (often dorsum of hands, forearms, face).
- Uroporphyrin and coproporphyrin significantly ↑ in plasma and urine.
- Dermatology opinion and skin biopsy may aid diagnosis.
- Elevated iron levels (e.g. serum ferritin) may be found.
- Sun-protection, phlebotomy, or desferrioxamine chelation for iron overload, and chloroquine may be effective.

Portal hypertension

Background

- If pressure gradient between hepatic and portal venous systems (hepatic venous pressure gradient (HVPG)) increases to > 10–12 mmHg (normal 4 mmHg), portosystemic collaterals (varices) may develop.
- Most commonly due to intrahepatic disease at the site of liver sinusoid (e.g. cirrhosis), but pre-sinusoidal, and post-sinusoidal causes also important (see table). Idiopathic non-cirrhotic portal hypertension common amongst young men in India.
- Increased intrahepatic vascular resistance important, due to fibrosis and disruption of microcirculation at sinusoid, but resistance may be dynamic, with likely role for myofibroblasts, derived from hepatic stellate cells. Increased portal blood flow also contributes.
- Bleeding due to varices occurs in 30–40% of patients with cirrhosis, with risk factors including variceal size and <u>Child–Pugh score</u>.
- Gastro-oesophageal region commonest site for varices, but stomach, rectum, duodenum, and surgical anastomoses (e.g. stomas) also affected.

Causes of portal hypertension

Pre-sinusoidal	Sinusoidal	Post-sinusoidal
Extrahepatic		*Extrahepatic*
Portal vein thrombosis	Cirrhosis Alcoholic hepatitis	Right heart failure/ valve disease
Splenic vein thrombosis	Nodular regenerative hyperplasia	Constrictive pericarditis
Arterio-venous fistula	Primary biliary cirrhosis	
Portal vein stenosis	Primary sclerosing cholangitis	
Intrahepatic		*Intrahepatic*
Schistosomiasis		Budd–Chiari syndrome
Sarcoidosis		Veno-occlusive disease
Early–primary biliary cirrhosis		
Early–primary sclerosing cholangitis		
Idiopathic non-cirrhotic portal hypertension		

Clinical features

- Bleeding from gastro-oesophageal varices usually presents with
  haematemesis ± malaena, with first bleeds carrying 25–50% mortality.
  Chronic blood loss and anaemia may occur due to portal hypertensive
  gastropathy (PHG).
- Left upper quadrant discomfort due to splenomegaly occasionally
  reported.
- Signs of chronic liver disease may be present (see Approach to GI
  examination), including ascites, splenomegaly, dilated superficial veins,
  and rectal haemorrhoids.

Investigation

- Aimed at defining type of portal hypertension, and underlying aetiology.
- Upper GI endoscopy showing varices confirms portal hypertension,
  and should be considered in all patients after diagnosing cirrhosis.
  Various grading systems for variceal size used (broadly: small=grade
  1 = < 25% lumen occluded on endoscopy; medium = grade 2 = 25–50%
  lumen occluded; large = grade 3 = >50% lumen occluded).
- Doppler ultrasound informs on abnormalities of hepatic and portal
  vein flow, portal vein thrombosis, and liver architecture. CT scanning
  with contrast and MRI also highly effective.
- Measurement of HPVG is invasive and rarely necessary to make
  diagnosis, but allows clarification of whether cause is pre-sinusoidal,
  post-sinusoidal, or sinusoidal. Transjugular liver biopsy and portal
  venography can be performed at same time.

- Other tests will depend on site of obstruction causing portal hypertension (e.g. see <u>Budd–Chiari syndrome</u>, <u>schistosomiasis</u>), and whether patient known to have liver disease (see <u>Approach to well patient with abnormal liver tests</u>). Liver function is usually excellent in pre-sinusoidal portal hypertension. Portal hypertension *per se* may cause ↓WCC, ↓ platelets, due to hypersplenism.

Management

- Acute variceal bleeding is an emergency (see <u>Acute upper GI bleeding</u>).
- Treat underlying cause of chronic liver disease (see <u>Approach to cirrhosis and chronic liver disease</u>).
- Prophylaxis—important, and often overlooked.
- **Primary prophylaxis** (to prevent 1st bleed) indicated when moderate–large varices found on screening endoscopy. Non-selective β-blockers (e.g. propanolol 40–80 mg bd PO) lower portal pressure, reduce risk of bleed (from 30% to 14% over 2 years in patients with large varices), and most hepatologists use these as 1st line therapy (but compliance may be poor, and side-effects preclude long term use in 30%). Adjust dose to maintain heart rate 60 bpm. Exact role of variceal band ligation (VBL) uncertain, as may effectively eradicate varices (e.g. with 2–4 weekly endoscopies until eradicated), but invasive, may precipitate bleeding in a few (e.g. post-banding ulcers), and no benefit for gastric variceal/PHG bleeding.
- **Secondary prophylaxis** (to prevent re-bleed) is essential, as 60% of patients re-bleed < 1 year. β-blockers and VBL both effective.
- Ongoing areas of debate: role of invasive HPVG measurement to assess response to β-blockers; role of adding nitrates (e.g. isosorbide mononitrate) to β-blockers in non-responders; and relative merits of VBL versus β-blockers as prophylaxis.
- Recurrent variceal bleeding that is difficult to control medically is an indication for transjugular intrahepatic portosystemic shunt (<u>TIPSS</u>) and consideration of <u>liver transplantation</u>.

Endoscopy and primary prophylaxis in compensated cirrhosis

Endoscopic finding	Action
No varices	Repeat endoscopy 2–3 years
Small varices	Repeat endoscopy 1 year
Medium–large varices	Life-long β-blockers
	Variceal band ligation if intolerant of β-blockers

Portal vein thrombosis (PVT)

Background

Thrombosis may involve only PV, or extend into splenic vein and splanchnic venous bed. Combination of local cause and systemic thrombotic predisposition important in development (see table).

Clinical features

- Acute PVT (usually defined as presentation within 2 months of thrombosis) may present with abdominal pain, fever, and signs of mesenteric infarction.
- Chronic PVT presents with complications of portal hypertension. Splenomegaly and hypersplenism common, but ascites rare (unless associated liver disease). Variceal bleeding occurs in 30%, but excellent prognosis, due to preserved liver function (the latter may also explain low rate of hepatic encephalopathy). 10 year survival > 80% in absence of cirrhosis.
- Biliary abnormalities (due to compression by varices or variceal mass around portal vein—'cavernoma') seen in 80%, but obstructive jaundice due to biliary stricture is rare.

Investigation

Aimed at defining cause (can be found in 80%) and extent of thrombosis.
- PVT accurately diagnosed with Doppler U/S, contrast CT, endoscopic ultrasound, and MRI. Formal angiography rarely required.
- Bloods may show signs of hypersplenism (↓WCC, ↓ platelets).
- Tests for prothrombotic tendency essential if no clear cause identified (see table).

Management

- No randomized trials to guide management.
- See Acute upper GI bleeding for management of variceal bleeding.
- Small studies suggest resolution of acute PVT in 80% of cases with prompt formal anticoagulation (heparin followed by warfarin) ± prior thrombolytic therapy. Duration of anticoagulation uncertain, but may be needed lifelong if thrombotic tendency persists (as for pulmonary embolism).
- In chronic PVT no clear consensus on variceal bleeding prophylaxis, as RCTs performed in patients with chronic liver disease, and low rate and severity of bleeding in isolated PVT, but secondary prophylaxis probably indicated (see portal hypertension). Recent large case series suggest that oral anticoagulation leads to no increase in frequency or severity of variceal bleeding, and may reduce mortality due to mesenteric infarction. Pragmatic approach may be consideration of warfarinization after eradication of gastro-oesophageal varices with endoscopic band ligation.
- Surgical portosystemic shunt and TIPSS considered for recurrent bleeding. Low rate of hepatic encephalopathy.

Causes of portal vein thrombosis

Cirrhosis	Post-surgical (e.g. liver transplantation)
Portal hypertension (any cause)	Umbilical vein catheterization
Prothrombotic tendency (see below)	PV compression by nodes (e.g. TB, lymphoma)
Malignancy (local/distant)	Drugs (e.g. oral contraceptive pill)
Sepsis (local/systemic)	Pregnancy/post-partum
Schistosomiasis	Pancreatitis (acute and chronic)

Prothrombotic factors associated with portal vein thrombosis

Myeloproliferative disorders (e.g. polycythaemia rubra vera, essential thrombocytosis, myelofibrosis)	G20210A prothrombin gene mutation
Anti-cardiolipin antibody	Hyperhomocysteinaemia
Protein C, S, anti-thrombin III deficiency	Paroxysmal nocturnal haemoglobinuria
Anti-phospholipid syndrome	Factor V Leiden deficiency

Positron emission tomography (PET) scanning

Background

- Most tumour imaging relies on demonstrating abnormal anatomy (e.g. a mass). Size is a limiting factor, as is homogeneity with surrounding tissue, and primary or secondary lesions < 1 cm often missed on CT/MRI/transabdominal U/S.
- PET scanning provides information on function, relying on the increased metabolic rate common to most malignancies. Glucose analogue (^{18}F)2-fluoro-2-deoxy-D-glucose (FDG) most commonly used as tracer.
- Combining FDG PET with CT allows functional and anatomical assessment.

Indications

- In GI disease, increasing role for PET CT in primary staging of colon cancer and oesophageal cancer, in particular identification of metastases.
- As well as primary staging, PET CT in colon cancer used for:
  - Differentiating local recurrence from post-treatment changes.
  - Excluding extrahepatic metastases in patients with apparently isolated (and therefore resectable) liver recurrence post-primary tumour resection.
  - Identifying site of recurrence in patients with rising tumour markers, and no sign of recurrence on anatomical imaging.
- Routine role in staging of pancreatic cancer less well defined. May be of use in characterizing benign versus malignant pancreatic lesions.
- PET using FDG of less use in carcinoid and pancreatic endocrine tumours, probably due to lower metabolic rate, but other tracers (e.g. ^{11}C-L-dopa , ^{11}C-5-HTP) provide better yields.

Limitations

- Differentiation between reactive and malignant lymph nodes difficult.
- False-negatives in tumours with low metabolic rate.
- False-positive uptake in colon (although may sometimes be first indication of undiagnosed colitis or colonic polyps).
- As with other imaging modalities, may fail to characterize lesions <1 cm.

Post-gastrectomy syndromes

Division of the vagal nerve, bypass or destruction of the pylorus, and resection of the stomach result in permanent anatomical and physiological changes resulting in:
- Reduced reservoir function.
- Altered gastric adaptation.
- Altered gastric emptying.
- Duodenal reflux into the stomach.
- Altered absorptive capacity.

Early complications of gastrectomy include:
- Delayed gastric emptying following widespread denervation of the stomach.
- Pain and distension 30–60 min after meals resulting from rapid emptying of the stomach and jejunal distension: this usually settles as the patient learns new eating habits.
- Most changes are long-lasting or **late complications**.

Delayed gastric emptying
- **Chronic gastroparesis** can occur following truncal vagotomy, and can be difficult to treat. Metoclopramide and erythromycin may help, but sometimes further surgery with a <u>Roux-en-Y anastomosis</u> is needed to return the patient to oral feeding.
- **Anastomotic ulcers** can occur due to decreased resistance to acid digestion of the jejunum, gastric stasis, and partial obstruction of the anastomosis due to scarring or oedema. Biopsy of the ulcer to exclude malignancy may be needed and revisional surgery is often needed.
- <u>**Afferent loop syndrome**</u> is described elsewhere.
- **Reflux of duodenal contents** (bile and pancreatic secretions) into the gastric remnant can cause pain and vomiting. Endoscopic biopsy may show features of a chemical gastritis. Treatment is operative, requiring conversion to a <u>Billroth I</u> or a a <u>Roux-en-Y</u> configuration.
- **Gastric cancer**. There is a twofold risk of gastric cancer 15 years after gastrectomy, probably due to reflux-stimulated increases in cell proliferation.

Rapid emptying
Post-vagotomy diarrhoea is poorly understood, but patients usually have rapid gastric emptying. Codeine and loperamide can help, as can <u>OCTREOTIDE</u> (see index of drugs).

<u>**Dumping**</u> is discussed elsewhere.

Metabolic complications
- **Iron deficiency** anaemia is common. Apart from recurrent ulceration, reduced gastric acid impairs absorption of ferric iron.
- **Intrinsic factor** is absent in patients with total gastrectomy, which can lead to B12 deficiency.
- **Steatorrhoea** can result from poor mixing of food with pancreatic enzymes or afferent loop syndrome.
- **Calcium deficiency** with <u>osteoporosis</u> and <u>metabolic bone disease</u> can result from steatorrhoea or impaired absorption at less acidic pH.

Pouchitis

Inflammation occurring in an ileal pouch after proctocolectomy with ileal pouch–anal anastomosis or Kock's continent ileostomy. Risk of pouchitis is highest in first 12 months after ileostomy, ranging from 20–35%. Patients with IBD (especially those with extra-intestinal manifestations) are more commonly affected than patients with familial adenomatous polyposis. After 10 years of a pouch, 50% of patients will have had at least one episode. Acute episodes of pouchitis do not affect long-term pouch function, but chronic pouchitis (affecting 10% of patients) is associated with dysplasia and carcinoma, probably via dysplasia in the rectal cuff.

Aetiology is unknown, but probably relates to anaerobic colonization of the pouch mucosa and subsequent colonic metaplasia. Exclusion of other superimposed infections is a concern, as is the possibility that the patient has had Crohn's disease all along.

Clinical features include diarrhoea, bleeding, urgency, abdominal pain. Accurate diagnosis requires a combination of endoscopic, clinical, and histological assessment: reliance on clinical assessment alone results in overdiagnosis and unnecessary treatment. Scoring systems have been developed to standardize evaluation and response to treatment: the best is the pouchitis disease activity index (PDAI, see table). Pouchitis is defined as a score over 7; remission is a score less than 7 in a patient with a history of pouchitis.

Treatment
Simple anti-diarrhoeal agents may help diarrhoea but for true pouchitis, antibiotics (metronidazole 400 mg tds for 5–7 days) are the first line of treatment. Topical treatment with 5-ASA enemas or steroid enemas can help. Treatment with bismuth subsalicylate (pepto-bismol) is not supported on current evidence. Oral probiotic therapy has been shown with at least one preparation (VSL-3) to maintain remission in patients with chronic pouchitis.

For a review see Mahadevan, U and Sandborn, WJ (2003) *Gastroenterology* **124**: 1636.

Pregnancy

See: Approach to GI problems in pregnancy and Approach to liver problems in pregnancy.

Pouchitis disease activity index (Adapted with permission from Sandborn, WJ et al. (1994). *Mayo Clin. Proc.* **69**: 409)

Criteria	Score
Clinical	
Stool frequency (usual: 1–2 more than usual: 3 or more more than usual)	0–2
Rectal bleeding (none/rare: present daily)	0–1
Faecal urgency/cramps (none: occasional: usual)	0–2
Fever	1 if present
Endoscopic	
Oedema, granularity, friability, loss of vascular pattern, mucous exudates, ulceration	1 for each if present
Histologic	
Polymorph infiltration: mild, moderate, severe	1–3
Average ulceration per low power field: < 25%, 25–50%, > 50%	1–3

Primary biliary cirrhosis (PBC)

Epidemiology + pathogenesis

Chronic, progressive cholestatic disorder, predominantly of middle-age women (90%). Prevalence 20–400/million. Aetiology unclear, but environmental trigger (e.g. bacteria, mycobacteria, viruses) in genetically susceptible individuals (familial link shown) suggested.

Clinical features

- Pruritis and lethargy classical presenting features, but 50% identified in asymptomatic stage. Associated autoimmune diseases (sicca syndrome (80%), thyroid disease, Raynaud's, arthralgia, Addison's disease). Osteoporosis is common. Increased risk of hepatocellular carcinoma (although lower than for chronic viral hepatitis and , haemochromatosis, and alcoholic liver disease).
- Clinical signs include xanthelasma around eyes, excoriations due to pruritis, clubbing, and signs of chronic liver disease (see Approach to GI examination).
- Median survival from presentation of 10–16 years for asymptomatic, 7–10 years for symptomatic patients.

Investigations

- ↑ALP, ↑GGT, with transaminases raised only mildly. Bilirubin ↑occurs late, and rise then usually inexorable. ↑ PT may be due to impaired synthetic function or vitamin K malabsorption. ↑serum IgM.
- Ultrasound performed in all cases to exclude biliary obstruction (see Approach to well patient with abnormal liver tests).
- Antimitochondrial antibodies (AMA) in 95% of cases of PBC. If negative, but histological features of PBC, and ↑ anti-nuclear antibody titres, likely 'autoimmune cholangitis', variant of PBC (see overlap syndromes).
- Role of liver biopsy debated, as little need when diagnosis clear (↑ALP, ↑IgM, AMA strongly +ve), as histology rarely changes management and of little prognostic value. Biopsy indicated where there is diagnostic uncertainty. Four histological stages:
  1. Florid bile duct lesion, portal hepatitis, granulomas.
  2. Periportal fibrosis ± hepatitis, portal tract enlargement, ductular Proliferation.
  3. Bridging necrosis, septal fibrosis, scarring.
  4. Cirrhosis; but staging again limited by the patchy distribution of lesions.
- DEXA scan (see bone densitometry), calcium, and parathyroid hormone levels to investigate bone disease. Measure fat soluble vitamins (vitamins A, D, E, K).

Management

- Complications of cirrhosis are managed along established lines (see Approach to cirrhosis and chronic liver disease).
- Wide range of immunomodulators tried in PBC (e.g. steroids, methotrexate, colchicine), without significant benefit shown to date.

- <u>URSODEOXYCHOLIC ACID</u> (<u>UDCA</u>) 10–15 mg/kg/day is safe and well-tolerated, and improves liver biochemistry, but its effect on disease progression and transplant-free survival is much debated
- For pruritis, give <u>CHOLESTYRAMINE</u> 4 g qds PO, and alternatives include UDCA, rifampicin, naloxone, phenobarbitone, and even extracorporeal liver support (e.g. MARS—see <u>liver support devices</u>).
- Treat <u>osteoporosis</u> and osteopenia if present (low threshold for giving calcium/vitamin D supplements, even without DEXA scan, e.g. Calcichew® D3 forte 1 tab bd).
- If vitamin deficient, give orally vitamin A 10000 IU/day, vitamin D + calcium (see above), vitamin E 400 IU/day, vitamin K 5–10 mg/day.
- <u>Liver transplantation</u> is highly effective (> 80% 5 year survival), and may be indicated for intractable pruritis and fatigue, as well as progressive liver failure, and serum bilirubin > 170 µmol/L.

Primary sclerosing cholangitis (PSC)

Epidemiology + pathogenesis

Cholestatic liver disease characterized by <u>biliary stricturing</u> and dilatation. Prevalence 60–80/million, and associated with <u>inflammatory bowel disease (IBD)</u> in 80% of cases (3–10% of patients with IBD, mainly <u>ulcerative colitis</u>, will get PSC). Immunogenetic factors (e.g. association with HLA A1, B8, DR3) and environmental factors (e.g. portal venous entotoxins/bacteria) likely to be important, but exact aetiology remains unclear.

Clinical features

Common presentation with fatigue, pruritis, intermittent jaundice, and right upper quadrant discomfort.

- Jaundice may result from intrahepatic stricturing, impaired liver function, 'dominant' extrahepatic biliary stricture (in 20%), biliary stone disease, or <u>cholangiocarcinoma</u> (lifetime risk 20–30%).
- Features of cholangitis (fever, pain, jaundice) usually occur following instrumentation (e.g. ERCP), rather than *de novo*.
- Signs of chronic liver disease and <u>portal hypertension</u> may be present (see <u>Approach to GI examination</u>).
- <u>Osteoporosis</u> and <u>metabolic bone disease</u> and steatorrhoea may occur.
- Time from symptomatic presentation to death or <u>liver transplant</u> 12–21 years.

Investigation

- LFTs show cholestatic pattern (↑ALP, GGT), but with AST/ALT ↑ < ×5 ULN. Bilirubin often fluctuates (unlike in <u>primary biliary cirrhosis</u>), with increases related to cholangitis/biliary stones/strictures.
- <u>ERCP</u> remains 'gold standard' for diagnosis, but <u>MRCP</u> may also show cholangiographic changes of multifocal intrahepatic ± extrahepatic stricturing and beading.
- <u>Liver biopsy</u> often not diagnostic, but histological features include bile duct proliferation, ductopenia, and concentric peribiliary fibrosis ('onion skin').
- p-ANCA is elevated in 65–85% of PSC patients.
- Diagnosis of <u>cholangiocarcinoma</u> in PSC always difficult at early stage, but combination of CT, biliary brush cytology at ERCP, and serum tumour markers CEA and CA19–9 used (although CA19–9 >180 U/ml reported to be > 95% specific, > 66% sensitive, high levels also seen in biliary obstruction).
- Surveillance colonoscopy programme in PSC patients with colitis is indicated (guidelines suggest yearly, although evidence base for this is weak) in view of markedly increased <u>colonic cancer</u> risk.

Management

- <u>URSODEOXYCHOLIC ACID</u> (<u>UCDA</u>) improves LFTs, but no effect on symptoms, histology, or survival at conventional doses (10–15 mg/kg/day). However, it may protect against colonic neoplasia, and at >20mg/kg/day improve liver histology.
- 'Dominant' extrahepatic biliary strictures endoscopically dilated ± stented.
- <u>ANTIBIOTICS</u> (e.g. <u>CIPROFLOXACIN</u>) for proven cholangitis, but no role for prophylaxis (except prior to ERCP).
- Pruritis managed initially with <u>CHOLESTYRAMINE</u> 4 g/day, with other options rifampicin 150 mg bd.
- Correct <u>vitamin A</u>, <u>D</u>, <u>E</u>, <u>K</u> deficiencies, if present.
- <u>Liver transplantation</u> provides 80–90% 5 year survival, but 20% recurrence at 5 years. <u>Cholangiocarcinoma</u> is absolute contraindication in most centres.

Differential diagnosis of PSC

- Biliary stone disease
- Post-cholecystectomy <u>biliary strictures</u>
- <u>Caroli's disease</u>
- HIV cholangiopathy
- <u>Cholangiocarcinoma</u>
- Ischaemic strictures
- Exposure to biliary toxins (e.g. formalin)
- <u>Autoimmune pancreatitis</u> with biliary involvement
- <u>Clonorchis</u> infection

Prokinetics

See: <u>PROKINETICS</u> in drug index.

Protein-losing enteropathy

Excess protein loss from the gut (which is non-selective and not limited to low molecular weight proteins as in the nephritic syndrome) can be due to:
- Increased mucosal permeability.
- Mucosal ulceration.
- Lymphatic obstruction.

Clinical features
- Oedema, diarrhoea, fat or carbohydrate malabsorption, signs of fat soluble <u>vitamin</u> deficiency, and consequences of reduced cellular immunity.
- **Laboratory abnormalities** may include ↓ serum albumin, Igs, proteins (e.g. caeruloplasmin, alpha-1 antitrypsin, transferrin, hormone binding proteins), and lymphocytopenia if there is lymphatic obstruction.

Diagnosis
The gold standard is measuring the loss of intravenously labelled albumin: this has disadvantages in terms of radioactive exposure and expense, so faecal measurement of alpha-1 antitrypsin is the preferred method. Note that because alpha-1 antitrypsin is degraded at pH < 3, it cannot be used to measure gastric protein loss and interpretation is difficult in patients with positive <u>faecal occult blood</u>.

Proton pump inhibitors

See: <u>PROTON PUMP INHIBITORS</u>.

Protozoa

See: amoebiasis, giardiasis, coccidia, microsporidia, and trypanosomiasis.

Pruritus ani

Perianal area is commonest site for intractable itching of the skin, due to:
- Benign anorectal condition such as haemorrhoids or anal fissure.
- Neoplasia such as Bowen's disease, Paget's disease, or anal cancer.
- Dermatological disease (dermatitis, lichen sclerosis).
- Infection: *Candida*, threadworm (more common with underlying systemic disease such as diabetes).
- Possible dietary components: coffee has been implicated as a common irritant.
- Before labelling the condition as 'idiopathic', consider faecal leakage; anorectal physiology and endoanal ultrasound will help to define a defect in the anal sphincters.

Treatment involves identifying the cause. An advice sheet may help (see box): most important single piece of advice is to avoid vigorous wiping or 'polishing'.

Pseudoachalasia

An appearance usually seen on barium swallow or endoscopy that can mimic achalasia, but in fact is due to malignant compression of the lower oesophagus. It accounts for about 5% of cases of manometrically defined achalasia, and should be suspected in the over-50 age group, if onset of symptoms is abrupt (< 1 year), or if there is early weight loss of over 7 kg. It should also be considered if there is a feeling at endoscopy of resistance or stiffness in crossing the lower oesophageal sphincter or if the patient tolerates endoscopic dilatation very poorly (in this case, stop the procedure and reconsider the diagnosis). Adenocarcinoma of the gastro-oesophageal junction is the commonest cause, but other tumours or infiltrative diseases have been reported (see oesophageal tumours).

Pseudomembranous colitis

See: clostridial infections of GI tract.

Advice sheet for pruritus ani

1. Avoid creams and ointments if possible. Short-term steroids (1% hydrocortisone ointment) can help: long-term use thins the skin
2. Wash the skin with water after each stool; pat dry, do not rub
3. Wear cotton underclothing. Try stockings rather than tights (note: this mainly applies to women)
4. Avoid hot and spicy foods that cause wind and loose stools
5. Wear a cotton pad or folded sheet of toilet paper to absorb any mucus or moisture seeping from the anus
6. Avoid scratching at all costs

Pseudomonas

- Can affect every portion of the GI tract. Most commonly affects very young children and adults with haematological malignancies and chemotherapy-induced neutropenia. Colonization of the GI tract is an important portal of entry for pseudomonal bacteraemia in patients who are neutropenic. Spectrum of disease can range from very mild symptoms to severe necrotizing enterocolitis with significant morbidity and mortality.
- Epidemics of pseudomonal diarrhoea can occur in nurseries. Young infants may present with irritability, vomiting, diarrhoea, and dehydration.
- The infection can cause enteritis, with patients presenting with prostration, headache, fever, and diarrhoea (Shanghai fever).
- *Pseudomonas* <u>typhlitis</u> typically presents in patients with neutropenia resulting from acute leukaemia, with a sudden onset of fever, abdominal distension, and worsening abdominal pain.

Pseudo-obstruction

Symptoms and signs of intestinal obstruction in the absence of an occluding lesion. Caused by disorders of smooth muscle, myenteric plexus or extra-intestinal nervous system. (See box.) <u>Ogilvie's syndrome</u> is acute pseudo-obstruction localized to the colon, precipitated by trauma, orthopaedic surgery, obstetric procedures, pelvic surgery, or electrolyte disturbances (e.g. $\downarrow K^+$).

Clinical features

Varying degrees of abdominal pain, distension, and vomiting, depending partly on which part of bowel is involved. Small bowel involvement with stasis and <u>bacterial overgrowth</u> may lead to steatorrhoea. This can lead to weight loss and malabsorption. There may be gastroparesis or oesophageal involvement. There may be a succussion splash and obstructive sounding bowel sounds.

Investigations

As well as blood tests directed to various diagnoses listed in the box, barium or cross-sectional imaging of the whole GI tract is indicated. The aim is to make a diagnosis where possible but mainly to exclude mechanical obstruction.

There may even be a need for brain MRI, electromyography, or nerve conduction studies, and autonomic function tests. There is an association with urinary tract involvement such as megacystis or megaureters.

Treatment

- **Electrolyte balance**, especially potassium, calcium, and magnesium is important. Drug treatment with <u>PROKINETICS</u> is attractive but <u>METOCLOPRAMIDE</u> and <u>DOMPERIDONE</u> rarely work: cisapride is more effective but is now restricted to a named patient basis. Erythromycin is a motilin agonist and is sometimes tried. <u>OCTREOTIDE</u> in small doses can induce migrating motor complexes in the small intestine. Broad spectrum antibiotics are useful in treating patients with <u>bacterial overgrowth</u> due to stagnant loop syndrome.

- **Diet** should be low fat, low residue, and low lactose.
- **Colonoscopic decompression** can be tried although is not universally effective.
- Treatment with neostigmine, 2.5 mg IV over 2–3 minutes (patient should be on a monitor with atropine ready in case of bradycardia) has been shown effective in a prospective controlled study (Ponec, RJ *et al.* (1999). *N. Engl. J. Med*: **341**: 137) and is probably underutilized.
- Surgery is rarely required and does not always remove symptoms. A small number ot patients need home <u>parenteral nutrition</u>.

Causes of chronic intestinal pseudo-obstruction
- Disorders of smooth muscle (either primary due to rare visceral myopathies, or secondary to amyloid, radiation, SLE, muscular dystrophy, or systemic sclerosis)
- Disorders of the myenteric plexus
- Neurological problems: Parkinson's, autonomic dysfunction
- Small bowel diverticulosis
- Endocrine: hypothyroidism, porphyria
- Drugs (<u>OPIATES</u>, phenothiazines, <u>ANTICHOLINERGICS</u>, tricyclics, calcium channel blockers)

Pyloric stenosis

Usually associated in adults with <u>peptic ulcer</u> disease or <u>gastric cancer</u>: hypertrophic pyloric stenosis is rare.

Symptoms are nausea, vomiting, early satiety, and epigastric pain after eating. Unlike in infants, physical exam is often not helpful because in adults the pyloric mass is difficult to palpate. A succussion splash may sometimes be elicited. Identical symptoms and signs may be found in gastric outlet obstruction due to duodenal structuring in <u>pancreatic cancer</u>.

Diagnosis can be via barium radiology, although imaging with ultrasound or CT is more effective at revealing any extraluminal pathology that may be contributing to luminal stenosis. Endoscopy is needed to diagnose peptic ulceration or tumour and to make a histological diagnosis.

Treatment. If malignancy has been excluded, <u>endoscopic dilatation</u> with a balloon can be effective, although there is a post-procedure recurrence rate of about 80%. Surgical pyloromyotomy or resection of the involved region can offer a long-term cure. Gastric bypass may be necessary.

Pyoderma gangrenosum

(see Colour Plate 24)
A papule, pustule, or nodule, most often seen on the leg but sometimes around a stoma, that progresses to an ulcer with undermined borders. Often displays pathergy (development of ulcers in response to minor trauma; shared with the skin lesion of <u>Behçet's syndrome</u>). Associated with both <u>ulcerative colitis</u> and <u>Crohn's disease</u>, but often not associated with intestinal disease activity and not unique to these disorders. Responds to topical steroid application and in the context of Crohn's disease responds very well to <u>INFLIXIMAB</u>.

Q

Quality of life scores

Monitoring and enhancement of a patient's health-related quality of life (HRQL) is an important element of research and medical care. Disease-specific instruments have been developed for inflammatory bowel disease, irritable bowel syndrome, dyspepsia, gastro-oesophageal reflux disease, liver disease, and GI malignancy. The structures and properties of the most commonly used generic and digestive disease-specific HRQL instruments have recently been reviewed (Yacavone, RF. et al. (2001). Quality of life in gastroenterology—what is available? *Am. J . Gastroenterol.* 96(2): 285).

R

Radiation damage to the GI tract

The bowel can be damaged by radiation treatment for a range of tumours, including cervical cancer, prostate cancer, or combined chemo-radiotherapy for rectal cancer. The effects of radiation on intestinal tissue depend on several factors.

- Rate of cell division (cell turnover is higher in the small intestine which is therefore more sensitive to radiation damage).
- Presence of genes regulating apoptosis (experimentally radiation-induced apoptosis depends on the presence of p53 and is inhibited by bcl2: the higher levels of bcl2 in the colon and rectum may explain the greater tolerance to radiation compared with the small intestine).
- Ionizing radiation activates inflammatory and fibrogenic cytokines. TGFβ promotes fibrosis by stimulating collagen synthesis and chemotaxis of fibroblasts.

Epidemiology

Acute radiation enteritis is common (incidence 20–70%), usually occurs in the third week of a fractionated course, and is rarely life-threatening unless there is pancytopenia and sepsis secondary to chemotherapy. It usually resolves 2–6 weeks after completion of radiotherapy.

Chronic radiation enteritis varies in incidence from 1–15% and the latency may range from 6 months to 25 years. Predisposing factors include older age, post-operative radiation, collagen vascular disease, combined chemotherapy, and poor radiation technique. Prolapse of small bowel into the pelvis after surgery exposes large volumes of bowel to radiation.

Pathology

Occlusive vasculitis and diffuse collagen deposition with fibrosis. Changes are progressive and result in mucosal ulceration, necrosis, and sometimes perforation.

Clinical features

- Fibrosis and vasculitis can lead to strictures and malabsorption.
- Fistulae and abscesses are serious complications that may need surgery.
- Bacterial overgrowth may be due to dilated bowel loops proximal to stricture.
- Patients with a history of pelvic irradiation can present with rectal bleeding due to mucosal friability or telangiectasia. They may have anorectal pain, tenesmus, or faecal urgency. Chronic inflammation can lead to reduced rectal capacity and diarrhoea.

Diagnosis

Not always straightforward.

- Analysis of the treatment plan and dose distribution may show areas of high dose and lesions found on imaging or endoscopy are usually localized to these areas.

Recurrence of cancer often needs excluding because the manifestations of chronic radiation colitis are non-specific. Mucosal ulceration and thickening of small bowel loops are radiological signs of radiation damage. Imaging requires adequate luminal distension: CT enteroclysis with infusion of contrast through a naso-enteric tube is probably the best single investigation, with good sensitivity and specificity for diagnosing recurrent tumour and low grade or intermittent obstruction. It can also help in suggesting the source of occult bleeding.

- Colonoscopy is helpful if there is rectal bleeding and can help in diagnosing the cause of stricturing as well as looking for recurrent or further new primary tumours.

Management

- Be as conservative as possible: surgery is difficult and associated with high morbidity rate. Management of pelvic fistulae is complex and requires diversion before corrective surgery.
- Diarrhoea can result from fast transit time, bile acid malabsorption, and lactose intolerance. Loperamide can help.
- Antibiotics can help if there is bacterial overgrowth.
- Laser therapy or argon plasma coagulation (APC) can control rectal bleeding due to radiation proctitis, and recent reports suggest that SUCRALFATE enemas (see index of drugs) or local formalin treatment (given under general anaesthetic) may be of help.
- Hyperbaric oxygen stimulates new blood vessel formation and is being evaluated. Small bowel transplantation might offer hope to a small number of paediatric patients with radiation enteritis.

Prevention is the best treatment.

- Surgical fixing of small bowel loops out of the pelvis and any radiation field is possible by placing a biodegradable mesh that supports the small intestine out of the pelvis.
- Pharmacological agents conferring protection against the effects of ionizing radiation (e.g. amifostine) are attractive but unproven.

Rectal cancer

Accounts for one-third of colorectal cancer. Epidemiology, aetiology, pathogenesis, and screening recommendations are common to colon cancer. Aspects meriting specific discussion include:

Imaging. Preoperative staging includes digital rectal examination, CT or MRI scanning of abdomen and pelvis, endoscopic evaluation with biopsy, and endoscopic ultrasound (EUS). EUS is accurate at evaluating tumour stage and perirectal node involvement.

Staging. Treatment decisions should be made with reference to the TNM classification (see tumour staging) rather than Dukes staging. The American joint committee on cancer has designated staging as stage I (T1 or T2, N0, M0), stage II (T3 or T4, N0, M0), stage III (any T, nodal involvement, M0), and stage IV (distant metastases).

Surgery. Resection is indicated for removal of primary tumour and regional lymph nodes for localized disease. Trans-anal excision can be used for early cancers confined to the rectal submucosa. The technique of excision can affect the rate of local recurrence: total mesorectal excision with colo-anal anastomosis is associated with low incidence of local recurrence (4%) but there is a risk of anastomotic dehiscence of up to 15%. Abdomino-perineal resection with end-sigmoid colostomy is indicated in patients with lower third rectal cancers who cannot undergo a sphincter-saving procedure because there is less than 2 cm disease-free distal margin.

Adjuvant therapy. Because of the increased risk of local recurrence (up to 50% for stage II or III disease), perioperative radiation has a greater effect in rectal cancer than, colon cancer. Pre- and post-operative radiation therapy decrease risk of tumour recurrence in stage II or III but increased patient survival has not been shown. Because pre-operative radiotherapy delays surgery and makes pathological staging difficult, post-operative radiotherapy may be preferable. Combined therapy with 5FU and radiation is widely used for stage II and III disease but further studies are needed to determine long-term results.

Palliative and experimental treatments. Endoscopic therapy using Nd:YAG laser can recanalize the rectum in patients with obstructing cancers who are unfit for surgery. Mesh metal stenting and photodynamic therapy have been used in small numbers of patients.

Prognosis. Overall 5 year survival rates are 72% for stage I, 54% for stage II, 40% for stage III, and 7% for stage IV.

Rectal prolapse

Intussusception of the rectum through the anal canal can vary from rectal mucosa only, to full thickness of rectum and sigmoid colon. Causal factors include any neurological or muscular disease leading to weakness of the pelvic floor, impaired function of the anal sphincters, chronic constipation with resultant straining, and colorectal tumours.

Clinical features and diagnosis. Presenting symptoms may include pain, incontinence, or a sensation of 'something coming down'. Demonstration can be helped by having the patient strain in a sitting position or by defecography; proctoscopy is important in excluding internal haemorrhoids and anal tumours. Colonoscopy to exclude a tumour is indicated, as is a complete pelvic floor examination because of the risk of associated bladder or uterine prolapse. Anorectal manometry, with testing of pudendal nerve function, may be necessary because the nerve can be injured by chronic traction by a prolapse.

Treatment. Surgery is central to managment. There are many different procedures depending on age and aetiology. Both abdominal (anterior repair and rectopexy) and perineal approaches (usually resection of the prolapse, possibly with pelvic floor repair) are possible: there is interest in laparoscopic repair of prolapse but long-term outcome data are needed.

Rectal ulcer

See: solitary rectal ulcer syndrome

Rectocele

In women, the anterior rectal wall above the perineal body is unsupported and the rectovaginal septum may bulge anteriorly to form a rectocele (see Fig. 2.25). This can give symptoms of incomplete evacuation of stool, a lump appearing at the introitus with straining, and sometimes having to support the posterior vaginal wall with finger or thumb, or digitally evacuate stool, to enable defecation. The rectocele is most easily demonstrated on a <u>defecography</u> study. Surgical repair can be done via endorectal, transvaginal, or transperineal approaches and is beneficial in about 75% of selected patients.

Refeeding syndrome

- Insulin secretion is reduced in starvation due to reduced carbohydrate intake: fat and protein are catabolized to produce energy. This results in intracellular loss of electrolytes, especially phosphate.
- Feeding results in increased insulin, which stimulates cellular uptake of phosphate. This usually occurs within 4 days of refeeding. Serum phosphate below 0.5 mM/l can produce clinical features of rhabdomyolysis, leucocyte dysfunction, respiratory failure, cardiac failure, hypotension, muscle weakness, arrhythmias, and seizures.
- Refeeding syndrome can occur with parenteral or enteral feeding: patients with <u>anorexia</u>, cancer, <u>alcohol dependency</u> and patients who have commenced <u>PEG</u> feeding after prolonged neurological dysphagia are at risk.

Treatment involves intravenous phosphate: give 50 mM IV phosphate over 24 h (Hearing, SD. (2004) *Br. Med. J.*; **328**: 908).

Acute vitamin and mineral deficiencies can be precipitated by feeding without appropriate micronutrients. Folate deficiency can result in megaloblastosis and thrombocytopenia: vitamin B12 deficiency can result in lactic acidosis.

Reiter's syndrome

Hans Reiter, 1916. A triad of arthritis, urethritis, and conjunctivitis occurring after bacillary dysentery or venereal disease. Urethritis can be mild or absent and periostitis, tendonitis, and plantar fasciitis can accompany arthritis.

- Commonest in males aged 20–40 years who are HLA-B27 positive (see box). Complicates 1–2% of cases of <u>*Shigella*</u>; also reported after <u>*Salmonella*</u>, <u>*Yersinia*</u>, and <u>*Campylobacter*</u> infection.
- Presentation is usually with symmetrical lower limb arthropathy 2–4 weeks after bacterial dysentery. Antibiotic therapy usually not indicated as the enteric infection has resolved. The arthritis tends to be chronic and relapsing: treatment involves symptomatic relief and nonsteroidals.

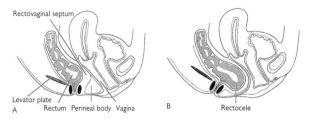

Fig. 2.25 Weakness of the levator plate and attenuation of the perineal body (A) predispose to formation of a rectocele (B). Reproduced from Feldman M, Friedman LS, and Sleisenger MH (2003). *Seleisenger and Fordtran's Gastrointestinal and Liver Deisease*, with permission from Elsevier.

HLA B27 and enteric arthropathy

- <u>Reiter's syndrome</u>. 80% are positive for HLAB27: conversely about 20% of HLA-B27 patients will develop Reiter's after bacillary dysentery
- Ankylosing spondylitis and <u>ulcerative colitis</u>
- Sacro-iliitis complicating <u>Whipple's disease</u>
- <u>Behçet's syndrome</u>

Retroperitoneal perforation

- Perforation of abdominal viscus into retroperitoneum may occur spontaneously (colonic <u>diverticular disease</u>, posterior <u>duodenal ulcer</u>), or be iatrogenic (complicates < 1% of biliary sphincterotomies (see <u>ERCP</u> and <u>endoscopic complications</u>) and also following rectal instrumentation).
- Air may rapidly track into mediastinum and soft tissues, presenting clinically with subcutaneous emphysema, with soft tissue swelling, and skin crepitus on palpation (like squeezing 'bubble wrap'). May be recognized clinically by air outlining kidney, bowel, or psoas muscle on plain X-ray, but CT confirms diagnosis. If not noted at time of ERCP, may present the following day with abdominal pain suggestive of <u>acute pancreatitis</u>, but without significantly raised amylase.
- Treatment includes strict NBM, IV fluids, and broad spectrum antibiotics (e.g. 3rd generation <u>CEPHALOSPORIN</u> and <u>METRONIDAZOLE</u>—see index of drugs). Surgery rarely necessary for sphincterotomy perforation, but involve surgeons early. Significant morbidity related to retroperitoneal abscess formation, which requires percutaneous drainage ± surgery. Large colorectal tears may require surgery.

Rheumatoid arthritis (RA) and the GI tract

GI manifestations of the disease

Temporomandibular arthritis can impair chewing. Oesophageal dysmotility results from low amplitude peristalsis and reduced lower oesophageal sphincter pressure. Vasculitis affects 1% of rheumatoid patients: in 10% of these GI involvement results in <u>cholecystitis</u>, colitis, or ruptured visceral aneurysm. <u>Amyloidosis</u> can result in <u>pseudo-obstruction</u> or malabsorption (see <u>Approach to malabsorption and steatorrhoea</u>). See also <u>Felty's syndrome</u> and <u>Still's disease</u>.

GI problems of drug therapy for RA

Endoscopic lesions are seen in 20–40% of rheumatoid patients who take NSAIDs: risk is increased by age over 60, history of peptic ulcer, use of steroids, and extra-articular manifestations. *Helicobacter pylori* is probably an independent risk factor for peptic ulceration in rheumatoid patients. In the past, use of gold was associated with GI toxicity, especially colitis. <u>METHOTREXATE</u> can cause hepatic fibrosis in cumulative doses over 1.5 g.

Rotavirus

See: <u>Approach to acute diarrhoea</u>.

Roundworm (nematode) infection

Think of four groups:

Infection confined to human GI tract

Organisms include *Tricuris* (whipworm), *Enterobius* (pinworm), *Capillaria* (important in Phillipines and Far East), and *Tricostrongylus* (human infection most prevalent in Middle East and Asia). Distribution is worldwide but commonest in areas of poor sanitation. Humans eat eggs, the larvae penetrate the intestinal mucosa and mature into adults that are confined to the gut. Heavy tricuris infestation can cause diarrhoea and rectal prolapse. Eosinophilia is common. Pinworm infestation is common in developed countries. Eggs are laid on the perianal skin, which causes intense pruritus.

Diagnosis is by finding eggs in the stool or worms attached to the mucosa: for pinworms, tape applied to the perianal area and then examined under the micsroscope may reveal eggs. Treatment is with albendazole or mebendazole. **Note**. *Tricuris* induces a strong Th2 response and minimizes Th1 response: this has led to experimental administration of the pig whipworm to patients with inflammatory bowel disease: initial results are promising.

Infection begins in the GI tract; larvae invade and reach the lungs, migrate to pharynx, are swallowed and mature in the gut

Adult *Ascaris* can be 10–25 cm long. Infection is common (1.2 billion worldwide: only cold dry climates are spared): clinical features can result from migration of larvae through the lung (bronchospasm, bronchiolar inflammation, urticaria, or other manisfestations of hypersensitivity) or in heavy infections, by blocking the gut or biliary tree. Diagnosis is by finding eggs in stool. Treatment is with albendazole or mebendazole.

Larvae invade the skin, migrate to the lungs, then are swallowed and mature in the gut

Hookworms (*Ankylostoma*, *Necator*) and *Stronglyoides*.

Hookworms secrete an anticoagulant and change their location often: they are a significant cause of iron deficiency anaemia. Spread is facilitated by walking barefoot and using human faeces as manure. Clinical features include a rash at the site of penetration and sometimes pulmonary hypersensitivity reactions. Iron deficiency anaemia and low albumin can occur. Eosinophilia is common. Diagnosis is by finding eggs in stool and treatment is with albendazole or mebendazole.

See separate entry for <u>Strongyloides</u>.

Intestinal nematodes of animals that can infect humans

Trichinella, cutaneous larva migrans caused by *Ancylostoma*, visceral larva migrans caused by *Toxocara*, and anisakiasis.

Trichinosis caused by *Trichinella* results from eating poorly cooked infected meat. Larvae burrow into the gut wall and migrate to skeletal muscle: extraocular muscles are often affected. Diagnosis is serological or rarely by muscle biopsy: CK is raised in 50%. Treat with albendazole or mebendazole.

Cutaneous larva migrans is a serpiginous dermatitis that is itchy and can be papulovesicular. In tropical and subtropical Africa, Caribbean, and Latin America. Hookworms of dogs and cats burrow through the skin. Treatment is with oral ivermectin or albendazole.

Visceral larva migrans results from ingestion of eggs of *Toxocara* living in dogs or cats. Larvae penetrate the intestine but cannot complete their life cycle in humans and wander through various organs. Clinical course is very variable: the classical triad is eosinophilia, hepatomegaly, and hyper-gammaglobulinaemia. There is an ELISA used to detect anti-*Toxocara* antibodies. Treatment is diethylcarbamazine or albendazole.

Anisakiasis is caused by nematode pathogens of fish and occurs if contaminated fish or squid are eaten raw or undercooked. Mucosal invasion of the stomach can cause severe gastritis or profuse haemorrhage within 12–24 h of ingestion.

Roux-en-Y anastomosis

- Procedure involves dividing jejunum approximately 15 cm from ligament of Trietze, and mobilizing a loop of jejunum. Proximal limb is anastomosed to the appropriate anatomic site (see figure). Divided end of jejunum is anastomosed to jejunal loop along its course.
- Indications for Roux-en-Y anastomosis include <u>biliary reflux</u> following partial <u>gastrectomy</u>, biliary reconstruction following bile duct injury (hepaticojejunostomy between jejunal loop and common hepatic duct); as anti-obesity ('bariatric') surgical intervention (jejunal anstomosis on to proximal stomach—see also <u>Approach to obesity</u>); and treatment of <u>post-gastrectomy syndromes</u>. See also <u>biliary bypass procedures</u>.

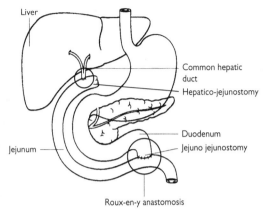

Fig. 2.26 Roux-en-Y anastomosis and hepatico-jejunostomy as part of <u>biliary byass procedure</u>.

S

Salmonella

A group of Gram-negative bacilli, causing food borne infection transmitted by 'flies, fingers, food, faeces, and fomites'. Recent pandemics in Western countries are especially due to infection of commercial eggs and poultry.

Salmonella penetrate the ileum and the colon, with haematogenous spread to other organs. There are 5 clinical syndromes of disease (box).

Salmonella gastroenteritis. Incubation period usually 6–48 hours. Symptoms include nausea and vomiting, cramps and diarrhoea. Diarrhoea usually lasts 3–4 days and can vary from a few loose stools to dysentery. Fever in 50%. Pain is central or right lower quadrant. 2–6 per 1000 become chronic carriers.

Risk increased by haemolytic anaemia, leukaemias, lymphoma, cancer, steroids, chemotherapy, gastric surgery or acid suppression, <u>schistosomiasis</u>.

Treatment. Most patients with uncomplicated salmonella should not have antibiotics (high rate of associated relapse and emergence of resistant strains). Indications for treatment include associated malignancy or immmnuosuppression, cardiovascular abnormalities, and presence of orthopaedic prostheses. Amoxicillin, co-trimoxazole, or a quinolone, such as <u>CIPROFLOXACIN</u>, are usual antibiotics, but there is some evidence of increasing drug resistance.

Clinical syndromes of *Salmonella* infection

- **Gastroenteritis**—seen in 75% of infections
- **Bacteraemia**—with or without gastroenteritis, associated with endocarditis and arteritis—10% of cases
- **Typhoid or enteric fever**—about 10% cases
- **Localized infection** (bones, joints, meninges)—5%
- **Carrier state** in asymptomatic people

Sarcoidosis

Inflammatory multisystem disease of uncertain origin. Within the GI system it particularly affects the liver, and sarcoid is one of important causes of <u>hepatic granulomas</u>.

Clinical features

- Often asymptomatic, with incidental liver function test abnormalities in patients with symptomatic lung, skin, or eye disease.
- Hepatomegaly, fever, right upper quadrant discomfort, in association with <u>hepatic granulomas</u> may occur.
- Rare presentations include severe intrahepatic cholestasis; <u>portal hypertension</u> due to cirrhosis/granulomas; and extrahepatic biliary obstruction due to portal lymph nodes, bile duct inflammation, and pancreatic sarcoid with distal <u>biliary stricture</u>.

Investigation

- Liver function tests often show ↑ALP/GGT ± mild ↑ AST/ALT. When previous diagnosis of sarcoid not made, elevated serum angiotensin converting enzyme (SACE) and lung changes (e.g. bilateral hilar lymphadenopathy) may aid diagnosis.
- CT or U/S findings non-specific, but granulomas may occasionally coalesce to form 0.5–3 cm nodules.
- Liver biopsy shows non-caseating granulomas in > 80%. Cirrhosis on biopsy has been reported in 6%.

Management

- URSODEOXYCHOLIC ACID may improve symptoms in intrahepatic cholestasis.
- Oral CORTICOSTEROID therapy induces clinical and biochemical improvement in patients with granulomatous hepatitis on biopsy. Duration of use uncertain, as relapse rate high if only short-term treatment given.
- Immunosuppression less effective in established cirrhosis and portal hypertension, and liver transplantation may rarely need considering.

Schatzki ring

See: oesophageal ring.

Schilling test

Used in vitamin B12 (cobalamin) deficiency to distinguish between causes due to intrinsic factor (IF) deficiency (i.e. gastric causes—pernicious anaemia, post-gastrectomy), and those due to impaired uptake of vita-min–IF complex (e.g. ileal Crohn's disease, small bowel bacterial over-growth, chronic pancreatitis). Test not affected by vitamin B12 replacement therapy.

Technique
- **Stage I.** Small dose of radiolabelled vitamin B12 (0.5–2.0 mCi) given orally in glass of water, followed 1 hour later by unlabelled vitamin B12 1 mg IM to saturate vitamin B12 carriers (so that radiolabelled dose excreted in urine, if absorbed). Vitamin B12 malabsorption diagnosed if < 7% of radiolabelled dose excreted in urine over subsequent 24 hours.
- **Stage II.** Needed to differentiate IF deficiency from other causes. Stage I repeated, but 60 mg of active IF administered orally with the oral test dose. Normalization of vitamin B12 excretion confirms IF deficiency.
- If vitamin B12 excretion low after stage II test, repeating stage I after 5 day course of antibiotic therapy (normalization suggests bacterial overgrowth), or with pancreatic supplements (normalization suggests pancreatic insufficiency), may help distinguish terminal ileal disease from other causes of malabsorption. Also see Approach to malabsorption and steatorrhoea.
- False positive results due to incomplete urine collection or renal impairment, and interpretation of excretion results may be difficult.

Schistosomiasis

Epidemiology + pathogenesis
- Schistosomes are blood flukes, with which 200 million people are chronically infected. Endemic areas include Africa, S. America, Far East, and S.E. Asia.

Schistosomiasis and hepatitis C—public health care link?

Up to 15% of the Egyptian population are infected with hepatitis C. This extraordinarily high rate may be linked to the mass population programme for schistosomiasis eradication carried out particularly in the 1960s and 1970s. Treatment with parenteral anti-schistosomal therapy (PAT) was sadly often given using multiply used, poorly steril-ized needles, so facilitating virus transmission

- Hepatosplenic schistosomiasis caused by *S. mansoni*, *S. japonicum* and *S. mekongi* (not *S. haematobium*, which causes urinary schistosomiasis).
- In life-cycle, eggs excreted into water in faeces, from where free-swimming miracidia infect freshwater snail, and develop into cercariae. These infect man through intact skin, enter the circulation, and mature into 1–2 cm adult worms within the portal venous system. Proportion of eggs produced may be retained within tissues, inducing a granulomatous inflammatory response that leads to <u>portal hypertension</u> ('pre-sinusoidal') but not cirrhosis.

Clinical features

- Acute schistosomiasis (Katayama fever) develops 3–6 weeks after primary infection, and coincides with egg laying. Fever, malaise, abdominal pain, and diarrhoea, which may last for several weeks. Associated hepatosplenomegaly may be found.
- Only small proportion of chronically infected people suffer significant clinical problems. Features are primarily due to <u>portal hypertension</u>, with varices, splenomegaly, and ascites. Stigmata of chronic liver disease and liver failure are rare, and as a result bleeding from gastro-oesophageal varices carries better outcome than in those with cirrhosis. Recurrent abdominal pain, bloody diarrhoea, and inflammatory colonic polyposis may also occur in chronic infection.

Investigation

- Peripheral eosinophilia characteristic of acute infection.
- Raised cholestatic liver tests (ALP, GGT) often seen.
- Stool analysis for ova often negative in acute infection. Yield for identifying ova improved by repeat stool samples and from biopsies at sigmoidoscopy.
- Schistosomal ELISA confirms exposure (and if negative reliably excludes infection), but not useful in distinguishing past from ongoing infection.
- <u>Liver biopsy</u> may show characteristic periportal fibrosis.
- Portal venous fibrosis may be seen on <u>CT scanning</u>.

Management

- Anti-schistosomal treatment (e.g. praziquantel 40 mg/kg/bd PO for 1 day) clears infection in 60–95% of cases, with reduction in egg burden in the others. It may prevent progression of chronic infection, but does not reverse portal hypertension.
- <u>Portal hypertension</u> may require standard management of its complications (e.g. primary/secondary prophylaxis).

Scleroderma and the GI tract

Connective tissue proliferation with fibrosis in the GI tract results in GI manifestations in 80% of scleroderma patients, often with more than 1 site affected. Treatment is symptomatic and supportive only, and often very difficult.

- **Oesophagus.** Abnormal peristalsis results in gastro-oesophageal reflux (GORD), intermittent dysphagia, and often stricturing. Oesophageal manometry shows lack of propagated swallows and low amplitude contractions. High dose PPIs needed to control reflux: dose–response curve is better for omeprazole than other PPIs in this context. Omeprazole 40 mg bd may be needed. Prokinetics theoretically increase lower oesophageal sphincter tone and speed gastric emptying but may not work.

- **Stomach.** Reduced gastric emptying is common and aggravates GORD. Prokinetics should be tried. Erythromycin is a motilin agonist and can speed gastric emptying. If there is intractable early satiety, low volume overnight PEG feeding can be very helpful: one useful manoeuvre is to place a jejunal extension through the PEG.

- **Small bowel.** Reduced motility, jejunal diverticulae, and consequent bacterial overgrowth may cause bloating, cramps, or signs of malabsorption. Barium studies useful (follow through shows a classical 'stacked coin' appearance). Bacterial overgrowth can be treated with low dose antibiotics (tetracycline 250 mg bd for 10 days or metronidazole 400 mg bd). Bacterial culture and sensitivities rarely useful. Prokinetics can be tried. Pseudo-obstruction sometimes seen and in worst cases parenteral nutrition needed. Malabsorption may be aggravated by pancreatic insufficiency (pancreatic exocrine output ↓ in 30%).

- **Large bowel.** Colon may be atonic and severe constipation is common. In our experience non-stimulant osmotic laxatives (e.g. movicol) are the best agents to help this. Thinning and fibrosis of anal sphincters is common and may explain an increased incidence of passive faecal incontinence.

Sclerosing cholangitis

See: primary sclerosing cholangitis.

Sclerotherapy

See: portal hypertension.

Sedation for endoscopy

- The degrees of sedation used for endoscopy include no sedation, conscious sedation, deep sedation, and general anaesthesia.
- Diagnostic upper GI endoscopy may be well tolerated with local anaesthetic throat spray only (e.g. xylocaine 2%), but conscious sedation (patient able to make purposeful responses to verbal/tactile stimuli, with spontaneous ventilation) is used for most endoscopies.
- The following required in patient undergoing conscious sedation:
  - Supplemental oxygen via nasal cannulae (e.g. 2 l/min).
  - IV access throughout procedure.
  - Pulse oximetry (but demonstrates only hypoxaemia, not hypoventilation, so clinical assessment remains vital).
  - Cardiac monitoring.
- Conscious sedation usually involves use of **benzodiazepine** (e.g. IV midazolam 2–10 mg) ± **opiate** (e.g. IV pethidine 25–50 mg, fentanyl 50–100 µg), administered by endoscopist. Opiate given first, because of slower rate of action, and careful titration of drug dosages to patient response is essential. In some countries, and for complex procedures (e.g. ERCP), anaesthetist-administered deep sedation with propofol (rapid action and recovery, but narrow therapeutic window) increasingly used.
- Sedation implicated in > 50% of endoscopic complications, including aspiration, over-sedation, hypoventilation, and airway obstruction. Risks crudely correlate with pre-procedure American Society of Anesthesiology (ASA) score (see box), and involvement of senior endoscopist ± anaesthetist essential in patients with ASA >3.
- Management of hypoxaemia/hypoventilation includes protection of airway (including 'jaw thrust'), administration of reversal agent (flumazenil 250–500 µg IV for benzodiazepines, naloxone 400 µg IV/IM for opiates), continued supplemental oxygen (via mask), and emergency mechanical ventilation as necessary. Jaw thrust and flumazenil sufficient in most cases, and addition of naloxone rarely needed, when combination of benzodiazepine and opiate have been used.
- Important that 'day case' patient warned before sedation that they must not drive, operate heavy or dangerous machinery, or sign any legally binding documents for rest of the day, and that they will require an escort home.
- General anaesthesia for endoscopy generally reserved for situations where cooperation is difficult (e.g. children), or where airway protection with endotracheal tube is important (see comments on variceal bleeding in Acute upper GI bleeding).

American Society of Anesthesiologists (ASA) status

Class 1 Patient has no organic, physiological, biochemical, or psychiatric disturbance. Condition for which procedure is to be performed is localized, with no systemic disturbance

Class 2 Mild to moderate systemic disturbance caused either by the condition to be treated, or by other pathological processes

Class 3 Severe systemic disturbance or disease from whatever cause, even though it may not be possible to define the degree of disability with finality

Class 4 Severe systemic disorders that are already life-threatening, not always correctable by intervention

Class 5 The moribund patient who has little chance of survival but is submitted to intervention/operation in desperation

Sengstaken–Blakemore tube (SBT)

Background

- Bleeding from gastro-oesophageal (GO) varices is primarily controlled by endoscopic and pharmacological therapy (see acute variceal bleeding in emergencies: <u>Acute upper GI bleeding</u> and <u>portal hypertension</u>). If these approaches are ineffective/unavailable, mechanical compression of varices at GO junction should be instituted.
- SBT insertion is one of the most effective emergency interventions in gastroenterology—**done right it saves, done wrong it may hasten the patient's demise.**

Technique

- Essential to be fully prepared before attempting SBT insertion:
    - ITU/HDU setting.
    - Enrol senior nursing/medical staff if available.
    - Anaesthetist in attendance, with very low threshold for endotracheal intubation and ventilation prior to insertion (in view of risk of aspiration, difficult insertion, bitten fingers).
- Mouthpiece in, lubricant jelly on SBT. Double glove (especially if any risk of <u>hepatitis C</u>). Left forefinger between mouthpiece and side of mouth, to guide tube. Slow, steady insertion, to limit of tube.
- Inflate gastric balloon to 250 ml with air, using 50 ml bladder syringe and then seal balloon port with 2 clamps. This should not elicit distress (if it does, this may suggest gastric balloon in oesophagus—risk of <u>oesophageal rupture</u>).
- Slow traction on tube, expecting resistance at about 35 cm from teeth.
- Secure tube to side of mouth, under light tension. To do this first release mouthpiece and leave on tube near ports. Then, maintaining traction, place 2 wooden tongue depressors either side of the tube at the mouth (at 90° to the line of the tube). Use Elastoplast to secure them firmly together and around tube. Place a piece of gauze between tongue depressors and side of mouth, to prevent trauma. Mark tube to detect slippage.
- Secure tube to side of mouth, under light tension. Mark tube to detect slippage. Never secure tube with bag hanging over end of bed.
- Check CXR (see gastric balloon in stomach, with 'nipple effect' due to slight traction into distal oesophagus).
- Aspirate oesophageal port quarter-hourly, gastric port half-hourly.
- Aim to deflate and remove SBT < 18 hours and rescope/watch response.

Lack of control of bleeding

- May be due to:
    - Ineffectively deployed SBT + gastric balloon. Attempt repositioning.
    - Varices feeding into mid-oesophagus (i.e. not controlled by pressure at GO junction). This may be treated by inflating oesophageal balloon.
    - Gastric or ectopic varices.
- Contact liver centre and consider emergency <u>TIPSS</u>.

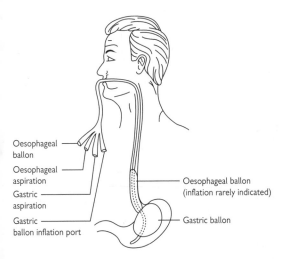

Oesophageal ballon

Oesophageal aspiration

Gastric aspiration

Gastric ballon inflation port

Oesophageal ballon (inflation rarely indicated)

Gastric ballon

Fig. 2.27 Sengstaken–Blakemore tube in place

Practice point
Forget the fridge!
The time honoured advice for insertion of SBT is to put tube in fridge beforehand. Even in the non-intubated patient this apparently ensures that the cool, stiffened tube gently glides into position without difficulty. Great, except that it doesn't work. By the time the tube has been in your warm, sweaty hands for 10 seconds, all stiffness has been lost. Safe, effective SBT insertion is achieved by having patient intubated beforehand. To aid insertion further, this author advises insertion of an 0.035 inch 'Tiger'/'JAG' wire down gastric aspiration port, with assistant ensuring that the wire tip does not pass out of tube through side holes at tip of SBT (so avoiding wire-related trauma). With wire in place tube insertion is easier, and it is virtually impossible for the tube to fold over in the oesophagus (which may result in oesophageal rupture if gastric balloon then inflated). The wire is removed after tube in place.

Seton suture

A seton is a suture, wire, or tubing that is used in the surgical management of anorectal fistulae (e.g. in perianal Crohn's disease). It is threaded though the fistulous tract, and secured outside the anus usually with a knot. It can be left loose to allow for drainage and subsidence of local infection, or tied tightly to slowly cut through the muscle—in theory maintaining muscle fibre alignment, allowing healing, and preventing abscess formation.

Shigella

An important cause of bacterial dysentery and food poisoning. The organism attacks the colon and terminal ileum; invasion beyond the intestinal mucosa and bacteraemia are rare. 4 subgroups: *S. dysenteriae,* (most severe) *S. flexneri, S. boydii, S. sonnei* (mildest).

Clinical features include lower abdominal pain, rectal discomfort, and diarrhoea (may be bloody). Fever present in 40%. Complications include intestinal perforation and arthritis (usually HLA-B27-associated—see Reiter's syndrome). Infection tends to be milder in children (1–3 days) than adults (approximately 7 days).

Diagnosis. Send stool for culture and sensitivity. Sigmoidoscopy shows a colitis and rectal biopsy may help in suggesting an infective cause rather than ulcerative colitis.

Treatment. Avoid opiate analgesics. Antibiotics are often not needed but are reasonable treatment if the diarrhoea is persisting by the time of positive stool cultures. Ampicillin and co-trimoxazole are most used but resistance has increased recently. Quinolone (e.g. CIPROFLOXACIN) resistance is < 1%.

Short bowel syndrome

- A malabsorption syndrome resulting from extensive intestinal resection. Major causes in adults are <u>Crohn's disease</u>, mesenteric infarction, and <u>radiation</u> injury. Degree of malabsorption is related to remaining length of small and large bowel. Nutrient absorptive capacity is higher in proximal small intestine than distal small bowel: intestinal failure can be avoided if there is 100 cm of jejunum with no colon or if there is 50 cm of jejunum with colon in continuity.
- **Water and electrolyte malabsorption.** Net sodium and fluid balance is related to jejunal length. Patients with <100 cm jejunum are often net secretors, while those with >100 cm are net absorbers. In these patients use of <u>oral rehydration solutions</u> can decrease stoma output and convert some patients from net secretors to net absorbers: sodium concentration should be in the range 90–120 mM. Importantly, sport drinks and commercially made liquid formula feeds contain too little sodium for maximal fluid absorption in patients with short bowel and a jejunostomy.
- **Site-specific transport processes.** Calcium and magnesium are absorbed in the duodenum and proximal jejunum but the malabsorption is potentiated by fat malabsorption because the mineral are precipitated intraluminally by long chain fatty acids. Ileal resection of more than 50 cm frequently impairs vitamin B12 absorption and resection of more than 100 cm cause bile acid malabsorption.

Short chain fatty acids (SCFA)

Contain 1–6 carbon atoms (acetate, proprionate, butyrate). Produced in the colon by bacterial fermentation of undigested carbohydrate (about 25 g/day: 90% can be metabolized to SCFA and absorbed). An important source of fuel for colonic mucosa; so reduced fibre intake with enteral feeding or diversion of faecal stream in ileostomy or colostomy can result in mucosal atrophy or <u>diversion colitis</u>.

Complications of short bowel

- **Cholesterol <u>gallstones</u>**. Reduced hepatic bile acid secretion leads to cholesterol supersaturation
- <u>**Oxalate kidney stones**</u>.
- **D-lactic acidosis.** If the colon is *in situ*, carbohydrate overfeeding can result in excess short chain fatty acids. This lowers colonic pH which promotes Gram-positive anaerobes that produce D-lactate. Humans lack D-lactate dehydrogenase. Absorbed D-lactate may produce nystagmus, ataxia, and confusion. Patients look drunk but blood alcohol is normal: D-lactate levels are high (>3 mM/l)

Sickle cell anaemia (SCA)

May be linked with a range of GI problems, due to the effects of haemolysis and ischaemia, or the consequences of recurrent transfusion.

Clinical features

- Chronic asymptomatic jaundice in SCA may relate to haemolysis and intrahepatic cholestasis.
- Acute abdominal pain due to range of causes (see box).
- Sickling or sequestration within liver presents with severe right upper quadrant pain, tender hepatomegaly, jaundice.
- Splenomegaly may occur due to sequestration or portal hypertension, but splenic infarction and hyposplenism usually develop by adulthood.
- Gallstones in > 30% of adults, with increased rates of cholecystitis, choledocholithiasis, and acute pancreatitis.
- Hepatitis B , hepatitis C, and HIV at increased frequency.
- Secondary haemochromatosis may result from recurrent transfusion.

Investigations

Diagnosis of SCA usually established in childhood. Specific investigations depend on clinical presentation. In those with jaundice, general rules apply (see Approach to recent-onset jaundice).

- FBC. Typical Hb 6–8 g/dl, reticulocytes 10–20%. Sickling test detects HbS. Marked ↓ Hb with abdominal pain may suggest sequestration crisis.
- LFTs. Bilirubin may be massively ↑ (> 600 µg/l); AST/ALT usually <1000 U/l) unless hepatic ischaemia/infarction or acute hepatitis.
- U/S or CT useful to exclude biliary obstruction, hepatic infarction, or vascular occlusion (e.g. Budd–Chiari syndrome, portal vein thrombosis).
- Iron studies (e.g. serum ferritin) may suggest overload (see haemochromatosis).
- Liver biopsy rarely necessary, but may show sinusoidal dilatation and sickling and/or fibrosis with cirrhosis.

Management

- Seek expert haematology input.
- Acute sickling crisis or sequestration treated with exchange transfusion (with aim to reduce HbS to < 30%), IV fluids, and adequate pain control (usually OPIATES). Keep warm, well oxygenated, and treat precipitant to crisis (e.g. infection).
- Specific management depends on diagnosis (e.g. see hepatitis B, hepatitis C, haemochromatosis, gallstones, choledocholithiasis).

Causes of acute abdominal pain in sickle cell anaemia

- Hepatic sickling/sequestration
- Splenic sickling/sequestration
- <u>Cholecystitis</u>
- <u>Acute pancreatitis</u>
- Renal vein thrombosis
- <u>Budd–Chiari syndrome</u>
- Hepatic artery thrombosis/hepatic infarction
- <u>Portal vein thrombosis</u>
- <u>Mesenteric ischaemia</u>/infarction

Sjögren's/sicca syndrome

Lymphocytic infiltration of salivary glands causes keratoconjunctivitis and dry mouth. Dysphagia occurs in 75%: mostly due to oesophageal dysmotility but there is also an increased incidence of <u>oesophageal rings</u>/webs. Chronic atrophic gastritis can occur, as can <u>acute</u> and <u>chronic pancreatitis</u> (perhaps as association with <u>autoimmune pancreatitis</u>); exocrine pancreatic secretion is often impaired. <u>Primary biliary cirrhosis</u> is more common in patients with Sjögren's.

Slimming diets

Increase in obesity in Western societies has been paralleled by range of slimming diets (also see <u>Approach to obesity</u> and <u>obesity surgery</u>). Traditional dietary advice centres on low calorie intake (800–1500 kcal/day) with 30–35% energy from fat, 50% from carbohydrate, and 10–15% from protein, although these figures are still debated.

- **Low fat/high carbohydrate diets** (< 30% energy from fat). Reducing dietary fat is an effective way of losing weight but the relative effectiveness of an unrestricted low fat/high carbohydrate diet compared with low fat/energy restricted diets is unknown. Low fat diets and modification of fatty acid composition reduce risk of type 2 diabetes and coronary heart disease.
- **Fixed energy deficit diets** involve a dietician individually calculating energy requirements based on basal metabolic rates and adjusting for physical activity. A diet providing an energy deficit of approximately 600 kcal/day will induce weight loss of about 0.5 kg/week.
- **Meal replacement** involves controlled portion products (shakes, bars, soups, pastas) replacing two meals per day (and snacks) while allowing one regular meal of 'healthy' foods. Calorie intake is about 1200–1600 kcal/day and there is support of efficacy in meta-analysis. Efficacy in real life, where meal replacement products need to be purchased, is lacking.
- **Very low calorie diets** provide 450–800 kcal/day and use formula foods to replace all meals and snacks. They induce rapid weight loss, but no evidence of long-term efficacy. <u>Gallstones</u> are an important complication of weight loss faster than 1–2 kg/week.
- **Low glycaemic index (GI) foods**. Low GI foods (wholegrain cereals, fruit, legumes) are more slowly absorbed than foods such as glucose or white bread and have a less acute effect on postprandial glucose and insulin levels, which has been proposed to reduce hunger and increase satiety. Some evidence suggests that low GI foods raise HDL cholesterol, suppress triglycerides, and decrease insulin resistance: they have a role as part of a conventional energy restricted diet.

- **High protein low carbohydrate diets** (e.g. Atkins) are popular (as of 2004) but possibly unhealthy. Severe carbohydrate restriction leads to dietary composition of 25% protein, 5% carbohydrates, and 70% fat: sharply contrasting with most dietary recommendations. Carbohydrate restriction leads to hepatic glycogenolysis and ketosis. This induces mild euphoria and loss of body water (which accounts for much of the weight loss). Evidence for long-term efficacy is lacking. The British Dietetic Association (www.bda.com) has issued warnings about adoption of long-term diets of this type.

Solitary rectal ulcer syndrome

Rare (incidence 1:100 000, equal in men and women, can be seen in all age groups) but also frequently misdiagnosed. The cardinal feature is isolated erythema or ulceration of part of the rectum, usually the anterior wall.

Clinical features

- Passage of blood and mucus PR with straining and a feeling of incomplete evacuation.
- Evidence of rectal prolapse.
- **Sigmoidoscopic appearances** are classically a single ulcer on the anterior rectal wall at 5–10 cm from the anal verge but a polypoid lesion may be seen in 25% or an isolated patch of hyperaemia in 20% (see Colour Plate 25).
- Histology shows distortion of glands with oedema and fibrosis of the lamina propria. The muscularis mucosae is thickened and muscle fibres extend up between the crypts.

Pathogenesis

Prolapse of rectal mucosa (possibly occurring internally and therefore not visible or palpable) and paradoxical contraction of the pelvic floor are thought to be important, possibly leading to ischaemia of the mucosa. Direct trauma due to rectal digitations has been implicated but many of the lesions are above the reach of a finger.

Investigations

Symptoms, sigmoidoscopic appearances, and histology are the most important. Endo-anal ultrasound may show thickening of the internal sphincter, and <u>defecography studies</u> may show abnormal patterns of defecation. Barium studies and anorectal physiology are not helpful.

Treatment

Topical treatments do not help. Dietary supplementation with fibre is disappointing, especially if there is associated rectal prolapse. <u>Biofeedback</u> may help those with paradoxical puborectalis contraction. Surgical options include rectopexy and resection of the prolapsing muscosa: rectopexy helps about 50% but increases symptoms in some. Surgery has a minor role and should be reserved for those with intractable symptoms and good evidence of prolapse.

Sphincter of Oddi dysfunction (SOD)

Definition + clinical features

Hypertension of biliary/pancreatic sphincter may cause episodic pancreatico-biliary-type pain, and biliary SOD is categorized into 3 clinical groups:

- **Type I:** biliary pain, plus <u>liver function tests</u> (LFTs) > ×2 ULN on > 1 occasion, and dilated common bile duct.
- **Type II:** biliary pain, and one of the above.
- **Type III:** biliary pain only.

Investigation

- Dilated CBD may be seen on U/S, CT, or MRCP (CBD normally < 7 mm in diameter, but may be slightly wider (up to approximately 9 mm) post-<u>cholecystectomy</u> and in extreme elderly, in the absence of other pathology.
- LFTs may be elevated during attacks of pain.
- Sphincter of Oddi manometry (SOM) at <u>ERCP</u> is the 'gold standard' investigation. Baseline sphincter pressure > 40 mmHg, or sustained peaks > 100 mmHg are consistent with the diagnosis, but the technique is technically difficult.
- <u>Hepatobiliary scintigraphy</u> (e.g. HIDA scan) may show delayed biliary emptying.

Management

- Definitive treatment for proven SOD is biliary (± pancreatic) sphincterotomy, but risks of <u>ERCP</u>-related complications are particularly high in this patient group (up to 20% <u>acute pancreatitis</u>). Safety of procedure, probability of abnormal SOM, and response to sphincterotomy are lowest for type III SOD. <u>Pancreatic stent</u> insertion may lower risks of procedure.
- Before ERCP/SOM, many physicians would try empirical medical therapy for SOD II/III (e.g. antispasmodics/tricyclic antidepressants), and consider <u>cholecystectomy</u> if any evidence of <u>gallstones</u>/sludge on transabdominal or <u>endoscopic ultrasound</u> (passage of microcalculi may mimic SOD).

SOD type	Frequency of abnormal manometry (%)	Benefit of sphincterotomy based on manometry findings (%)	
		Abnormal	Normal
I	75–95	90–95	90–95
II	55–65	85	35
III	25–60	55–65	<10

Spontaneous bacterial peritonitis (SBP)

Background

- SBP is present in 10–30% of hospitalized cirrhotic patients with ascites.
- Increased risk related to gastrointestinal bleeding, ascitic protein: <10 g/l, advanced liver disease, and previous episodes.
- Bacterial translocation, bacteraemia, and impaired antimicrobial activity of ascitic fluid contributes to its development. Gram-negative bacilli (especially *Escherichia coli*) cause 80% of infections.

Clinical features

Majority present with fever, systemic signs of sepsis, but few abdominal features. Abdominal pain and rebound tenderness occur in minority. Asymptomatic in 10%. Liver decompensation, with worsening hepatic encephalopathy, and renal failure are important associations.

Investigation

Diagnostic ascitic tap mandatory in all patients admitted to hospital with ascites, because of high rate of SBP (see Approach to ascites).

- Ascitic white count: WCC > 500 cells/μl, neutrophils > 250 /μl strongly suggestive of SBP, unless intra-abdominal source of infection.
- Ascitic protein: < 10 g/l merits antibiotic prophylaxis.
- Microscopy and culture: 5–10 ml of fluid should be inoculated into blood culture bottles with media for aerobes and anaerobes (not just into specimen bottles). Despite this, 20–40% of presumed SBP (i.e. ↑WCC) are culture negative. Isolation of multiple organisms raises possibility of contamination or intra-abdominal source (e.g. diverticular perforation).

Management

- Treat on finding ascitic neutrophils > 250 cells/μl, without waiting for microbiological confirmation. Give 3rd generation CEPHALOSPORIN (e.g. cefotaxime 2 g bd IV). In non-severely ill, oral quinolones (e.g. ofloxacin 400 mg bd, CIPROFLOXACIN 500 mg bd) may be considered (see index of drugs).
- Continue antibiotic until clinical sepsis resolved, and ascitic neutrophils < 250 cells/μl.
- Routine infusion of human albumin (1.5 g/kg at time of diagnosis) advised by some (may ameliorate renal failure), but controversial (see albumin (use in liver disease)).
- Resolution of infection in 75–90%, but hospital mortality remains at 20–40% (predicted by degree of renal failure (also see hepatorenal syndrome), and largely due to hepatic decompensation).
- Antibiotic prophylaxis with a quinolone (e.g. norfloxacin 400 mg od PO, ciprofloxacin 750 mg/week PO) reduces risk of SBP over next year from 70% to 20%.
- Episode of SBP predicts 50% 2 year mortality. Its occurrence requires consideration of suitability for liver transplantation.

Steatorrhoea

See: <u>Approach to malabsorption and steatorrhoea</u>.

Still's disease

The adult form of rheumatoid arthritis often has GI manifestations such as weight loss (75%), sore throat, hepatomegaly (45%), abnormal liver blood tests (75%), and abdominal pain (50%). Liver failure can be associated with aspirin or NSAID therapy.

Stool microscopy

A very useful test to establish an inflammatory cause of diarrhoea. Invasive pathogens such as *Shigella* and *Campylobacter* produce many polymorphs and red blood cells. Toxigenic organisms, viruses, and food poisoning bacteria produce a watery stool containing few formed elements. An acute exacerbation of <u>ulcerative colitis</u> can also produce leucocytes and erythrocytes in the stool, giving appearances that resemble bacillary dysentery.

Strongyloides

Strongyloides stercoralis is one of the most important intestinal nematode infections. Endemic in tropical areas, but may persist for decades following exposure, due to autoinfection. Adult worms (3 mm long) usually reside in duodenum/jejunum. Eggs may hatch in stool prior to defecation, and larvae may then penetrate bowel wall, circulate to lung, and mature into more adults. See <u>roundworms</u>.

Clinical features
- Local rash (cutaneous larva migrans) due to skin penetration by larvae.
- Chronic intestinal infection may be asymptomatic, or associated with abdominal discomfort, bloating, bulky loose stools linked to small bowel infection (i.e. similar to <u>giardiasis</u>).
- Heavy infestation (e.g. associated with immunosuppression) may cause asthma, pulmonary haemorrhage, profuse diarrhoea, bowel wall thickening, and fatal Gram-negative sepsis.

Investigations
- FBC: eosinophilia in 50%.
- Stool microscopy may show larvae or eggs (but only 25% sensitivity, and always negative in early infection).
- Serological test using ELISA available.
- Endoscopy: subtotal villous atrophy, lymphocytic infiltrate, eggs, and larvae in submucosa may be seen on low duodenal histology.

Management
Ivermectin 150 µg/kg PO × 1 dose, or thiabendazole 50 mg/kg/day for 2 days (extended to 10 days if hyperinfection) are effective.

Superior mesenteric artery syndrome

Rare but real condition (3 cases seen by a very youthful author). The superior mesenteric artery comes off the aorta at a right angle and crosses over the duodenum just to the right of the midline. Rarely, the artery may obstruct the duodenum as it crosses over: an acute angle between the SMA and aorta might be relevant, and it only seems to happen in very thin patients.

Symptoms include epigastric fullness and bloating after meals and bilious vomiting. Barium or CT may reveal a dilated stomach and duodenum with a sharp cutoff to the right of the midline (don't forget other causes of duodenal dilatation: scleroderma, diabetes, distal duodenal stricture).

Treatment is by decompression, possibly surgical—most commonly duodeno-jejunostomy.

Systemic lupus erythematosis (SLE) and the GI tract

Clinical features

- Anorexia, nausea, and vomiting occur in 50% but may be due to disease or treatment. Mouth ulcers are common and usually painless. Sjögren's syndrome and dry mouth occur in 20%.
- Oesophageal symptoms are common, but do not correlate well with results of oesophageal manometry. In contrast to scleroderma, lower oesophageal sphincter is rarely involved.
- Risk of peptic ulceration is increased by combined NSAID and steroid use. PPIs are indicated for gastroprotection.
- Most dangerous manifestation of intestinal involvement is vasculitis (2% prevalence, mortality 50%: commonest in territory of superior mesenteric artery, though classically small vessels are involved), which can progress to ulceration, haemorrhage, perforation, and infarction. Although rare overall in SLE, an acute abdominal presentation may often reflect vasculitis, especially if there active disease elsewhere. A smaller proportion of acute abdominal presentations are caused by intra-abdominal thrombosis, either secondary to vasculitis or to anti-phospholipid syndrome (see portal vein thrombosis). There is an increased incidence of inflammatory bowel disease in patients with SLE, most often ulcerative colitis. Protein-losing enteropathy and fat malabsorption can also occur.

Investigation. Look for thumbprinting on a plain X-ray which suggests ischaemic bowel. Check inflammatory markers. A CT can show abscesses, lymphadenopathy, serositis, bowel wall thickening, pancreatic pathology, and hepato-splenomegaly. Visceral angiography usually does not help but colonoscopy with biopsy can diagnose vasculitis.

Management. Treatment of vasculitis with IV pulsed steroids can be effective, but vital to exclude infection (e.g. with stool and blood cultures) beforehand.

Systemic mastocytosis

Results from excessive histamine and prostacyclin release from inappropriate mast cell proliferation in skin, bones, lymph nodes. The classic skin sign is multiple red-brown papules or urticaria pigmentosa. 80% have GI symptoms of nausea, vomiting, diarrhoea, or abdominal pain. May present with steatorrhoea (see Approach to malabsorption and steatorrhoea). Symptoms are often bought on by alcohol. There may be hepatomegaly and portal hypertension. Diagnosis is by measuring urinary histamine levels.

T

Tapeworms (cestodes)

Fish tapeworm. *Diphyllobothrium latum* is acquired by people eating raw or undercooked fresh water fish. Disease is endemic in northern Europe, Russia, and Alaska. Worm is not invasive and causes no direct symptoms. It absorbs nutrients through its surface including <u>cobalamin</u> and can cause vitamin B12 deficiency. Diagnosis made by finding eggs in stool. Treatment with praziquantel (single dose, 10 mg/kg) or albendazole 400 mg/day for 3 days.

Beef and pork tapeworms. Colonization occurs by eating raw or undercooked meat infested with cysticerci of *Taenia saginata* or *T. solium*. 50 million people are affected in areas where livestock are exposed to untreated human waste and humans eat raw or undercooked meat. Most people are asymptomatic. Most feared complication is cysticercosis, which occurs when people consume *T. solium* eggs. These release oncospheres that penetrate the intestinal wall and produce inflammation in the brain, spinal cord, eye, and heart. Diagnosis is by finding eggs or proglottids in stool. Treatment is with praziquantel (single dose, 10 mg/kg) or albendazole 400 mg/d for 3 days.

Other tapeworms. The commonest tapeworm affecting humans is the dwarf tapeworm or *Hymenolepis nana*, which can be transmitted from person to person without an intermediate host.

Telangiectasia

See: <u>hereditary haemorrhagic telangiectasia (Osler–Weber–Rendu syndrome)</u>.

TIPSS (transjugular intrahepatic portosystemic shunt)

Technique
- Involves formation of artificial track between portal vein and hepatic vein, through liver, using radiologically placed mesh metal stent (see figure).
- Used in treatment of complications of <u>portal hypertension</u>, and aims to reduce hepatic venous pressure gradient (HVPG) to < 12 mmHg.
- Procedure usually performed in specialist liver units. Stent insertion does not preclude <u>liver transplantation</u>, provided not sited too far down portal vein.

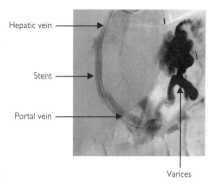

Hepatic vein ⟶

Stent ⟶

Portal vein ⟶

Varices

Fig. 2.28 Transjugular intrahepatic portosystemic shunt (TIPPS).

Indications

- Uncontrolled acute variceal bleeding (see : Acute upper GI bleeding), where drug/endoscopic therapy has failed, is main indication for TIPSS. Sengstaken–Blakemore tube may be inserted prior to TIPSS. Especially useful for gastric and ectopic (e.g. rectal) varices.
- Secondary prevention of recurrent variceal bleeding (but only where medical/endoscopic prophylaxis has failed).
- Refractory ascites (see Approach to ascites). Reduces need for large volume paracentesis , but no comparative reduction in mortality, and increases risk of hepatic encephalopathy.
- Efficacy of TIPSS reported in Budd–Chiari syndrome, type 2 hepatorenal syndrome, and portal hypertensive gastropathy, but few controlled studies.

Contraindications

- Intrahepatic lesions (e.g. cysts, tumours).
- Vascular obstruction (complete hepatic or portal vein thrombosis).
- Cardiopulmonary disease (severe pulmonary hypertension, congestive cardiac failure).
- Severe bleeding risk (INR > 1.5, platelets < 20×10^6/l—but consider in clinical context).
- Biliary obstruction (risk of biliary puncture/fistula).

Complications

- TIPSS blockage. Early thrombosis in 10–15%, but dysfunction in 80% by 1 year (thrombosis or intimal hyperplasia). Covered stents may reduce TIPSS dysfunction. Blockage clinically suggested by further portal hypertensive complications. Doppler U/S within 1 week of insertion, and formal venography at 1 year suggested to exclude occlusion.
- New/worsened hepatic encephalopathy in 10–44% limits use of TIPSS (particularly in Child–Pugh C disease). May necessitate stent occlusion.
- Direct procedure-related complications (e.g. haemobilia, intraperitoneal bleed, hepatic infarction, arteriovenous fistulae, sepsis) in <15%, but major complication in < 3%.
- Haemolysis in 10–15%, due to flow through shunt, but usually resolves in < 4 weeks.

TNM classification

See: tumour staging.

Toxic megacolon

- Defined as a transverse colonic diameter of > 6 cm with loss of haustration in a patient with colitis. It occurs in about 5% of cases of severe attacks and can be triggered by opiates or hypokalaemia.
- Feared complication of fulminant inflammatory bowel disease that can also complicate infectious colitis (e.g. *Campylobacter, Shigella*) and acute distal obstruction (e.g. volvulus). Can occur in patients without obvious colonic disease or mechanical obstruction (see Ogilvie's syndrome).

Treatment. If dilatation occurs during treatment of an acute attack of colitis surgery is indicated. If the dilatation is present when the patient is first seen, medical treatment with IV fluids and steroids can be tried. Many clinicians try and decompress the colon with a colonic tube: air accumulates in the transverse colon because it is the most anterior portion of the colon, and rolling of the patient into a prone position for 15 min every 2 h is also advocated. 50% respond with therapy: urgent colectomy is required for those who do not improve after 24–72 h of medical therapy.

TPMT (thiopurine methyltransferase)

Plays a key role in metabolic pathway of AZATHIOPRINE/6 mercaptopurine (6-MP; see index of drugs). Variations in TPMT (largely determined genetically) allow for shunting of 6-MP into 6-methylmercaptopurine when levels are normal or high. Patients homozygous for a recessive mutation resulting in inactivation of TPMT (1 in 300 people) produce very high levels of 6 thioguanine nucleotides that make them unlikely to tolerate thiopurines at all (with high risk of side effects, such as significant neutropenia). People heterozygous for the TPMT mutation (10% of people) require lower doses of thiopurines. Normal range 25–55 nmol/g Hb/h.

TPN

See: parenteral nutrition.

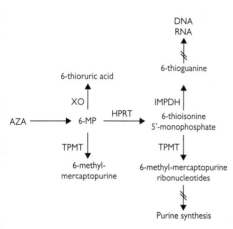

Fig. 2.29 Metabolism of <u>AZATHIOPRINE</u>/6-MP. Azathioprine is converted to 6-MP nonenzymatically. AZA, azathioprine; 6-MP, 6-mercaptopurine; XO, xanthine oxidase; HPRT, hypoxanthine phosphoribosyltransferase; TPMT, thiopurine methyltransferase; IMPDH, inosine monophosphate dehydrogenase.

Tracheo-oesophageal fistula (TOF)

Background
- Congenital causes.
  - Commonly trachea communicates with abnormal, atretic, distal oesophagus (due to failure of lung bud to separate from foregut).
- Acquired causes.
  - Tumour invasion (e.g. bronchial or <u>oesophageal tumour</u>).
  - Instrumentation (e.g. <u>endoscopic dilatation</u> or ablation of malignant stricture).

Clinical features
- Congenital TOF usually presents in infancy with regurgitation and aspiration of feed (due to associated atresia as well as TOF).
- In adulthood TOF presents with features of <u>oesophageal rupture</u>, recurrent pneumonia, and systemic sepsis.

Investigation
- In congenital TOF diagnosis often confirmed by failure to pass NG tube into the stomach ± injection of 1 ml of barium down tube.
- CXR may show air-filled upper oesophagus ± air–fluid level.

In adulthood, CT may show fistula, with diagnosis confirmed using oral non-ionic contrast, if necessary.

Management
- Congenital TOF treated surgically with resection of oesophageal atresia and TOF, with end-to-end anastomosis, or interposition of colon, dependent on length of defect. Surgery 90% successful, but patients may develop significant reflux and oesophageal motility problems in adulthood.
- Endoscopically placed covered metal stents may be effective in sealing the defect in > 70% of cases of TOFs related to oesophageal cancers.

Traveller's diarrhoea

See: <u>Approach to acute diarrhoea</u>

Trematodes

See: flukes (flatworms, trematodes).

Tropical sprue

Initially described by Hilary in 1759 who wrote observations of chronic diarrhoea in Barbados. Characterized by chronic diarrhoea and malabsorption in residents or visitors to the tropics. Recently redefined as **malabsorption of at least two different substances in people in the tropics when other causes have been excluded.**

Epidemiology

Restricted to Southern and South-east Asia, the Caribbean, and Central South America. Usually occurs in long-term visitors or residents of over 6 months but epidemics have occurred in India and Burma. The prevalence may be decreasing due to increasing self-medication with antibiotics.

Clinical features

Chronic diarrhoea with steatorrhoea, anorexia, cramps, and bloating. There may be lactose intolerance, vitamin B12 or vitamin A deficiency, hypocalcaemia, anaemia, stomatitis, glossitis, and oedema.

Pathological features

Includes atrophic gastritis (although this may relate to co-infection with *Helicobacter*) and mild changes in colonic epithelial cells, but the major changes are in the small intestine. There is reduced disaccharidase activity and reduced fat absorption: the latter may account in part for altered transit time through the small bowel. Aetiology still uncertain but likely to involve chronic infection with enteropathogens.

Diagnosis

Requires demonstration of partial villous atrophy, exclusion of specific cause of diarrhoea and malabsorption, and presence of fat and B12 malabsorption.
- Search carefully for intestinal pathogens; three stool specimens for microscopy, with particular attention to looking for microsporidia and *Isospora* in the immunocompromised. Faecal microscopy is insensitive for *Giardia* and *Stronglyoides*.
- Duodenal biopsy or serological ELISAs may be helpful to diagnose giardiasis and *Stronglyoides*.
- Coeliac serology is important to exclude gluten-sensitive enteropathy.
- Contrast examination or capsule endoscopy of the small bowel may be needed to exclude lymphoma.

Treatment

'Simple' general measures (restoring water and electrolytes, replacing nutritional deficiencies of iron, folate, B12) have reduced mortality of epidemic tropical sprue. The use of antibiotics is controversial, but overland travellers improve on tetracycline 250 mg qds, usually given for several months.

Prognosis is good, particularly in expatriates returning from the tropics. There is some evidence of recurrence in indigenous populations of the tropics.

Trypanosomiasis

Trypanosoma cruzi is endemic in central Brazil, Venezuela, and Argentina, and spread between humans by the reduviid bugs of the *Triatominae* group. The name reduviid comes from the Latin reduvia, meaning hang-nail, and relates to the curved, powerful beaks adapted to suck blood from mammals. The bugs defecate when biting and the parasite is introduced when the bite is scratched. Chronic disease results from widespread destruction of autonomic ganglion cells in the heart, gut, respiratory tract, and urinary tract. It is thought that autoimmune damage occurs to cardiac or nerve epitopes cross-reacting with *T. cruzi* antigens. Resulting cardiac arrhythmias can be fatal. GI involvement can produce megaduodenum or megacolon as well as megaoesophagus, which helps to distinguish the disease from idiopathic achalasia. Small bowel dilatation and lack of peristalsis can also be found.

Diagnosis can be made by demonstration of trypanosome forms on blood smears but is more usually made by a serological complement fixation test.

Treatment of the infection uses the drugs nifurtimox and benznidazole; treatment of the achalasia syndrome in Chagas' disease is similar to that of idiopathic achalasia.

Tuberculosis and the GI tract

Historically related to the severity of pulmonary involvement, especially pulmonary cavitation and positive sputum smears (increased risk of swallowed organisms). In modern series, chest X-ray is unremarkable in most patients seen with intestinal TB.

Location and pathology. Can affect any part of the GI tract, including gut lumen, liver (see <u>hepatic granulomas</u>), and pancreas (mass may mimic pancreatitis or tumour). Ileocaecal area and jejunum are the commonest sites affected. Incompetence of the ileocaecal valve (due to disease on either side), said to distinguish TB from <u>Crohn's disease</u>. Key pathological features are thickening of the bowel wall, transmural granulomas (caseation is often seen in regional lymph nodes but not always in mucosal granulomas), mesenteric lymphadenopathy, serosal tubercles easily visible on laparotomy or laparoscopy but not (currently, in 2005) on <u>CT scanning</u>.

Clinical features. Abdominal pain in 90%. Weight loss, fever, altered bowel habit can occur. Two-thirds have a mass in the right iliac fossa. Intestinal obstruction is commoner than perforation.

Diagnosis. Often delayed and difficult. Acid-fast bacilli are seen in a minority of cases: the organism can be cultured from infected tissues but takes 6–12 weeks: PCR can help. A positive tuberculin skin test does not always mean active disease and where the immune response is impaired (old people, those with substantial weight loss/malabsorption, HIV positive) skin testing can be negative in active disease. Laparoscopy can be useful in allowing biopsy of serosal nodules. Differential diagnosis includes <u>Crohn's disease</u>, *Yersinia* infection, caecal involvement with cancer or <u>amoebiasis</u>. Syphilis and lymphogranuloma vernereum are quoted but now vanishingly rare.

Treatment. No controlled studies but 3 drug regimen for 12/12 recommended.

Tumour staging

TNM classification widely applied to staging of solid tumours (e.g. <u>colorectal</u> (but also see <u>Dukes classification</u>), <u>oesophageal</u>, <u>gastric</u>, <u>pancreatic cancer</u>), as is of prognostic value and guides management.

T—Primary tumour

T0   No evidence of primary
Tis Carcinoma *in situ*
T1   Invasion of lamina propria or submucosa
T2   Invasion of muscularis propria
T3   Invasion of adventitia
T4   Invasion of adjacent structures

N—Regional lymph nodes

N0   No regional nodal metastases
N1   Regional nodal metastases

M—Distant metastases

MX   Cannot be assessed
M0   No distant metastases
M1   Distant metastases

Tumour staging (TNM classification)

Stage	T	N	M
0	Tis	N0	M0
IA	T1	N0	M0
IIA	T2,T3	N0	M0
IIB	T1, T2	N1	M0
III	T3	N1	M0
	T4	Any N	M0
IV	Any T	Any N	M1

Turcot's syndrome

A syndrome of familial colonic polyposis with primary tumours of the CNS. The commonest group has a germline mutation, and the CNS tumours tend to be medulloblastomas. The second group has germline mutatons in mismatch repair genes typical of HNPCC and is associated with glioblastoma multiforme.

Tylosis

- Autosomal dominant disease characterized by hyperkeratosis of palms and the soles of feet.
- Associated high incidence of oesophageal, bronchial, and laryngeal cancer, often at a younger age than usual (oesophageal cancer in > 90% of cases by 65 years—see <u>oesophageal tumours</u>).
- Endoscopic surveillance suggested from age 30 years, repeating every 3 years.

Typhlitis

Background
- From Greek 'typhlon', meaning caecum, but also known as ileocaecal syndrome and neutropenic enterocolitis.
- Occurs almost exclusively in immunocompromised patients (e.g. HIV, post-bone marrow transplant).
- Rarely diagnosed by gastroenterologists, but accounts for 10% of deaths in children with leukaemia during chemotherapy.
- Aetiology unknown, but important factors may include mucosal injury due to cytotoxics, *cytomegalovirus* or bacterial infection, and mucosal ischaemia. <u>*Pseudomonas*</u> has been implicated.

Clinical features
- Nausea, vomiting, fever.
- Generalized or right-sided abdominal pain + tenderness.
- Diarrhoea (± blood).
- Shock, due to secondary sepsis or caecal perforation.

Investigations
- Important to exclude other causes (e.g. <u>*Clostridium*</u> *difficile* toxin for pseudomembranous colitis).
- Neutrophil count almost always < 0.1 × 10^9/l.
- Abdominal X-ray may show free air (perforation) or 'thumb-printing'.
- CT scan may show caecal distension, and caecal, right colon, or terminal ileum wall thickening (> 3 mm), ± perforation.

Management
- NBM (± TPN), NG tube, and gastric decompression.
- IV fluid replacement.
- Broad spectrum antibiotics (e.g. 3rd generation <u>CEPHALOSPORIN</u> + <u>METRONIDAZOLE,</u> see index of drugs).
- Surgery necessary for perforation (and some advocate it at diagnosis in view of 40–50% mortality associated with caecal perforation, bowel necrosis, and sepsis).

U

Ulcerative colitis

First recognized as different from infectious colitis in 1859 by Samuel Wilks.

Definition. An inflammatory condition that affects the rectum and extends proximally to affect a variable amount of the colon.

Epidemiology

Found worldwide but incidence varies about 10-fold between high incidence areas (UK, USA, Northern Europe, Australia: approximate incidence 10 per 100 000 per year, approximate prevalence 100 per 100 000 population) and low incidence areas (Asia, Japan, South America). In contrast to the rising incidence of <u>Crohn's</u>, the incidence has remained steady over the last 50 years. Affects men and women equally, with peak incidence age 20–40 and a second smaller peak in older adults. Said to affect (Ashkenazi) Jews more frequently, but the lower incidence among Jews in Israel compared to the USA suggests that environmental factors play a role.

Genetics

There is a genetic component (concordance rates for identical twins are 13% and 2% for monozygotic and dizygotic twins: more than allowable by chance but less than occurs in <u>Crohn's</u>) but inheritance is not simply Mendelian: several genes may be involved in disease susceptibility. Several linkage studies suggest a susceptibility locus on chromosome 12 and other loci on 2, 3, 6, and 7 have been implicated. Other genes may influence disease behaviour independently of susceptibility.

Aetiology

Unknown; hypotheses include infection, sensitivity to food components (no evidence to support this), immune response to bacterial or self-antigens, and the role of the central nervous system ('stress') and a possible abnormality in colonic epithelial cells. Few attempt to explain the mainly left-sided nature of the disease.

- **Infection.** No specific pathogen has been identified. There may be differences in adhesions of *E. coli* from patients compared to controls and attempts at altering the luminal environment with probiotic bacteria suggest that the luminal microflora are relevant to disease pathogenesis.
- **Immunopathogenesis.** There are increased IgG1- and IgG3-secreting plasma cells. There are autoantibodies to components of epithelial cells and also to p-ANCA in 60–80% patients. Changes in T cells and intraepithelial lymphocytes are confusing and have an uncertain relevance to pathogenesis. There is strong epithelial expression of MHC class II antigens in active colitis which may relate to antigen expression to local T cells. Many of the changes in immune cell function may be secondary to increased levels of pro-inflammatory cytokines (IL-1, IL-6, interferon gamma).

Clinical features

Symptoms. Bloody diarrhoea, and mucus per rectum. Urgency of defecation is common and may give abdominal discomfort but pain is not usually a prominent symptom (although abdominal cramps may accompany severe disease). Symptoms do not always correlate with endoscopic severity of disease. Onset is classically slow and insidious but acute onset can happen and UC can be precipitated by an acute infectious colitis.

Blood and pus are usually mixed with the stool but pure blood alone may be seen in disease localized to the rectum (proctitis). Diarrhoea is common but patients with proctitis may complain of constipation or hard stools.

Systemic symptoms are common in severe attacks: there may be anorexia, vomiting, fever, and symptoms of anaemia.

Signs. Affected bowel may be tender. Bowel sounds are usually normal.

Signs of dehydration, fever, evidence of weight loss, tachycardia are evidence of a severe attack.

There may be extraintestinal manifestations of colitis (see below).

Assessing disease severity. Although there are endoscopic and histological scoring systems, the clinical criteria of Truelove and Witts (Truelove, SC and Witts, LJ (1995). *Br. Med. J.* **2**: 1041) are still used as a guide to decide on admission and intravenous therapy.

- **Mild**: less than 4 stools per day, no systemic disturbance.
- **Moderate**: 4–6 stools/day, minimal disturbance.
- **Severe**: over 6 stools per day, with blood and systemic disturbance (fever, tachycardia, anaemia, or ESR over 30). Note that it is unclear how many systemic features are required.

Laboratory markers of severity include ↑ CRP, ↑ platelet count, ↓ albumin.

Diagnosis and differential diagnosis

The diagnosis rests on the clinical picture, especially the history, the endoscopic appearance, histologic appearance of colonic biopsy specimens, and microbiological exclusion of infectious colitis. The endoscopic appearances vary with severity of disease from mild (oedema, loss of vascularity, and patchy subepithelial haemorrhage) to severe (loss of vascular pattern, haemorrhage, mucopus, ulceration, and loss of epithelium, sometimes with small islands of residual mucosa that can be mistaken for polyps and are therefore called 'pseudopolyps') (see Colour Plate 26).

Always consider <u>Crohn's</u> colitis in the differential diagnosis: ileoscopy or radiological small bowel evaluation is often necessary (especially if inflammation appears confined to the rectum but there are raised inflammatory markers, low albumin, or anaemia). Exclude other forms of segmental colitis such as ischaemia, <u>radiation colitis</u>, <u>microscopic colitis</u>, and drug-induced colitis.

Investigations

Laboratory tests. Check for anaemia or iron deficiency. Thrombocytosis, eosinophilia, leucocytosis may all reflect active disease. Hypokalaemia, hypoalbuminaemia, and abnormal liver blood tests may be associated with severe disease. Liver blood tests may be abnormal reflecting <u>primary sclerosing cholangitis</u> in about 5% of cases.

Colonoscopy is not usually necessary for diagnosis (sigmoidoscopy, either rigid or flexible, is often sufficient for this) but can be helpful for determining the extent of disease. Although colonoscopy is safe in expert hands, in severe disease it cannot be recommended for general use. In the assessment of chronic colitis and in surveillance for dysplasia as a complication of long-standing colitis, colonoscopy is still essential.

Radiology. A plain abdominal X-ray is useful in excluding a perforation, assessing the amount of faecal loading, excluding toxic dilatation, and giving some evidence of extent of disease. Contrast barium radiology has very little role in assessing ulcerative colitis. In the case of an acutely tender abdomen, CT with contrast gives much more information and can show colonic wall thickening and hyperaemia.

Biopsies. Always take a biopsy since there is often disparity between endoscopic appearance and histology.

Pathology

50% have disease confined to the sigmoid or rectum, 30% have disease beyond the sigmoid but not affecting the whole colon, and 20% have a pan-colitis. Rectal sparing can be seen as a result of topical treatment with steroids or 5-ASA. Although shortening and narrowing of the colon can occur as a result of chronic colitis, fibrosis and stricturing is uncommon. Microscopic features: inflammation is confined to the mucosa, with neutrophils, lymphocytes, macrophages, and eosinophils. There is inflammation of the crypts and depletion of goblet cells.

Extraintestinal manifestations

See box. There is an important association between UC and thrombo-embolism (DVT and PE). Hospitalization, immobility, and malnutrition contribute, but in addition platelets can be high and many clotting factors are increased. There is no independent association with factor V Leiden. Treatment with prophylactic anticoagulants is safe and effective.

Histological differentiation of infective from ulcerative colitis

This is difficult, but the following features suggest chronicity and help to make the diagnosis with a probability of more than 80%:
- Distorted crypt architecture
- Crypt atrophy
- Irregular mucosal surface
- Basal lymphoid aggregates
- Chronic inflammatory infiltrate

Extraintestinal manifestations of ulcerative colitis

Related to activity of colitis
- Peripheral arthropathy
- Erythema nodosum
- Episcleritis
- Aphthous mouth ulcers

Usually related to activity of colitis
- Pyoderma gangrenosum
- Anterior uveitis

Unrelated to colitis
- Sacroiliitis
- Ankylosing spondylitis
- Primary sclerosing cholangitis

Rare
- Pericarditis
- Amyloidosis

Management

Medical

<u>CORTICOSTEROIDS</u> (see box) have reduced mortality of acute attacks from over 35% to under 1% and are effective in about 70% of acute attacks. 5-ASA (see 5-<u>AMINOSALICYLATES</u>) has significantly reduced relapse rate and improved quality of life. Immunosuppressant drugs (azathioprine/6-mercaptopurine, methotrexate) have been introduced for the management of chronic active disease, because they have a steroid-sparing effect, and to maintain remission. <u>CYCLOSPORIN</u> is being increasingly used in severe ulcerative colitis. Suggested treatment regimens for proctitis, mild disease, severe disease, chronic active disease, and maintenance therapy are shown in the box. Recent data suggest <u>INFLIXIMAB</u> may be useful in moderate – severe colitis.

Surgical

Indications for surgery in ulcerative colitis include:
- Severe attacks not responding to medical therapy.
- Complications of a severe attack (perforation, acute colonic dilatation).
- Chronic continuous disease with impaired quality of life.
- Dysplasia or carcinoma.

Choice of operation
- Total colectomy with permanent ileostomy.
- Total colectomy with ileo-anal pouch formation.

Colectomy with pouch formation is the operation of choice except for the elderly, those with impaired sphincter pressures, and those who do not wish to have a restorative proctocolectomy.

Complications, course, and prognosis

Most (80%) patients have intermittent attacks with varying lengths of remission. A few have chronic continuous disease and the remainder have a severe first attack with toxic megacolon or disease refractory to medical treament which requires colectomy. The extent of the disease can change with time: about 20 patients with proctitis will extend their disease after 10 years. Disease extending past the rectosigmoid is associated with a risk of malignant transformation: this risk relates principally to the duration and extent of disease of disease.

Colitis in pregnancy

Fertility is normal. Pregnancy is not a risk factor for relapse. Disease has no adverse effect on developing fetus. Steroids, 5-<u>ASA</u>, and even <u>AZATHIOPRINE</u> appear safe in pregnancy. <u>METHOTREXATE</u> is teratogenic and is contraindicated.

Treatment regimens for ulcerative colitis

Proctitis

Most respond to topical 5-ASA or steroid enemas or a combination of both (e.g. colifoam enema in the morning and 5-ASA enema at night. Suppositories are effective for pure proctitis. If symptoms continue, add in oral 5-ASA. **Remember to check for proximal constipation above the inflammation:** this is common and stops patients improving. Most clinicians treat proximal constipation with fibre but there is emerging evidence that this is poorly tolerated: an osmotic laxative such as movicol should be used instead

Mildly active disease

Use oral mesalazine, oral steroids in moderate doses (prednisolone 20 mg/day) and consider topical therapy if the disease is confined to the left colon

Severe disease

Admit to hospital, replace fluid and electrolyte losses. Give IV steroids (hydrocortisone 100 mg qds). Continuing oral nutrition appears not to influence outcome of a severe attack.

Treatment with IV steroids should be continued for 5–7 days if the patient is improving. If the patient does not improve then decision often lies between starting cyclosporin or sending the patient for surgery (total colectomy with a view to ileo-anal pouch formation).

Chronic active disease

2 flares within 12 months or disease that relapses rapidly on tapering steroids is an indication for starting second-line treatment with an immunosuppressive agent. Persistent chronic disease in patients receiving steroids and immunosuppressive drugs is an indication for surgery

Maintenance treatment

Use mesalazine indefinitely in a dose of 1200–1600 mg/day. Monitor renal function yearly because of the low risk of interstitial nephritis

When to start cyclosporin? When to refer for surgery?

Difficult and controversial. Data from the 1980s suggested that if mucosal islands, colonic dilatation, or small intestinal loops were visible on abdominal X-ray, there was an over 70% chance of the patient needing colectomy.

The best recent data on prognosis in severe colitis comes from Travis, SP *et al.* (1996) *Gut* **38:** 905): the following factors if present at day 3 give an 85% prediction of needing surgery:

- Stool frequency > 8 × per day
- CRP > 45 in those passing 3–8 stools per day

These factors are used by many to allow a decision on day three after admission on starting cyclosporin. Trials are underway to assess whether cyclosporin on admission confers added benefit

Ultrasound

- Widely available imaging modality with the great and unique property of enabling imaging of flow and soft tissues in real time. It is a complex and challenging technique and results are dependent on user expertise, particularly for specialist work. Extracorporeal (transabdominal) ultrasound is not very useful in imaging the gastrointestinal wall (this is also true of CT) because resolution is insufficient to reveal the cause of wall thickening or the depth of localization of a specific abnormality. This led to the development of combining endoscopy with ultrasound and more recently the capability of EUS-guided tissue sampling to differentiate benign from malignant lesions (see endoscopic ultrasound (EUS)).
- Technique works by sending out high-frequency (1–20 MHz) sound waves from a transducer. These waves reflect back to differing degrees dependent on underlying tissue, are converted into electric pulses, and sent back to analyser, which provides image of tissues and distance from skin. Higher frequency waves produce more detailed images, but penetrate less deeply into the body (2–5 MHz generally used for abdominal U/S, with 7.5–12 MHz used for EUS). Doppler sonography, integral in modern machines, allows real time information on flow within the morphological image.
- Most useful information provided when a specific question is asked (e.g. 'is there biliary dilatation?' rather than 'abdo U/S').

Indications

Hepatobiliary

- U/S used as first-line imaging modality for most diffuse and focal hepatobiliary abnormalities. Ideal for studying cystic lesions, and > 90% sensitive and specific in identifying gallstones.
- Many advocate liver biopsy to be done under U/S control, and widely used (alternative is CT) for targeted biopsies in general.
- Doppler facility allows flow in large blood vessels (e.g. see portal vein thrombosis, Budd–Chiari syndrome) and even vascularity of large lesions to be assessed.

Pancreatic

- In acute pancreatitis, U/S can help with detecting gallstones and biliary dilatation, although CT is more sensitive in evaluating pancreatic disease overall.

Luminal GI tract

- Useful for evaluation of the patient with right lower quadrant pain and possible appendicitis. U/S may also help in diagnosis of terminal ileal inflammation or stricturing, diverticulitis, small bowel obstruction, and bulky mesenteric nodes or GI neoplasms.
- Excellent in diagnosing intraperitoneal fluid collections such as ascites, abscesses, or haemorrhage and also in guiding percutaneous needle, aspiration for definitive diagnosis.

Strengths and weaknesses of ultrasound as an imaging modality

Strengths
- Unique ability to display flow and soft tissue in real time
- Spatial resolution superior to CT and MRI
- Safe and well tolerated: no ionizing radiation
- Can be performed at the bedside

Weaknesses
- Technically challenging
- Not good in fat or gaseous patients
- Inability to see beyond gas/soft tissue or bone/soft tissue interface
- Relatively poor contrast resolution—this may improve with the development of media for contrast-enhanced ultrasound
- Findings less reliable the farther area of interest is from skin probe (e.g. retroperitoneal structures, pancreas)

Urea breath tests

See: *Helicobacter pylori* (HP).

V

Vaccine use in the immunocompromised

- In general live vaccines should not be given to immunocompromised people or pregnant women.
- Immunocompromised people should probably not receive yellow fever vaccine because of a (theoretical) risk of vaccine-induced encephalomyelitis. This includes patients with HIV (see HIV and the gut).
- Inactivated hepatitis A vaccine is safe and effective and should be given to all travellers to endemic areas.
- If indicated (health care workers, long stay in endemic area, high risk of sexual transmission, high risk of hospitalization in endemic area), hepatitis B vaccine is safe in immunocompromised persons.
- In general cholera vaccination is not recommended for most travellers: exceptions are those with reduced gastric acid or the immunocompromised.

Variceal bleeding

See: Acute upper GI bleeding and portal hypertension.

Varices

See: portal hypertension.

Vasculitis and the GI tract

- Inflammation and necrosis can affect splanchnic blood vessels of all sizes from capillaries to larger arteries. Involvement of medium or large arteries (by e.g. polyarteritis nodosum, rheumatoid arthritis) may be confused with ischaemic insults (thrombosis or embolism) but look for systemic features (renal involvement, cutaneous nodules, rheumatoid factor).
- Typically vasculitis is caused by deposition of immune complexes in the walls of vessels, leading to complement activation and an inflammatory reaction that can result in aneurysm formation, vessel rupture, vascular occlusion, and fibrosis.

Veno-occlusive disease (VOD)

- Hepatic VOD occurs in 10–50% of patients following bone marrow transplantation, usually within first 20 days, and severe cases carry a 90% mortality. Pathogenesis involves fibrosis and obliteration of terminal hepatic venules, due to deposition of coagulation factors, red cells, and haemosiderin-laden macrophages.
- Presentation may be similar to that of acute Budd–Chiari syndrome (BCS), with jaundice, tender hepatomegaly, and ascites. Acute liver failure and multiorgan involvement may occur.

- Liver function tests often show ALT/AST (deranged LFTs >20 days post-BMT also require consideration of <u>graft versus host disease (GVHD)</u>). Doppler U/S may show reversal of portal vein flow, but hepatic venous flow is normal. Transjugular liver biopsy (with portal pressure measurements) may make the diagnosis.
- Treatment has traditionally been supportive, but defibrotide shows considerable promise. This drug binds to vascular endothelial cells, enhancing factors that contribute to fibrinolysis and suppressing those that promote coagulation.

Diseases involving GI vasculitis
- <u>Behçet's syndrome</u>
- <u>Polyarteritis nodosa</u>
- <u>Rheumatoid arthritis</u>
- <u>Scleroderma</u>
- <u>Systemic lupus</u>

Visceral arteridides: Churg-Strauss, Henoch–Schönlein, Wegener's, cryoglobulinaemia, <u>familial Mediterranean fever</u>, Henoch–Schönlein purpura.

Video capsule endoscopy

See: enteroscopy

VIPoma

See: pancreatic endocrine tumours.

Viral hepatitis

See: hepatitis A–G.

Vitamins

Defined as organic compounds required in small (<100 mg/day) quantities.

Vitamin A (retinol)

The precursor beta carotene contains 2 molecules of retinol and is found in green vegetables and carrots. Retinol is found in milk, eggs, and fish oils. Retinoids are stored in hepatocytes and hepatic fat storage cells (Ito cells) and function as regulators of many embryonic and adult genes through binding to the RXR and RAR transcription factors. Deficiency causes night blindness because retinol is a precursor of rhodopsin.

Vitamin B

- **B1** is thiamine: see beriberi.
- **B2** is riboflavin: deficiency causes sore tongue and mouth. Measure by red blood glutathione levels.
- **B3** is niacin: see pellagra.
- **B5** is pantothenic acid.
- **B6** is pyridoxine. Deficiency leads to dermatitis and glossitis.
- **B7** is biotin.
- **B9** is folic acid.
- **B12** See cobalamin (and pernicious anaemia).

Vitamin C (ascorbic acid)

Water soluble. Dietary source (fresh fruit, liver) essential. Deficiency causes scurvy: look for bent or coiled body hair, perifollicular haemorrage and bruising, and gingivitis. Scurvy is common in alcoholics but can occur in severe Crohn's or other mucosal enteropathies.

Vitamin D

Needs bile acids for solubilization and absorption. Enterocytes package it in chylomicrons. Low levels lead to osteomalacia. Apart fom low plasma levels, biochemical evidence for low vitamin D includes 24 chylomicrons urinary calcium of less than 100 mg/day, a high PTH level, and elevated urinary hydroxyprolene.

Vitamin E (tocopherol)

Found in grains, vegetables, meats. Absorption requires intraluminal bile salts and pancreatic esterases. The vitamin is packaged in chylomicrons and stored in liver and fat. The main role is as antioxidant. Chronic cholestasis causes clinical deficiency in children and can lead to retinopathy, cerebellar ataxia, reduced vibraton sense, and areflexia (abetalipoprotein-aemia causes similar syndrome because of failure to secrete chylomicrons). In adults symptoms take years to develop, but any disease impairing fat absorption can lead to deficiency (ileal disease, impaired bile secretion, intrahepatic disease like PBC).

Vitamin K

Main dietary source is green vegetables. About 50% comes from gut bacterial synthesis. Diets deficient in Vitamin K do not cause deficiency unless gut-sterilizing antibiotics are given. Vitamin K deficiency may arise due to a range of GI diseases, including chronic cholestasis (e.g. primary biliary cirrhosis) and coeliac disease. Diagnosis suggested by finding elevated prothrombin time (PT) in right clinical setting. In patient with suspected liver failure, vital to give parenteral vitamin K to exclude deficiency of this as cause of elevated PT.

Volvulus

A twisting of the gut around one axis causing lumen occlusion and sometimes strangulation. Can affect the stomach or colon.

Gastric volvulus

Most common in 5th decade, affects men and women equally. In 60% the stomach twists about its long axis. This is usually associated with a diaphragmatic hernia and is commonly an acute event: classically there is upper abdominal or retrosternal pain and unproductive retching. Gastric infarction can occur. In 40% the stomach twists about its short axis. This is more likely to be incomplete, intermittent and to present with chronic symptoms.

Acute gastric volvulus is an emergency and has a high mortality if untreated. Nasogastric intubation is indicated and if there is no infarction upper GI endoscopy is indicated to attempt detorsion. Surgery if necessary can be open or laparoscopic: repair of associated hiatus hernia is necessary.

Colonic volvulus

Can occur where there is a loop of bowel that is movable in the peritoneal cavity with close approximation of the fixation points. Commonest in the sigmoid colon (75%) and caecum (20%). Rarely may affect the transverse colon and splenic flexure. A history of chronic constipation and laxative abuse is common: patients with sigmoid volvulus are often elderly and abdominal tenderness is present only in a minority.

Management of colonic volvulus. Sigmoidoscopic decompression of the colon with placement of a rectal tube into the obstructed segment works in about 60% patients with sigmoid volvulus. The risk of recurrence is 40–50%, which suggests elective resection of the volvulus following successful decompression. Strangulated sigmoid volvulus requires emergency laparotomy with end colostomy.

Colonoscopic decompression of caecal volvulus can be successful but the risk of perforating the thinned often ischaemic caecum is higher. The best surgical option is controversial but right hemicolectomy is often performed.

Overall mortality approaches 10%, the major predictive factor being the presence of gangrenous bowel, which occurs in of about 20%.

Vomiting

See: Approach to nausea and vomiting.

(a)   (b)

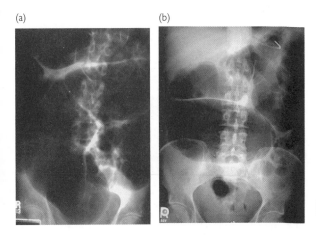

Fig. 2.30 Abdominal X-ray of sigmoid (left) and caecal (right) volvulus. On the left the dilated segment comes from the pelvis towards the right upper quadrant. On the right the caecum extends from the right lower abdomen across the midline. Reproduced from Feldman M, Friedman LS, and Sleisenger MH (2003). *Sleisenger and Fordtran's Gastrointestinal and Liver Disease*, with permission from Elsevier.

W

Weil's disease

See: leptospirosis.

Wernicke's encephalopathy (WE)

- Results from <u>vitamin</u> B1 (thiamine) deficiency. Predominantly found in malnourished patients with <u>alcohol dependency</u> or <u>alcohol-related liver disease</u> (reduced hepatic thiamine storage capacity). May be mistaken for drunkenness (see <u>Approach to agitation and confusion in the GI patient</u>).
- Clinical triad (only present in 30%) of ophthalmoplegia (horizontal nystagmus, conjugate gaze palsy, fixed pupils, paralysis of lateral rectus muscles), ataxia (wide based cerebellar gait, with vestibular dysfunction), and cognitive impairment (apathy, spatial disorientation, global confusion).
- Diagnosis is usually clinical, but red cell transketolase low.
- Potentially fatal if untreated, and 80% subsequently develop Korsakoff psychosis, characterized by retrograde and anterograde amnesia.
- Give parenteral vitamins B and C for rapid correction of severe depletion (e.g. Pabrinex® I and II tds IV—in 100ml N-saline over 30 min for 3/7, followed by thiamine 100 mg bd PO + VitB Co strong 2 tabs bd PO for 10 days. Address nutritional state, but maintainence thiamine 100 mg od required.
- Acute WE may be precipitated by high carbohydrate load (e.g. IV dextrose in hospital), so vital to administer thiamine if any clinical suspicion of deficiency. Check serum magnesium, and treat if low as thiamine may be ineffective with hypomagnesaemia.

Whipple's disease

> **George Whipple, 1878–1976. Described disease in 1907. Suggested role of bacteria, but this was not proven until 1997. Won Nobel prize for work on <u>pernicious anaemia</u>.**

- A systemic infection caused by the Gram-positive bacterium *Tropheryma whippelii*. A rare disease (incidence about 0.5 per million per year), it tends to affect middle-aged men: 30% are in farming-related trades. Acquisition is presumed to be oral but this has not been proven.
- The nature of the bacterium was obscure until the 1990s when 16S ribosomal sequencing revealed bacterial DNA related to actinomycetes. The doubling time of the bacterium is very long (18 days).
- Infected people have subtle immune defects in Th1 function, but whether this predisposes them to disease or is a consequence of infection is unclear.

Clinical features

Whipple's disease may affect several organ systems.

- **GI tract.** Malabsorption syndrome with gradual weight loss, diarrhoea (steatorrhoea or watery stool), and abdominal pain. Occult blood loss is common. Mesenteric and retroperitoneal lymphadenopathy are common.
- **Central nervous system .** Progressive dementia, ophthalmoplegia, and psychiatric symptoms. (Of note, CSF usually normal on examination, although PCR for *T. whippelii* can be positive.)
- **Cardiovascular system.** Endocarditis, myocarditis, or pericarditis.
- **Musculoskeletal system.** Seronegative polyarthralgia is common.

Investigation

Endoscopy. White or yellow patches due to lipid deposits may be seen at upper GI endoscopy. Multiple duodenal biopsy essential, and biopsy shows swollen macrophage cytoplasm, which contains many lysosomes stuffed with *T. whipplei*; these stain positive with PAS. Specific PCR-based assays have been developed. Disorders mimicking the histology of Whipple's are uncommon and include infection with *Mycobacterium avium* and histoplasmosis.

Treatment and prognosis. Initial response to antibiotics is rapid (diarrhoea resolving within days, arthralgia within weeks, weight gain within 1–2 months). Tetracyclines were initially used but CNS relapses were common and difficult to treat: current recommendations are for benzylpenicillin plus streptomycin or a third-generation cephalosporin to induce remission (success rate over 90%), followed by an antibiotic that crosses the blood–brain barrier for at least 1 year. Relapse rate approoximately 5% in retrospective studies.

Whipple's procedure

> Allen Oldfather Whipple (1881–1963). American surgeon. Medical historian on Middle East after retirement. Also reported Whipple's triad in insulinoma (see <u>pancreatic endocrine tumours</u>), but did not describe <u>Whipple's disease</u>.

- Procedure (also called pancreatoduodenectomy) involves excision of head of the pancreas, gallbladder, distal common bile duct, duodenum ± distal stomach. Anastomoses result in gastrojejunostomy, choledochojejunostomy, and pancreaticojejunostomy (see figure).
- Indications include <u>ampullary</u>, duodenal, and <u>pancreatic cancer</u> (procedure possible in < 15% of patients with pancreatic cancer, with subsequent approximate 25% 5 year survival), <u>cholangiocarcinoma</u> of distal bile duct, duodenal <u>familial adenomatous polyposis</u>, and occasionally <u>chronic pancreatitis</u>.
- Surgical morbidity > 30% (e.g. biliary leak, pancreatic fistula, secondary haemorrhage, <u>post-gastrectomy syndrome</u>), surgical mortality 3–5%.
- Pylorus-preserving pancreaticoduodenectomy (PPPD) has been advocated as alternative to Whipple's procedure, as means of reducing early satiety and biliary reflux. Analysis to date suggests no significant differences in surgical morbidity/mortality, or prognosis with <u>pancreatic cancer</u> after PPPD or Standard Whipple's procedure.

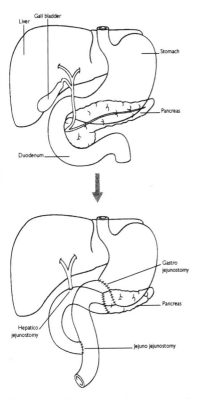

Fig. 2.31 Whipple's procedure (pancreatico-duodenectomy).

Whipworm

- *Trichuris trichiura* is a roundworm of the phylum *Nematoda*. The adult worm usually reaches 3–5 cm in length and has a lifespan of 1–3 years. Estimated worldwide infection rate of 800 million.
- Organism spread via the faecal–oral route, and humans only hosts. Embryonated (mature) eggs are ingested.
- Usually asymptomatic, but heavy worm infestation may result in lower abdominal discomfort, flatulence, and altered bowel habit.
- *Trichuris* dysentery syndrome characterized by bloody diarrhoea, tenesmus, and anaemia, but is rare.
- Diagnosis made by identifying *T. trichiura* eggs on stool microscopy.
- Treatment with mebendazole 100 mg bd for 3/7.

Wilson's disease

Background

- Autosomal recessive disorder, incidence 1:30 000.
- In normals approximately 10% of the 1–2 mg/day of ingested copper is absorbed, and bound to albumin in serum. After transport to the hepatocyte, copper is either incorporated into caeruloplasmin and excreted into plasma (90% of circulating copper in this form), or bound to ATPase Wilson's disease protein (WDP) and excreted in bile.
- The *ATP7A* gene encodes for WDP, with mutations resulting in retention of copper in the liver and impaired incorporation of copper into caeruloplasmin.

Clinical features

- Disease may present at age 3–40 years, with range of features (first table).
- Liver disease most common presentation in childhood. Chronic hepatitis may be similar to autoimmune hepatitis, and acute liver failure often associated with haemolysis. First presentation may be with complications of cirrhosis. Gallstones occur due to recurrent haemolysis.
- Neuropsychiatric presentation usual in adolescence/early adulthood.
- Kayser–Fleischer rings are rarely absent in patients with neurological disease (brown-green discolouration around periphery of cornea).

Investigations

Diagnosis rarely made unless considered, and biochemical parameters may be inconsistent particularly in patients with liver disease (see caveats opposite). No test result should be viewed in isolation, and diagnosis usually made through combination of clinical picture and highly suggestive results. **Unexplained liver disease in young person with Coomb's negative haemolytic anaemia should raise suspicion.**

- LFTs non-specific, but ALT usually < 1500 U/l, even in acute liver failure.
- Slit lamp examination to exclude Kayser–Fleischer rings.
- Plasma caeruloplasmin < 200 mg/l in 85% of cases.

Clinical features of Wilson's disease

System	Features
Liver	Acute hepatitis
	Acute liver failure
	Decompensated cirrhosis
	Portal hypertension
	Gallstones
Neurological	Behavioural change
	Parkinsonism/tremor
	Cognitive impairment
	Dysarthria, dystonia, dysphagia
Renal	Renal tubular acidosis
	Renal calculi
Musculoskeletal	Arthropathy
	Osteoporosis
	Osteomalacia
Haematological	Haemolytic anaemia
Ophthalmic	Kayser–Fleischer rings

Caveats in diagnosing Wilson's disease

Kayser–Fleischer rings	Copper deposition in other cholestatic liver diseases (e.g. primary biliary cirrhosis, primary sclerosing cholangitis)
↓ Caeruloplasmin	Acute phase reactant, so may be falsely ↑ in Wilson's with active liver inflammation. Falsely ↓ in chronic liver disease due to ↓ synthesis
↓ Serum copper	May ↑ due to leakage of non-caeruloplasmin bound copper from necrotic liver in acute Wilson's
Liver histology	Copper staining may be negative, despite raised liver copper concentrations
Genetic analysis	3 commonest mutations in UK patients only account for 30% of patients

- Serum copper < 11 μmol/l.
- 24 hour urinary copper > 3 μmol (found in 65% of Wilson's, but penicillamine challenge (500 mg 12 hourly × 2) leads to diagnostic elevation
  of > 25 μmol/24 hours in 90%).
- <u>Liver biopsy.</u> Hepatic copper > 250 μg/g dry weight (normal
  < 50 μg/g). Liver histology may show necrosis, chronic hepatitis, or
  cirrhosis, depending on clinical presentation. Suggestive features
  include fatty change, Mallory hyaline, copper staining, and
  vacuolated nuclei.
- Genetic analysis.

Management

- Acute liver failure:
  - Manage as for <u>acute liver failure</u> and transfer to specialist liver unit
    for <u>liver transplantation</u>.
- Liver disease without liver failure:
  - Avoid high copper-containing foods (e.g. chocolate, shellfish).
  - Penicillamine (20 mg/kg/day) with pyridoxine 25 mg/day leads to
    urinary copper excretion and good prognosis. Trientine (300 mg
    tds) is an alternative. Zinc (150–300 mg/day) may be used for
    maintenance.

Y

Yersinia

A genus of Gram negative rods. *Yersinia pestis* is reponsible for plague—a disease with an important role in human history. Other species (e.g. *Yersinia enterocolitica)* produce a self-limiting gastroenteritis.

Y. enterocolitica causes damage by invading epithelium overlying Peyer's patches, (especially in the terminal ileum) then spreading to the lamina propria.

Epidemics relate to consumption of contaminated milk and ice cream. Rare (1 culture confirmed case per 100 000 people per year in the USA). Two-thirds of cases are of enterocolitis: children under 5 are most commonly affected. Associated mesenteric adenitis is common and the condition may be confused with appendicitis: ultrasound can be helpful in separating these conditions.

In adults erythema nodosum, erythema multiforme, and reactive polyarthritis can occur, usually 1–2 weeks after onset of diarrhoea.

Diagnosis. Antigens can be found in mucosal biopsies. Specific IgA antibodies may be found in the blood. *Y. enterocolitica* may be grown in culture.

Treatment. Although the disease is usually diagnosed late when antibiotics probably do not alter the course of the gastrointestinal infection, treatment with chloramphenicol, septrin, or a quinolone is indicated in severe infections.

Z

Zieve's syndrome

(Also see Piccini, J et al. (2003) Am. J. Med. **115**: 729.)

First described in 1957 by Leslie Zieve, who reported a triad of jaundice, hyperlipidaemia, and transient haemolytic anaemia in a cohort of 20 male patients with alcoholic steatohepatitis. Most patients have upper abdominal/right upper quadrant pain and macrocytic anaemia. The hypercholesterolaemia and jaundice both resolve within 3 weeks if the patient stops drinking. The exact mechanism of haemolysis is not known, but may involve several acquired intracellular defects (unstable pyruvate kinase, membrane alterations).

Zollinger–Ellison syndrome

See: gastrinoma.

Drugs used in gastroenterology and hepatology

Acyclovir

GI indication	Herpes simplex (usually stomatitis or perianal: oesophageal or colonic in the immunocompromised) and varicella–zoster (also some efficacy *in vitro* against Epstein–Barr virus and cytomegalovirus)
Mode of action	Purine nucleoside analogue. Not a substrate of normal cellular thymidine kinase, so non-toxic to mammalian host cells. Phosphated acyclovir is a substrate for and inhibitor of herpes specified DNA polmerase, which prevents further viral DNA synthesis
Dose/duration	200 mg (400 mg in immunocompromised) 5 times a day for 5 days. IV dose is 5 mg/kg tds for 5 days
Side-effects	Impairment of renal function; usually reversible with rehydration.
Practice points	Reduce dose in renal impairment (creatinine clearance < 50 ml/min)

Adefovir dipixol (Hepsera®)

GI indication	Replicating chronic <u>hepatitis B</u>
Mode of action	Antiviral nucleotide reverse transcriptase inhibitor. Inhibits HBV DNA polymerase, so reduces HBV DNA
Dose/duration	Adefovir 10 mg PO od if creatinine clearance (CrCl) > 50 ml/min Dose adjustment in renal failure: If CrCl 20–49 ml/min: 10 mg PO every 48 hours If CrCl 10–19 ml/min: 10 mg PO every 72 hours Haemodialysis: 10 mg PO weekly, following haemodialysis
Contraindication	Drugs that alter renal tubular secretion may affect adefovir renal elimination
Side-effects	Renal dysfunction, diarrhoea, anorexia, pharyngitis may occur, but rare at lower 10 mg dose. Symptomatic hepatitic flare possible following drug discontinuation
Practice points	Present main role as additional drug in patients who develop treatment-resistant YMDD variant on lamivudine, but adefovir also shown to be effective as monotherapy

5-Aminosalicylates (5-ASA)

(e.g. mesalazine, olsalazine, balsalazide, sulfasalazine)

GI indication	Treatment of mild to moderate inflammatory bowel disease (<u>ulcerative colitis</u>, <u>Crohn's disease</u>, <u>collagenous colitis</u>), and the maintenance of remission of <u>ulcerative colitis</u>
Mode of action	Complex and not fully understood. *In vitro* low concentrations stimulate prostaglandin production while higher concentrations inhibit PGE2 production. *In vitro* inhibition of leukotrienes may not be relevant physiologically. May be important in attenuating damage caused by reactive oxygen metabolites. They also reduce IL-1 release and alter HLA-DR expression
	Rapid drug absorption in the upper GI tract has led to development of several carrier systems to allow 5-ASA drug delivery to different sites in colon and small intestine (see table)
Dose/duration	Confusing because of the many preparations but also conflicting practice in Europe and USA. In Europe the treatment dose for mesalazine is 2.4 g /day in three divided doses. In USA treatment doses are higher and there is evidence of superiority of 4.8 compared to 2.4 g/day with no difference in adverse event profile. Maintenance dose is 1.2–1.6 g/day
Contraindication	Sensitivity to salicylates. Use with caution in established renal impairment
Side-effects	May cause diarrhoea and headache. Renal toxicity is well reported, usually due to idiosyncratic interstitial nephritis. May cause aplastic anaemia, agranulocytosis, or thrombocytopenia. Very rarely associated with pancreatitis, allergic lung reactions, and lupus-like syndrome
Practice points	Choice of preparation depends largely on differences in site of action of the drug (see table). Sulfasalazine is effective and cheap but side effects are quite common (15% headache, photosensitive skin rash, reversible oligospermia in men) and mostly due to the sulfapyridine component. The newer 5ASAs have a better side effect profile but olsalazine may cause a secretory diarrhoea (an effect that may possibly be useful if there is proximal constipation associated with distal colitis). Pentasa® is the 5-ASA of choice for small intestinal involvement in Crohn's disease. Balsalazide may be more effective in left-sided colitis

Classification of the aminosalicylates	
pH dependent	
Asacol	Mesalazine coated in Eudragit-S, dissolving at pH > 7. Used for colonic disease
Salofalk	Mesalazine coated in Eudragit-L, dissolving at pH > 6. May release in terminal ileum
Microspheres	
Pentasa	Microgranules of 5-ASA. Release starts in stomach and duodenum. 60% released in small intestine; remainder should be available in the colon.
Prodrugs	
Sulfasalazine (salzopyrine)	5-ASA conjugated by a di-azo bond to sulfapyridine, thought responsible for many side effects
Olsalazine (dipentum)	2 5-ASA molecules linked by a di-azo bond
Balsalazide (colazide)	5-ASA linked to 4-aminobenzoylalanine

Antacids and alginates

- Often used in ulcer dyspepsia and non-erosive gastro-oesophageal reflux. Evidence of efficacy in non-ulcer dyspepsia is uncertain.
- Usually contain compounds of aluminium (tend to be constipating) or magnesium (tend to be laxative). Bismuth-containing antacids should be avoided because bismuth absorption can cause neurotoxicity and is often constipating. High doses of calcium-containing antacids can cause hypercalcaemia and alkalosis.
- A few antacids contain simeticone, which is an antifoaming agent that can reduce flatulence (asilone, maalox plus).
- Alginates are antacids that form a raft that floats on the surface of stomach contents to reduce reflux.
- The sodium content of antacids varies widely and may be a factor affecting prescribing in chronic liver disease.

Antibiotics

Antibiotic selection should be based on prior culture and sensitivity, in order to optimize response, and reduce ever-increasing problem of resistance. Many GI-related infections are due to Gram-negative or anaerobic bacteria. The choice of antibiotics is wide, and only a commonly used selection in gastrointestinal practice is given here. See METRONIDAZOLE, CIPROFLOXACIN, CEPHALOSPORINS, GENTAMICIN, PIPERACILLIN.

Anticholinergics (e.g. hyoscine hydrobromide)

GI indication	General nausea; motion sickness; premedication
Mode of action	Anticholinergic action
Dose/duration	Hyoscine hydrobromide (buscopan) 300 µg PO before journey, or transdermal patch (Scopodem TTS®) 1 mg/72 hours
Contraindication	Urinary retention, GI obstruction, porphyria, cardiovascular/liver/renal disease, closed angle glaucoma
Side-effects	Drowsiness, dry mouth, blurred vision, urinary retention

Anti-diarrhoeal agents

- Mostly include antimotility agents such as codeine, loperamide, and morphine. Absorbents such as kaolin are not recommended for acute diarrhoea.
- Antimotility agents should not be used where inhibition of peristalsis may be dangerous, as in acute <u>ulcerative colitis</u> or <u>antibiotic-associated diarrhoea</u>.
- In severe secretory diarrhoea, <u>OCTREOTIDE</u>, <u>PROTON PUMP INHIBITORS</u>, and clonidine may be tried, in addition to conventional antimotility agents. <u>CLONIDINE</u> is a receptor agonist that may be used for diarrhoea related to opiate withdrawal and diabetic diarrhoea. It may induce postural hypotension.

Anti-diarrhoeal drugs in mild to moderate diarrhoea

Drug	Mechanism of action	Side effects
Bismuth subsalicylate (Denol)	Is bactericidal: suspended in clay that might bind enterotoxins	Black stools and black tongue: salicylate toxicity
Opiates (morphine, codeine phosphate)	Alter motility, possibly anti-secretory: loperamide has calmodulin-binding and calcium channel blocking activity	May precipitate toxic megacolon, CNS and respiratory depression, delayed gastric emptying; addictive potential
Bulk forming agents (ispaghula, methylcellulose)	Hydroscopic and increases stool viscosity: used in controlling faecal consistency in ileostomy effluent	Bloating and flatus
Adsorbents (kaolin)	Hydroscopic, may bind enterotoxins. However not recommended for acute diarrhoea	
Antimotility (loperamide) and anticholinergics (e.g. lomotil: a mixture of diphenoxylate and atropine 100:1)	Reduce motility	Similar to opiates; atropine toxicity; no CNS or respiratory depression
Cholestyramine, aluminium hydroxide	Binds bile acids	Binds drugs and vitamins

Anti-emetics/anti-nausea drugs

- ANTIHISTAMINES can be effective but may cause drowsiness and antimuscarinic effects. Phenothiazines act to block the chemoreceptor trigger zone and are useful in treating nausea associated with cancer, radiation, and drugs such as anaesthetic agents, opioids, and cytotoxics.
- Metaclopramide and domperidone (see DOPAMINE RECEPTOR ANTAGONISTS) are very useful in treating nausea and vomiting associated with gastroduodenal and biliary disease.
- SEROTONIN (5HT₃) RECEPTOR ANTAGONISTS are very useful in managing post-operative nausea and cytotoxic-associated nausea.

Antifungals

- Gastroenterologists often treat candidal infections, and may be involved in treating patients infected with *Cryptococcus*, *Histoplasma*, and *Aspergillus*. They may also be involved in the treatment of patients with drug-induced hepatotoxicity due to some antifungal drugs (itraconazole, ketoconazole).
- Amphotericin and nystatin belong to the polyene family: neither are absorbed when given orally but are useful in the treatment of oral or intestinal candidiasis. Fluconazole is well absorbed orally and also penetrates the CSF, which makes it useful for treating fungal meningitis.
- For *Candida*, use **fluconazole** 50–100 mg/day PO for 7–14 days or **nystatin** 500 000 units every 6 hours.

Antihistamines

(e.g. cinnarizine, cyclizine, promethazine)

GI indication	General nausea; motion sickness, vestibular disorders
Mode of action	Antagonism of histamine H1 receptors
Dose/duration	Cinnarizine 15–30 mg PO tds
	Cyclizine 50 mg PO/IV tds
Contraindication	Avoid promethazine in patients with porphyria, and cyclizine in severe heart failure
Side-effects	Drowsiness, enhanced effect of alcohol, dry mouth, blurred vision
Practice points	Important to advise patients of potential effects on driving and skilled tasks

Antispasmodics

- Drugs used for gastrointestinal smooth muscle spasm include antimuscarinics (atropine, dicyclomine, hyoscine) and direct relaxants (alverine, mebeverine, peppermint oil). All of these may relieve pain in <u>irritable bowel syndrome</u> and <u>diverticular disease</u>.
- Antimuscarinics should be avoided in angle-closure glaucoma, myasthenia, paralytic ileus, pyloric stenosis, and prostatic enlargement.

Azathioprine

GI indication	Steroid-dependent inflammatory bowel disease, fistulating <u>Crohn's disease,</u> and other autoimmune conditions such as <u>autoimmune hepatitis</u>
Mode of action	Metabolized *in vivo* to 6-mercaptopurine, then metabolized to 6-thioguanine nucleotides that inhibit DNA synthesis. See <u>thiopurine methyltransferase (TPMT)</u>
Dose/duration	Dose of azathioprine in inflammatory bowel disease is 2–2.5 mg/kg/day or 6-MP 1–1.5 mg/kg/day. Both agents take up to 3–4 months to become fully effective. Intravenous loading does not speed time to response. The duration of therapy is not established. Maintenance therapy for at least 4 years in patients with IBD is safe. Early fears over the incidence of immunoproliferative disorders have not been substantiated
Contraindication	Hypersensitivity: absent TPMT levels
Side-effects	Nausea, malaise, dizziness, myalgia in about 15%. Leucopenia in 4%, severe (WCC < 2) in 1%; not solely related to TPMT genotype. Can cause acute hepatitis (usually cholestatic: centrizonal changes on histology) and pancreatitis (5%). Also associated with hepatic <u>veno-occlusive disease</u>
Practice points	At least some intolerance (nausea, malaise, dizziness) relates to the nitroimidazole ring that differentiates azathioprine from 6-MP. Arguably all patients should be given 6-MP rather than azathioprine
	Reduce dose by 30–50% if giving concurrent xanthine oxidase inhibitors like allopurinol
	Leucopenia can develop after prolonged therapy. Measure white cell count weekly for 4 weeks, monthly for 3 months, then every 3 months. Low white count will usually respond to stopping treatment for a few weeks and adjusting dose
	TPMT levels should be measured prior to starting drug, and low levels necessitate dose reduction. 1 in 300 patients has undetectable levels of TPMT due to homozygous deficiency and in these patients azathioprine should probably be avoided, although some would consider extremely low doses

Bismuth

Effective in healing gastric and duodenal ulcers when given as tripotassium dicitratobismuthate (denol: dose 2 tablets twice a day). It also has a role as a second-line agent in _Helicobacter_ eradication, usually as part of quadruple therapy with 2 antibiotics (e.g. amoxicillin, clarithromycin) and a PROTON PUMP INHIBITOR. It may darken the tongue and blacken the faeces. Should not be given for longer than 12 weeks.

Botulinum toxin (Botox®)

GI indication	Achalasia
Mode of action	Produced by gram-positive anaerobic bacterium _Clostridium botulinum_. Blocks acetylcholine release from presynaptic neuromuscular junction. Reduces tone at gastroesophageal junction when given for achalasia
Dose/duration	In achalasia, injection using sclerotherapy needle of 80 units of botulinum toxin A (20 unit per ml injected into each of 4 quadrants) at level of lower oesophageal sphincter
Contraindication	Hypersensitivity
Side-effects	Transient chest pain in 25%. Gastro-oesophageal reflux. Oesophageal perforation or mediastinitis rare. Long-term safety unknown
Practice points	Intrasphincteric botulinum provides short-term relief in 60% of achalasia patients, but majority of patients have recurrence < 1 year. Subsequent injections less effective. Generally reserved for older patients, and poor candidates for endoscopic dilatation or surgery

Bowel cleansing solutions

See: bowel preparation

Cannabinoids (e.g. nabilone)

GI indication	During cytotoxic chemotherapy, particularly if unresponsive to conventional treatments
Mode of action	Unclear. May act on brainstem nuclei
Dose/duration	Nabilone 1–2 mg PO bd
Contraindications	Pregnancy/breast feeding, severe liver impairment. Caution in those with psychiatric disease
Side-effects	Drowsiness, vertigo, mood disturbance, psychosis, abdominal pain. Enhanced effects of alcohol
Practice points	Important to advise patients of potential effects on driving and skilled tasks

Cephalosporins

(e.g. Cefotaxime®, Ceftazidime®, Ceftriaxone®)

GI indication	<u>Spontaneous bacterial peritonitis</u>, intraabdominal sepsis, <u>oesophageal rupture</u>, <u>cholangitis</u>, <u>pyogenic liver abscess</u>. Often in combination with <u>METRONIDAZOLE</u>
Mode of action	Bactericidal β-lactam antibiotic. Inhibits synthesis of peptidoglycan layer of bacterial cell wall. Active against Gram-negative and (to lesser extent) Gram-positive bacteria.
Dose/duration	E.g. Cefotaxime 1–2 g IV bd
	Ceftriaxone 1–2g IV od (over 2–4 minutes)
Contraindications	Penicillin hypersensitivity—10% cross-reactivity with cephalosporin. However, always check what is meant by 'penicillin allergy'—history of urticaria/angio-oedema clearly more relevant than diarrhoea, and may influence use of cephalosporin. <u>Porphyria</u>. Caution in renal impairment.
Side-effects	Nausea, vomiting, <u>pseudomembranous colitis</u>, rash, headache, fever, arthralgia, abnormal liver function tests
Practice points	Calcium salt of ceftriaxone may deposit in gallbladder, occasionally giving symptoms, but usually resolves on stopping

Cholestyramine (e.g. Questran®)

GI indication	Pruritis related to biliary obstruction (e.g. <u>primary biliary cirrhosis</u> (PBC), <u>primary sclerosing cholangitis</u> (PSC)); diarrhoea/steatorrhoea due to <u>bile acid malabsorption</u>, (e.g. <u>Crohn's disease</u>, radiation ileitis, ileal resection), <u>obstetric cholestasis</u>
Mode of action	Anion-exchange resin. Binds <u>bile acids</u>, forming insoluble complex, and preventing reabsorption
Dose/duration	Pruritis: cholestyramine 4 g sachet 1–2/day, mixed with water. Bile acid diarrhoea: 3–6 sachets/day, in 2–4 divided doses
Contraindications	Complete large duct biliary obstruction, as this requires instrumental relief (e.g. <u>ERCP</u>). Pruritis due to this is unlikely to respond to cholestyramine. Absorption of wide range of drugs affected by cholestyramine (e.g. oral contraceptive, digoxin, thyroxine), so give these > 1 hour before, or > 4 hours after drug.
Side-effects	Abdominal discomfort, nausea, constipation, diarrhoea. Interference with fat soluble vitamin absorption (<u>vitamins A, D, E, K</u>) may requires monitoring (e.g. vitamin K dependent prothrombin time) and supplementation
Practice points	Cholestyramine most effective given before and after breakfast (time of maximal gallbladder emptying and thus bile acid binding). Cholestyramine may paradoxically worsen diarrheoa if > 100 cm ileum resected (see <u>bile acid malabsorption</u>) Pruritis alone may be indication for liver transplantation in PBC (if all measures failed (e.g. rifampicin, naloxone)

Ciprofloxacin

GI indication	Traveller's diarrhoea (e.g. _Salmonella, Shigella, Campylobacter_), cholangitis/biliary tract sepsis, spontaneous bacterial peritonitis prophylaxis
Mode of action	Quinolone, active against Gram-negative and (to lesser extent) Gram-positive bacteria. Bactericidal, blocks bacterial DNA replication by binding to DNA gyrase
Dose/duration	E.g. ciprofloxacin 500 mg PO bd , 200 mg IV bd
Contraindications	Caution in pregnancy/breast feeding, myasthenia gravis
Side-effects	Nausea, vomiting, dyspepsia, pseudomembranous colitis, photosensitivity, rash (rarely Stevens–Johnson syndrome), urticaria. Increases blood levels of theophyllines, and enhances effects of warfarin
Practice points	Few indications for intravenous, rather than oral administration, but bioavailability of oral preparation may be significantly reduced by concomitant use of enteral feeds

Corticosteroids

(e.g. prednisolone, hydrocortisone, budesonide)

GI indication	Autoimmune hepatitis, acute ulcerative colitis, Crohn's disease, unresponsive coeliac disease, liver transplantation
Mode of action	Immunosuppressive and anti-inflammatory. Inhibit proinflammatory cytokines (e.g. interleukin-1 (IL-1), IL-2, interferon-α (IFN-α) , tumor necrosis factor (TNF)), adhesion molecules, MHC class II molecules, elastase, collagenase, and nitric oxide synthase
Dose/duration	Preparation, dose, route, and duration depend on clinical indication. Examples: Prednisolone 30–40 mg PO od (initial treatment acute ulcerative colitis, autoimmune hepatitis) Hydrocortisone 100 mg IV qds (severe acute ulcerative colitis) Budesonide (Entocort®) 9 mg PO od, reducing dose over 8 weeks (active ileal/right colon Crohn's disease) Rectal prednisolone (Predsol®, Predfoam®) PR od (proctitis, rectosigmoid ulcerative colitis)
Contraindications	Ongoing sepsis (unless specific antimicrobial therapy given). Avoid live vaccines if taking high dose steroids
Side-effects	Most side-effects relate to dose and duration. Fewer systemic effects with rectal steroids (and budesonide) than with oral prednisolone, but occur with all GI: dyspepsia; peptic ulceration (causative role of steroids still debated, but prophylactic PROTON PUMP INHIBITORS often given if long-term steroids used); oral/oesophageal candidiasis. Infection: may mask systemic sepsis/TB (but negligible increased risk if equivalent of prednisolone < 10 mg/day). Musculoskeletal: growth impairment (but in children with Crohn's this is more due to disease than treatment); bone loss (additional risk with GI disease, e.g. Crohn's disease, coeliac disease); proximal myopathy. Endocrine: adrenal suppression; Cushing's syndrome; amenorrhoea; diabetes mellitus. Skin: bruising; atrophy; striae; acne. Endocrine: diabetes mellitus; hypertension. Eye: glaucoma; cataract. CNS: euphoria; depression; psychosis; insomnia

Practice points	Patients should be given steroid card
	Exclude bone loss and consider prophylaxis in patients on long-term steroids (see <u>bone densitometry</u> and <u>osteoporosis</u>).
	Rectal steroids best self-administered just before going to bed, as more likely to be retained.
	Steroid-sparing agents (e.g. <u>AZATHIOPRINE</u>) often indicated after disease remission obtained (e.g. <u>autoimmune hepatitis</u>).
	Step-wise withdrawal of steroids if taken for > 3 weeks
	Increased neutrophil count during steroids may relate to increased immature cells from the bone marrow, increased circulating half-life, and reduced vascular margination of cells, but always consider sepsis

Cromoglycate

- A mast cell stabilizer that has been proposed for use in hypersensitivity reactions to food and some cases of <u>irritable bowel syndrome</u> (IBS). It is also used by some paediatricians in the management of inflammatory bowel disease where there is a predominance of eosinophils or an allergic component.
- Role in treating IBS is controversial as there is no good evidence that symptoms in IBS are caused by type I hypersensitivity reactions or that there is an increased incidence of IBS in atopic patients. However, sodium cromoglycate (e.g. 100–200 mg before meals, has been used with and without exclusion diets in the treatment of patients with reported food intolerance and higher success rates have been found in patients with positive skin prick reactions to food extracts. These studies were neither blinded nor adequately controlled and the principle remains unsubstantiated.

Cyclosporin (ciclosporin)

GI indication	Severe <u>ulcerative colitis</u> in hospitalized patients. Commonly used in those not responding to steroids by third day of admission but studies ongoing to determine optimal timing of administration. Not effective in <u>Crohn's disease</u>. <u>Liver transplantation</u>.
Mode of action	Prevents T cell activation by inhibiting the calcineurin parthway
Dose/duration	In IBD: initial trials used 4 mg/kg IV/day: recent data shows 2 mg/kg IV/day equally effective. Oral preparation (Neoral®) 5 mg/kg/day may be as effective
Contraindication	Renal impairment. Monitor cholesterol and magnesium levels before starting
Side-effects	Main toxicities are renal and neurological. Can cause hypercholesterolaemia, eosinophilic colitis, hypertension, hyperuricaemia, hypertrichosis, and gingival hyperplasia
Practice points	Opportunistic infections can occur and some centres use prophylactic co-trimoxazole. Cyclosporin may delay but not prevent the need for colectomy: many centres couple its use with long-term azathioprine started on discharge from hospital. Patients on steroids, cyclosporin, and azathioprine are heavily immunosuppressed and need very close supervision: steroids should be weaned over 6 weeks, followed by weaning cyclosporina as azathioprine takes effect. Dose reduction of 25–50% required if creatinine increases by > 30% above baseline on treatment

Dopamine (D$_2$) receptor antagonists

(e.g. prochlorperazine, domperidone, metoclopramide)

GI indication	Nausea, vomiting, especially in association with non-ulcer dyspepsia/GORD where prokinetic effects may be beneficial (e.g. domperidone, metoclopramide)
Mode of action	Anatagonize D$_2$ receptor within central chemoreceptor trigger zone. Metoclopramide also antagonizes 5HT$_3$ + 5HT$_4$ receptors, and has both central and peripheral action
Dose/duration	E.g. domperidone 10–20 mg PO tds
	metoclopramide 10 mg PO/IM/IV tds
	prochlorperazine 10 mg PO tds, 12.5 mg IM stat
Contraindications	Pregnancy/breast feeding, phaeochromocytoma
Side-effects	Drowsiness, dystonic reactions (less prominent with domperidone), hyperprolactinaemia, rashes, neuroleptic malignant syndrome (metoclopramide, prochlorperazine)
Practice points	These drugs increase lower oesophageal sphincter tone and speed gastric emptying. They can be helpful in treating functional symptoms of early satiety and bloating

Ganciclovir

GI indication	Active cytomegalovirus infection
Mode of action	Synthetic analogue of guanine that inhibits herpes virus replication
Dose/duration	5 mg/kg IV bd for 14–21 days
Contraindication	Pregnancy, hypersensitivity
Side-effects	Leucopenia, anaemia, thrombocytopenia. Myelosuppression particularly severe when given with zidovudine
Practice points	Do not give if neutrophils less than 0.5 × 10^9/l. Dose needs to be reduced in renal impairment (creatinine > 130 µmol/l)

Gentamicin

GI indication	Severe intraabdominal infection/septicaemia, <u>cholangitis</u> (usually in addition to other agents, e.g. 3rd generation <u>CEPHALOSPORIN</u> and <u>METRONIDAZOLE</u>)
Mode of action	Bactericidal aminoglycoside, which binds to bacterial ribosomal subunit, leading to misreading of t-RNA, with impairment of bacterial protein synthesis. Particularly effective against Gram-negative bacteria
Dose/duration	3–7 mg/kg/day IV od. Doses up to 240 mg given by slow injection in 3–5 minutes, larger doses by 30–60 minute infusion.
Contraindications	Caution and dose reduction in renal impairment
Side-effects	Dose-related hearing, vestibular and renal toxicity. Nausea, <u>pseudomembranous colitis</u>, rash
Practice points	Monitoring of dose essential. Take plasma concentration 6–14 hours after 1st dose. Comparison made of drug level and time after dose, to plan further dose adjustments. Repeat daily if varying renal function, otherwise every 3–5 days. Liaise closely with pharmacy/microbiology departments. Extending dosing interval (24, 36, 48 hours) ± dose reduction may be necessary

H2 receptor antagonists (H2RA)

(e.g. cimetidine, ranitidine, nizatidine, famotidine)

GI indication	Peptic ulceration
	Gastro-oesophageal reflux: less effective than PROTON PUMP INHIBITORS (PPIs), but may have synergistic effects on resting parietal cell acid output and so are often combined with PPIs in difficult or refractory cases
	H2RAs reduce incidence of bleeding gastric erosions in acute liver failure, and of acid aspiration in obstetric patients at delivery
Mode of action	Reduce gastric acid output by histamine receptor blockade
Dose/duration	Ranitidine 150 mg bd PO; 300 mg at night, or cimetidine 400 mg bd PO; 800 mg at night for reflux
Contraindication	Caution in severe liver and renal impairment
Side-effects	Diarrhoea, altered liver function. Cimetidine can be associated with gynaecomastia. Cimetidine binds hepatic cytochrome p450 and should be avoided in patients on warfarin, phenytoin, and theophyllin. Hepatotoxicity
Practice points	In clinical practice PPIs have replaced H2RAs as first-line agents in controlling gastric acid

Infliximab (Remicade®)

GI indication	Severe active <u>Crohn's disease</u> in patients not responding to steroids and a conventional immunosuppressant, or who are intolerant of them. Also licensed for the management of refractory fistulating Crohn's disease. Maintenance therapy can be considered for those responding to the initial induction course. Recent trials (ACT-1, ACT-2) suggest efficacy in <u>ulcerative colitis</u> but more data needed
Mode of action	A chimeric monoclonal antibody (25% murine, 75% human) of IgG4 subclass that binds to circulating and membrane bound tumour necrosis factor alpha (TNFα). It facilitates antibody-dependent cellular cytoxicity, which may explain its effectiveness in Crohn's compared with other TNF antibodies like etanercept and onercept
Dose/duration	Initially 5 mg/kg by IV infusion, with further doses at 2 and 6 weeks. In patients on maintenance therapy, 5 mg/kg every 8 weeks is probably better than intermittent dosing
Contraindication	Active infection, tuberculosis. Patients must be evaluated for active or latent TB before treatment (e.g. CXR).
	Heart failure: discontinue if symptoms develop or worsen: avoid in moderate/severe heart failure
Side-effects	Acute hypersensitivity reactions (fever, chest pain, hypotension, dyspnoea, angio-oedema). Antibodies to infliximab develop in 30% of patients: but are clinically significant with lupus-like syndrome in very few
Practice points	Prophylactic hydrocortisone 100–200 mg IV can be given to minimize risk of acute reaction. Risk of hypersensitivity increased if there has been an interval of more than 16 weeks between infusions
	Contraindicated in stricturing Crohn's disease because of the possible risk of rapid healing inducing obstruction: data from the ACCENT 1 study do not support this and suggest that higher doses of infliximab may be associated with lower rates of stricturing

Interferon alpha

GI indication	Replicating chronic hepatitis B, hepatitis C
Mode of action	Immunomodulator. Possible direct antiviral effects
Dose/duration	Hepatitis B: e.g. pegylated interferon (PEG-IFN) α2a 180 g/week for 48 weeks. Traditional regimen: standard IFN α9MU SC ×3/week, for 4 months)
	Hepatitis C: usually in combination with ribavirin
	e.g. PEG-IFN α2a 180 µg/week or PEG-IFN α2b 1.5 µg/kg/week, plus ribavirin 15 mg/kg/day (duration dependent on viral and patient factors).
Contraindication	Severe depression, decompensated cirrhosis, autoimmune disease, ischaemic heart disease, diabetic retinopathy, pregnancy, renal transplant
Side-effects	Influenza-like symptoms (fatigue, fever, arthralgia, head-ache), psychiatric problems, weight loss, myelosuppression (usually neutropenia), hypotension/arrhyhthmias, hair loss, abdominal pain (also see hepatitis C)
Practice points	Influenza symptoms 6–8 h after dose, responds well to paracetamol, and usually improves on repeat doses. Blood monitoring (especially neutrophils) needed weekly for first 3 weeks, then monthly. Neutrophils $< 1.5 \times 10^9$/l requires dose reduction, $<1 \times 10^9$/l requires cessation

Lamivudine

GI indication	Chronic hepatitis B
Mode of action	Nucleoside analogue. Inhibits viral reverse transcriptase, so suppressing HBV replication
Dose/duration	100 mg PO od. Duration at least 12/12 (discontinue 3/12 after HBeAg seroconversion, if achieved?)
Contraindication	None, but use with other antiretrovirals if patient co-infected with HIV, to avoid HIV escape mutants
Side-effects	May lead to ALT flare on discontinuation
Practice points	Drug reduces serum HBV DNA, improves serum ALT and liver histology. HBeAg seroconversion increases with duration of use (and high baseline ALT), as do treatment-resistant YMDD variants (approximately 20%, 40%, 55% for both at 1, 2, 3 years). Addition of other agents (e.g. ADEFOVIR) may reduce effects of these variants

Laxatives

Bulking agents (bran, methycellulose, ispaghula) relieve constipation by increasing faecal mass which stimulates peristalsis.

Stimulant laxatives include bisacodyl, docusate, senna, and picosulphate. Prolonged use can cause an atonic non-functioning colon and hypokalaemia.

Stool softeners. Paraffin can cause anal seepage and possibly a granulomatous reaction following absorption of small amounts.

Osmotic laxatives increase the amount of water in the large bowel. Includes saline purgatives like magnesium hydroxide, but also phosphate enemas. Lactulose is a disaccharide that is not absorbed: it produces an osmotic diarrhoea of low faecal pH, which inhibits proliferation of ammonia-producing organisms and is therefore used in hepatic encephalopathy. Macrogols (e.g. movicol) are inert polymers of polyethylene glycol that sequester fluid in the bowel.

Laxatives—uses and effects of abuses

Type	Usual dose	Side effects and comments
Bulk-forming Psyllium, methylcellulose	4–7 g	Useful in those with small hard stools. Need to increase fluid intake. Impaction can occur above strictures
Emollient Mineral oil	15–45 ml	May decrease fat soluble vitamin absorption, can cause lipid aspiration pneumonia: do not give in dysphagia, the debilitated, or at bedtime
Docusate salts		Anionic surfactants that soften the stool and stimulate fluid secretion
Hyperosmolar Polyethlene glycol solutions	Movicol 1–3 sachets per day Kleenprep 1–4 litres per day 15–60 ml PO	Often used as bowel prep for colonoscopy, but can be very useful in treating intractable constipation
Lactulose	5–15 ml enema	Metabolized by colon bacteria to low molecular weight compounds that increase stool osmolarity
Glycerine		Given intrarectally—may produce rectal irritation
Saline Magnesium salts		Avoid in renal failure due to magnesium absorbption and possible toxicity
Stimulant Castor oil		Hydrolysed by lipases to ricinoleic acid which stimulates secretion and motility
Diphenylmethane (bisacodyl) Anthraquinones		Cause fluid and electrolyte accumulation in the colon. Absorbed by the small intestine, metabolized by the liver. Can cause melanosis coli and degeneration of myenteric plexus

Methotrexate

GI indication	Steroid-dependent <u>Crohn's disease</u>, often in those unable to tolerate <u>AZATHIOPRINE</u>/6-MP. Possible role in steroid-dependent <u>ulcerative colitis</u>
Mode of action	Its action as a folate antagonist is unlikely to be relevant as it is usually given with folic acid. It inhibits IL-1, IL-2, IL-6, IL-8
Dose/duration	Best trial used 25 mg IM once a week for 16 weeks: if effective this can probably be converted to 15 mg per week for maintenance
Contraindication	Pre-exisiting liver or pulmonary disease (seek advice). Methotrexate is teratogenic. Both men and women should be infomed of the risks to gametogenesis. Crosses into breast milk
	Extensively protein bound; can be displaced by salicylates, diuretics, sulphonamides, tetracyclines. NSAIDs reduce renal excretion and may enhance toxicity
Side-effects	Can cause hepatic fibrosis and interstitial pneumonitis
Practice points	Monitor full blood count and LFT before starting treatment, weekly until stabilized, then every 3 months
	Routine liver biopsy on methotrexate no longer advised
	Give folic acid 5 mg/day for 5 days of the week (avoiding methotrexate day and day after) to prevent stomatitis and nausea

Metronidazole (e.g. Flagyl®)

GI indication	<u>Pseudomembranous colitis</u>, <u>amoebiasis</u>, pyogenic <u>liver abscess</u>, perianal <u>Crohn's disease</u>, <u>giardiasis</u>, <u>cholangitis</u>, <u>diverticular</u> abscess, <u>*Helicobacter pylori*</u> infection (usually used in combination with other agents)
Mode of action	Imidazole ring-based antibiotic. Active against anaerobic bacteria and protozoa
Dose/duration	E.g. pseudomembranous colitis: 400 mg tds PO 10 days Cholangitis: 500 mg IV tds 7–10 days (with 3rd generation <u>CEPHALOSPORIN</u>)
Contraindications	Alcohol—see below
Side-effects	Nausea, vomiting, metallic taste, rash, headache, drowsiness, dizziness, abnormal liver function tests, jaundice, peripheral neuropathy (with prolonged use), leucopenia. May increase toxicity of warfarin, phenytoin, lithium. Disulfiram reaction may occur with alcohol
Practice points	In patients with <u>*Helicobacter pylori*</u>, approximately 20% metronidazole resistance in UK (lower in rural than urban areas), and common reason for failure of eradication therapy. Drug not usually included in first-line treatment regimens

Misoprostol

Synthetic prostaglandin analogue with antisecretory and gastroprotective properties. It can prevent NSAID-associated <u>peptic ulceration</u> but its use is limited by its side-effect profile (diarrhoea very common with doses over 200 µg).

N-acetylcysteine (NAc)

GI indication	<u>Paracetamol overdose</u>
Mode of action	Precursor of reduced glutathione, so replenishes hepatic glutathione stores. Antioxidant effects
Dose/duration	In paracetamol overdose: 150 mg/kg in 200 ml 5% dextrose over 15 min, then 50 mg/kg in 500 ml over 4 hours, then 100 mg/kg in 1000 ml over 16 hours
Contraindication	Known hypersensitivity
Side-effects	Rarely causes anaphylaxis, allergic reactions (urticaria, angio-oedema). Nausea, vomiting reported
Practice points	Give drug following paracetamol according to tomogram (see <u>paracetamol overdose</u>), but if any doubt about timing of overdose, or cause of <u>acute liver failure</u>, give anyway. Emerging data on role of NAc in non-paracetamol <u>acute liver failure</u>

Nitrates

The use of a topical nitrate (glyceryl trinitrate ointment 0.2–0.3% ointment) speeds healing of anal fissures but can cause systemic effects from vasodilatation such as headache in about 30%. Nitrates have also been used in the management of oesophageal spasm: in uncontrolled trials they can reduce pain and improve manometric parameters in some patients. Diltiazem ointment 2% is also effective in anal fissure, with fewer side-effects. There are currently no data showing convincing difference between GTN and diltiazem.

Octreotide (e.g. Sandostatin®, Lanreotide®, Somatostatin®)

GI indication	Metastatic <u>carcinoid</u>, <u>pancreatic endocrine tumours</u> (especially VIPoma), acute variceal bleeding
Mode of action	Mimics action of natural hormone—inhibits insulin, splanchnic blood flow, and gut hormones (e.g. glucagon, gastrin), and reduces gut motility
Dose/duration	Depends on drug formulation + indication: e.g.
	Metastatic carcinoid: octreotide 50 μg SC tds reduces diarrhoea in 50–83% patients and flushing in 50–100%. May be increased, depending on response. Long-acting octreotide LAR 10–30 mg monthly SC also effective
Contraindications	Contraindicated with cyclosporin. May require adjustment of dose of hypoglycaemic drugs
Side-effects	Abdominal symptoms in 5–10% (diarrhoea, pain, nausea), with increased risk of gallstones and biliary complications due to gallbladder hypomotility; hypo/hyperglycaemia; cardiac arryhythmia (e.g. bradycardia) reported.
Practice points	Case reports of benefit in managing pancreatic fistulae.
	Evidence of benefit in acute variceal bleeding inconclusive (most hepatologists only use as pharmacotherapy if contraindication to <u>TERLIPRESSIN</u>)

Opiates

(e.g. codeine, tramadol, pethidine, fentanyl, morphine)

GI indication	The many causes of <u>acute abdominal pain;</u> severe chronic pain not controlled by other measures (e.g. <u>chronic pancreatitis,</u> abdominal malignancy). Sedation for endoscopy. Weak opiates may help control diarrhoea
Mode of action	Act at various sites centrally (eg periaqueductal gray matter) and peripherally (e.g. peripheral afferent terminal) on a range of opiate receptors, and thought to facilitate endogenous release of endorphins and enkephalins, Neurotransmitter action of opioid peptides is inhibitory
Dose/duration	Preparation and dose depend on severity and cause of pain. Stepwise approach to <u>pain control</u> may include increasing from milder (e.g. codeine, tramadol), to more potent opiates (e.g. fentanyl, morphine): E.g.: • Codeine phosphate 30–60mg PO 4 hourly • Tramadol 50–100mg 4–6 hourly • Morphine sulphate 2.5 to 20 mg IM, IV, SC 2–6 hourly as required. IV/SC continuous infusion: 0.8–10 mg/hr. Morphine sulphate controlled release (e.g. Oramorph®) 15–16mg PO bd/tds • Fentanyl 25–100ug IV, 25–75ug transdermal patch (lasts 72 hours)
Contraindication	Known hypersensitivity. Caution in respiratory depression. Use may precipitate <u>hepatic encephalopathy</u> in patients with significant liver disease
Side effects	Respiratory and central nervous system depression. Vomiting. Reduced gastric emptying and gut hypomobility. Dry mouth. Itching. Addiction
Practice points	Involve <u>pain control</u> team early—in most hospitals in UK, now they are the most experienced in advising appropriate regimens. Dosing requirements may vary widely in an individual patient, and dose of opiate given should only be that sufficient to relieve pain. There is little literature to support traditional advice to avoid morphine in <u>acute pancreatitis</u> because it may worsen condition due to increased <u>sphincter of Oddi</u> contraction

Orlistat (Xenical®)

A lipase inhibitor that reduces absorption of dietary fat. Used in conjunction with a low calorie diet in obesity management. Indications are <u>body mass index</u> over 30 kg/m^2 or BMI over 28 kg/m^2 in the presence of other risk factors such as type 2 diabetes, hypertension, or hypercholesteraemia. Not licensed for longer than 2 years. Dose is 120 mg with each meal: max 360 mg/day. Side-effects include steatorrhoea, incontinence, and pain if fat intake is not reduced.

NICE guidance (2001) recommends:
- Only use if patient has lost 2.5 kg by diet/exercise in the previous month.
- Only use 18–75 years.
- Only continue beyond 3 months if weight loss is over 5% from start of treatment.

Pancreatic enzyme supplements

(e.g. Creon®, Pancrease®, Nutrizym®)

GI indication	Pancreatic insufficiency (e.g. due to chronic pancreatitis, cystic fibrosis, or extensive pancreatic resection)
Mode of action	Replaces deficient pancreatic enzymes, allowing digestion of starch, fat, protein
Dose/duration	E.g. Creon® 10 000 1–2 capsule with meals. Smaller dose with snacks Adjust dose according to response (e.g. resolution of steatorrhoea)
Contraindications	Fibrosing colonopathy using high dose supplements in children with cystic fibrosis, but not seen in adults, or with Creon® 25000 or less.
Side-effects	Nausea, abdominal discomfort. Perianal irritation at high dose
Practice points	Give pancreatic supplements with PROTON PUMP INHIBITOR, to reduce inactivation by gastric acidity. Faecal elastase measurement (see pancreatic function tests) provides good indicator of exocrine insufficiency, and assay not affected by concomitant pancreatic supplements

Piperacillin (Tazocin®)

GI indication	Severe intraabdominal infection/septicaemia (usually used as second-line therapy). Infective episodes after liver transplantation. Active against Gram-positive and Gram-negative aerobic and anaerobic bacteria
Mode of action	Bactericidal through inhibition of cell wall synthesis. Tazocin® also contains beta-lactamase inhibitor tazobactam
Dose/duration	4.5 g tds slow IV (over 3–5 minutes)
Contraindications	Penicillin hypersensitivity (but check what is being meant by this—non-specific antibiotic-related diarrhoea should not preclude using piperacillin for life-threatening sepsis, but angio-oedema/anaphylaxis clearly should).
Side-effects+ Interactions	Rash, urticaria, anaphylaxis, nausea, vomiting, diarrhoea, pseudomembranous colitis, abnormal liver function tests
Practice points	High doses may lead to ↑ serum Na^+

Prokinetics

- Metoclopramide and domperidone are dopamine-receptor antagonists that stimulate gastric emptying and small intestinal transit, and increase lower oesophageal sphincter tone. They are useful in some patients with non-ulcer dyspepsia, and are also effective anti-emetics. Domperidone does not cross the blood–brain barrier and has fewer side-effects than metaclopramide.
- Newer drugs. Prucalopride, a 5-HT4 agonist. facilitates cholinergic and non-adrenergic , non-cholinergic neurotransmission. It increases small and large bowel transit and results of a placebo-controlled trial suggest efficacy in both slow and normal transit constipation. Tegaserod is a partial 5-HT$_4$ agonist and improves symptoms in constipation-predominant IBS.

Propanolol

GI indication	Prophylaxis against first/recurrent variceal bleed in patients with <u>portal hypertension</u>
Mode of action	Non cardioselective β-blocker. Reduces portal pressure through reduction in portal and collateral blood flow
Dose/duration	40–80 mg bd PO (start at low dose and increase)
Contraindication	Congestive cardiac failure, bradycardia, hypotension, first degree heart block
Side-effects	Depression, impotence, nightmares, cold hands. Reduces warning signs of hypoglycaemia
Practice points	Effective primary + secondary prophylaxis (cheaper/safer/easier than variceal band ligation, but compliance uncertain). Checking resting heart rate useful means of assessing drug response /compliance (aim for 25% reduction in heart rate).

Proton pump inhibitors (PPIs)

(e.g. omeprazole, esomeprazole, lanzoprasole, rabeprazole, and pantoprazole)

GI indication	Effective short-term treatments for gastric and duodenal <u>peptic ulceration</u>
	Used in combination with antibiotics for <u>*Helicobacter*</u> eradication
	Useful in treating symptoms of gastro-oesophageal reflux and in maintenance treatment of ulcerative or stricturing oesophagitis, as well as in <u>Barrett's oesophagus</u>
	Used to prevent and treat NSAID-induced ulcers
	Effective in the treatment of hyperacidity in patients with <u>gastrinoma</u> (Zollinger–Ellison syndrome)
Mode of action	Irreversible blockade of the hydrogen–potassium adenosine triphosphatase system (the 'proton pump') of the gastric parietal cell
Dose/duration	Omeprazole 20 mg/day, lansoprazole 30 mg/day, pantoprazole 40 mg/day, rabeprazole 20 mg/day
	There is some evidence of dose response with high doses of omeprazole, which leads some to favour this agent in difficult reflux or in gastrinoma
Contraindication	No evidence of safety in pregnancy
Side-effects	Mild to moderate hypergastrinaemia has not been shown to predispose to gastric <u>carcinoids</u>
	Diarrhoea (some evidence that profound acid suppression can predispose to bacterial overgrowth)
	Abnormal liver function has been reported rarely
Practice points	All PPIs metabolized by cytochrome P450. Omeprazole has the greatest potential for drug interactions, and delays clearance of warfarin, diazepam, and phenytoin. Rabeprazole and pantoprazole interact to a lesser degree
	Best given immediately before meals (70% of proton pumps are secreting acid). Efficacy is relatively limited if administered in the fasting state (only 5% of proton pumps are active). 70% patients on bd PPI have nocturnal acid breakthrough (pH < 4 for > 1 h) which can be abolished in the short term by adding a histamine receptor antagonist

Ribavirin

GI indication	Hepatitis C
Mode of action	Guanosine analogue. No antiviral action given alone. Mechanism of benefit with <u>INTERFERON ALPHA</u> uncertain
Dose/duration	15 mg/kg or 800–1200 mg/day PO, with IFN/PEG IFN
Contraindication	Pregnancy, haemoglobinopathies (due to haemolysis, but use may be possible with careful monitoring), renal failure
Side-effects	Haemolysis (fall in Hb <10 g/dl in 14% of patients), teratogenicity, depression
Practice points	Ribavirin should not be given to female patient during or within 4 months of planned pregnancy, and males given ribavirin should use condoms during and for 6 months after treatment, and if partner pregnant

Serotonin (5HT$_3$)-receptor antagonists

(e.g. ondansetron, granisetron)

GI indication	Severe nausea and vomiting (e.g. associated with cancer therapy), post-operative, nausea/vomiting associated with <u>carcinoid</u> tumours
Mode of action	Blocking of 5HT$_3$-receptor dependent afferent impulses to vomiting centre in medulla
Dose/duration	Ondansetron: e.g. 8 mg PO tds during delayed phase of chemotherapy-induced nausea. 16 mg slow IV 1 hour pre-op Granisetron 2–9 mg PO/day in divided doses
Contraindication	Pregnancy/breast feeding, severe liver impairment
Side-effects	Constipation; headache; abdominal discomfort; prolonged QT on ECG.
Practice points	5HT$_3$-receptor antagonist-induced constipation may be severe, particularly in patients already on <u>OPIATES</u> for pain

Sucralfate

GI indication	<u>Gastritis</u>; <u>peptic ulceration</u>; post-variceal sclerother-apy/banding ulcers; radiation proctitis (see <u>radiation damage to the GI tract</u>)
Mechanism	A complex of aluminium hydroxide and sulphated sucrose and may act by forming a protective barrier against acid and other mucosal irritants
Dose/duration	For gastro-esophageal disease: 1 g qds PO Radiation proctitis: 2 g qds as enema
Contraindications	Caution in renal failure
Side-effects	It may rarely cause gastric bezoars and binds to some drugs including phenytoin and warfarin
Practice points	Separate administration from feed by > 1 hour

Tacrolimus/FK 506

GI indication	<u>Liver transplantation</u>. Possible alternative to <u>CYCLOSPORIN</u>. Has been used on trial basis in inflamma-tory bowel disease
Mode of action	Powerful immunosuppressant. Prevents T-cell activation by inhibiting the calcineurin pathway
Dose/duration	Oral tacrolimus (Prograf®) taken twice daily (usual dose 0.1 mg/kg/day, but doses vary based on maintaining trough blood levels at 5–10 ng/ml)
Contraindication	Avoid concomitant anti-lymphocyte therapy
Side-effects	Tremor, headache, paraesthesia. Renal toxicity. GI side-effects of diarrhoea, abdominal pain, and nausea. Like cyclosporin can cause eosinophilic colitis
Practice points	Tacrolimus is extensively metabolized via the hepatic micro-somal cytochrome P450. Concomitant inhibitors or inducers of cytochrome P450 may affect tacrolimus blood levels

Terlipressin (Glypressin®)

GI indication	Acute variceal bleeding (see Acute upper GI bleeding + portal hypertension). Type 1 hepatorenal syndrome in patients with decompensated liver disease
Mode of action	Longer-acting synthetic analogue of vasopressin. Peripheral and splanchnic vasoconstrictor. Reduces splanchnic blood flow and portal hypertension. Increased systemic vascular resistance may improve renal blood flow
Dose/duration	1–2 mg IV 4–6 hourly (slow peripheral injection)
Contraindication	Documented hypersensitivity; coronary artery disease; severe arrhythmias; MI; stroke. Drug effect may be potentiated by carbamazepine, chlorpropamide
Side-effects	Vascular complications (e.g., myocardial infarction, arrhythmia, mesenteric/peripheral ischaemia, pulmonary oedema, stroke). Vertigo, migraine, bronchoconstriction, abdominal cramps, nausea, and vomiting
Practice points	Reduces mortality in acute variceal bleeding. Avoid in patients with known arteriosclerosis or coronary artery disease (check ECG prior to administration in all). If contraindicated, OCTREOTIDE is an alternative

Ursodeoxycholic acid (UCDA)

(e.g. UrsoFalk®)

GI indication	Primary sclerosing cholangitis (PSC), primary biliary cirrhosis (PBC), obstetric cholestasis, Biliary stone disease (see practice points)
Mode of action	Displaces endogenous bile acids from enterohepatic circulation, and stabilizes hepatocellular membranes. Promotes bile flow
Dose/duration	15–30 mg/kg/day in divided doses
Contraindications	May reduce absorption of aluminium-based antacids, cholestyramine, or oral contraceptive pill
Side-effects	Fatigue, headache, rash, nausea, vomiting, dyspepsia, metallic taste, abdominal pain, biliary pain, diarrhoea, myalgia.
Practice points	UCDA improves liver biochemistry, but ongoing debate as to whether it improves natural history of PSC and PBC. In PSC, higher dose (e.g. 20 mg/kg/day) may be associated with reduced progression of liver fibrosis and colonic dysplasia/malignancy. Low rate of stone dissolution, but often used in patients with recurrent intrahepatic biliary stones

Emergencies

Acute abdominal pain

Acute abdominal pain is a common reason for casualty presentation ('the acute abdomen') and for patients to require review on the wards. The duration of pain that defines it as acute is ill-defined, but would usually be no more than a few days. With a huge range of causes of GI and non-GI causes of abdominal pain (see box), many of which may present acutely, the challenge is in making a differential diagnosis on the basis of history and examination, so allowing investigations to be tailored to the specific clinical setting.

Clinical assessment

- Ask about the following aspects of the pain:
    - **Site.** Particular intra-abdominal organs and diseases tend to produce pain localized to particular abdominal segments (see figure in <u>Approach to chronic or recurrent abdominal pain</u>).
    - **Character.** Colic tends to wax and wane, in a regular manner, due to spasm in a muscular viscus (e.g. gallbladder, ureter, small bowel); in peritonitis the pain is often constant and unremitting, and the patient wishes to lie still. Pain arising from the abdominal viscera tends to be largely midline, dull in nature, and poorly localized. Inflammation of the parietal peritoneum tends to be sharper, well localized, and exacerbated by movement.
    - **Onset, severity, and duration.**
    - **Radiation.** Right shoulder tip in <u>cholecystitis</u>; through to the back in <u>acute pancreatitis</u>.
    - **Relieving and exacerbating factors.**
- Ask about associated symptoms.
    - Is there a history of faeculent vomiting and absolute constipation, suggesting bowel obstruction?
- Take a full genitourinary and gynaecological history.
- Have there been previous episodes, and has a diagnosis been made? Any previous surgery (e.g. adhesions, <u>Crohn's disease</u>)?
- Do other medical problems provide hints to diagnosis (e.g. arteriopathy with AF and acute abdominal pain:may suggest <u>intestinal ischaemia</u>).

A full **examination** is essential, including assessment of vital signs and evidence of hypovolaemia or shock. See <u>Approach to GI examination</u>. In generalized peritonitis there may be rigidity, guarding, and rebound tenderness. **Never forget** to examine for inguinal and supraclavicular lymph nodes, hernial orifices, femoral pulses, external genitalia, bowel sounds (may be absent in peritonitis/ileus, tympanitic in obstruction), bruits, and to do a rectal examination.

Causes of acute abdominal pain

Note: some conditions can present recurrently!

Generalized parietal pain due to peritonitis

- Perforated viscus–<u>peptic ulceration</u>, gallbladder (see <u>gallbladder empyema</u>), <u>diverticulum</u>
- Bacterial peritonitis (and <u>spontaneous bacterial peritonitis</u>)
- Ruptured intra-abdominal cyst
- <u>Familial Mediterranean fever</u>

Localized peritoneal pain

- <u>Appendicitis</u>, <u>cholecystitis</u>, regional enteritis, colitis, abdominal abscess, <u>acute pancreatitis</u>, hepatitis, lymphadenitis, endometriosis, <u>diverticulitis</u>.

Pain from increased tension in viscera

- Intestinal obstruction (mechanical, intussusception, internal herniation)
- Intestinal hypermotility
- Biliary obstruction (<u>choledocholithiasis</u>)
- Ureteric obstruction
- Hepatic capsule distension (e.g. <u>liver abscess</u>, <u>hepatocellular carcinoma</u>)
- Renal capsule distension
- Ectopic pregnancy
- Abdominal aortic aneurysm

Ischaemia

- <u>Intestinal ischaemia</u> (arterial stenosis, embolism, inflammation)
- Splenic infarction, hepatic infarction
- Torsion (gallbladder, cyst, omentum, <u>volvulus</u>, appendix)
- Tissue necrosis

Retroperitoneal causes

- Tumours (e.g. <u>pancreatic cancer</u>)
- Retroperitoneal abscess
- <u>Acute/chronic pancreatitis</u>

Extra-abdominal

- Thoracic (pulmonary embolus, empyema, myocardial infarction, <u>oesophagitis</u>, basal pneumonia)
- Neurological (neurogenic tumours, spinal degenerative disease, herpes zoster)
- Metabolic (diabetic ketoacidosis, acute intermittent <u>porphyria</u>, uraemia, hypercalcaemia)
- Haematological (<u>sickle cell anaemia</u>, <u>Henoch–Schönlein purpura</u>, vasculitis)
- Poisoning (e.g. lead)

Investigations

Specific investigations will be tailored to the differential diagnosis arising from initial assessment, but in most cases will include:

- Blood tests
  - FBC + differential (raised neutrophils suggest inflammation, infection, mesenteric infarction, but may be normal in elderly).
  - U&Es, glucose.
  - <u>Liver function tests</u>: AST/ALT > 1000 IU/l usually due to drugs (e.g. paracetamol), acute viral <u>hepatitis</u>, or hepatic ischaemia.
  - <u>Amylase</u> (elevated in many causes of abdominal pain; only indicative of <u>acute pancreatitis</u> if > 5× ULN).
  - ESR/CRP. If significantly elevated suggests inflammation/infection. Also classically elevated in <u>familial Mediterranean fever</u>. CRP of prognostic use in <u>acute pancreatitis</u>.
  - Arterial blood gases (metabolic acidosis?).
  - Blood cultures.
  - Group + save if laparotomy or transfusion requirement possible.
- Urine β-HCG pregnancy test in women of child-bearing age (ectopic pregnancy?).
- Urinalysis ± MSU.
- Erect CXR (air under diaphragm due to viscus perforation?).
- Supine AXR (often non-contributory, but may show bowel dilatation (2.5 cm small bowel, 6 cm colon) ± air–fluid levels in obstruction).
- Abdominal U/S. Useful in patients with acute abdominal pain for exclusion of acute cholecystitis and biliary obstruction, detection of abdominal fluid and collections, and assessment of organomegaly, masses, and aortic aneurysms.
- Abdominal CT. More sensitive than U/S in most circumstances (except <u>gallstones</u>), and allows much better views of pancreas and retroperitoneum.
- Diagnostic laparoscopy may have a role in the investigation of acute abdominal pain associated with abdominal trauma, or in women with unexplained right iliac fossa pain, but is contraindicated in peritonitis, obstruction, or intra-abdominal adhesions.

Management

A clear diagnosis may not possible on basis of initial assessment and investigations. Specific treatment will be largely determined by differential diagnosis (see A–Z section according to diagnoses) and process underlying acute abdominal pain.

- If evidence of peritonitis, viscus perforation, or obstruction, need urgent surgical involvement. If laparotomy may be required, ensure that blood available, and CXR/ECG performed beforehand.
- Keep NBM.
- Obtain IV access and resuscitate with colloid/crystalloid/blood according to degree of hypovolaemia, and blood loss. If evidence of shock, give 500 ml colloid (e.g. Haemaccel) or crystalloid (e.g. 0.9% N saline) stat, and monitor response (HR, BP, CVP). Repeat as necessary.

- Insert central line if evidence of shock, requirement for significant fluid replacement, and/or underlying cardiovascular disease.
- Pass nasogastric tube if evidence of obstruction, and keep on free drainage.
- Insert urinary catheter and monitor hourly output.
- After taking blood cultures, give 3rd generation CEPHALOSPORIN (e.g. cefotaxime 1 g tds IV) and METRONIDAZOLE 500 mg tds IV.
- Pain of peritonitis may be severe, and analgesia should not be withheld for fear of 'masking' clinical features. Opiates (e.g. diamorphine 5–10 mg IV 4 hourly or pethidine 50–100 mg IM 4 hourly, given with METOCLOPRAMIDE 10 mg IV/IM or cyclizine 50 mg IV/IM tds) may be required.
- Laparotomy is generally indicated for patients with generalized peritonitis related to a viscus perforation (e.g. duodenal ulcer), or following organ rupture (e.g. spleen, aorta).

Where a definitive diagnosis cannot be made, a fundamental aspect of management is patient review and reassessment of clinical course and response to initial treatment.

Acute diarrhoea

Diarrhoea can constitute an emergency in three clinical situations.

Acute watery diarrhoea. This is usually due to infection (see Approach to acute diarrhoea).

Common causes
- Viruses. Rotavirus in infants and young children can cause profound dehydration. The illness typically lasts about 7 days. Adenovirus infection can last longer
- In adults, enterotoxigenic *Escherichia coli* (ETEC).
- Food borne pathogens (see food poisoning).
  - Bacteria that colonize the gut: *Salmonella*, *Campylobacter*, entero-haemorrhagic *E. coli*, *Vibrio parahaemolyticus*, *Yersinia*, *Clostridium perfringens*.
  - Preformed toxins: *Staphyllococcus aureus*, *Bacillus cereus*, *Clostridium botulinum*.
- Invasive pathogens and protozoa can produce watery diarrhoea in the initial stages.

Diarrhoea with blood
Making a diagnosis is important because of the importance of differentiating infection from inflammatory bowel disease and other disorders. Differential diagnosis includes:
- Invasive infectious diarrhoea (dysentery): *Shigella*, *Salmonella*, *Campylobacter*, EHEC, and the protozoan *Entamoeba* histolytica.
- Inflammatory bowel disease (ulcerative colitis, Crohn's).
- Ischaemic colitis.
- Radiation colitis.
- Colorectal cancer.
- Diverticular disease.
- Intussusception.

Toxic dilatation
Acute dilatation of the colon (**transverse colon diameter > 6 cm on plain abdominal X-ray**) occurs in
- Severe ulcerative colitis or colonic Crohn's disease.
- Infectious colitis.
- Acute distal obstruction (volvulus or carcinoma).
- Acute pseudo-obstruction (see Ogilvie's syndrome).

Management

Resuscitate the patient

- Oral rehydration is the mainstay of managing acute watery diarrhoea (see oral rehydration solutions). The World Health Organization oral rehydration solution (sodium concentration 90 mM, osmolality 331 mOsm/kg) is recommended to give adequate glucose source for the sodium–glucose co-transporter and may be necessary if there is a short bowel or jejunostomy: in children with acute diarrhoea, the recommendation is for a sodium concentration of about 50 mM (see Approach to acute diarrhoea).

Making a diagnosis

Clinical examination

This may not yield the diagnosis but it's important to look for signs of **dehydration** and **metabolic acidosis** (textbooks always say look for a dry tongue, loss of skin turgor, and tachycardia, but these are unreliable: the best sign to look for is a **postural drop in BP**). Look also for signs of inflammatory bowel disease (perianal disease, pyoderma, oral ulceration) or signs of immunosuppression (oral candidiasis, Kaposi's sarcoma, leucoplakia). A toxic dilated colon is usually accompanied by fever, tachycardia, and neutrophilia.

Investigations

Blood tests

- Distinguishing infection from non-specific inflammatory bowel disease is important but can take several days. Most cases of acute infective diarrhoea are self-limiting, providing attention is paid to restoring fluid balance.
- **Dehydration:** haemoconcentration with raised haemoglobin, increased packed cell volume, and a raised blood urea.
- **Acidosis:** raised venous bicarbonate, decreased arterial pH, and base excess.
- **Inflammation:** anaemia, raised neutrophil count, and elevated inflammatory markers (ESR, CRP, platelets).
- **Magnesium and potassium** losses can become significant in severe diarrhoea.
- **Eosinophilia** accompanies helminthic infections of the gut, although only stronglyoides, trichinella and schistosoma are associated with diarrhoea (see eosinophilia and the GI tract).

Microbiological examination of the stool

This is the usual way of making a diagnosis of infection, but the delay is always 1–2 days and often longer for slow growing organisms.

- Faecal antigen ELISAs are available for _Giardia_ and rotavirus.
- DNA probes often do not work on crude faecal extracts but can help in characterizing bacterial isolates.
- Stool culture, faecal _Clostridium difficile_ assay (ask for both A and B toxins: see Clostridial infections of the GI tract) and blood cultures should be sent.
- Anti-microbial chemotherapy is indicated for dysenteric infections such as amoebiasis, shigellosis, and pseudomembranous colitis: see Approach to acute diarrhoea.

Radiological imaging

A **plain abdominal X-ray** can help in assessing intestinal inflammation and is also useful in excluding free air as a result of bowel perforation.

- A gas-filled colon devoid of faeces suggests a total colitis.
- Loss of haustration and dilatation indicate severe inflammation.
- There may be mutiple small bowel fluid levels and small bowel dilatation (indicating partial ileus rather than obstruction).

Abdominal ultrasound can reveal bowel wall thickening and enlarged lymph nodes.

Endoscopy

Sigmoidoscopy can be highly informative, demonstrate a colitis, and allows biopsy, which may be of help in differentiating infection from inflammation; appearances of amoebic colitis, ischaemic colitis, radiation colitis, and pseudomembranous colitis can be diagnostic. **Total colonoscopy** is usually not necessary and may be risky.

Common mistakes and important points in early management

- Always think of **acute megacolon due to toxic dilatation.** If there is any abdominal tenderness or sign of systemic upset, get a plain abdominal X-ray.
- If the patient is unwell **frequent review** by a senior clinician is essential, as is a **surgical opinion**.
- Intravenous fluids. Keep **potassium** above 4.0 mmol/L.
- Monitor FBC, electrolytes, and colonic diameter on daily X-rays.
- Stop any drugs that may be contributing to colonic paralysis, especially opiates and anti-diarrhoeal agents.
- **Avoid NSAIDs.** They can aggravate diarrhoea and have profound effects on reducing renal cortical blood flow, which can precipitate renal failure in hypovolaemia or patients with pre-existing kidney disease.
- In cases of fulminant colitis or toxic dilatation of the colon, the decision to proceed to colectomy can be difficult: useful indicators are:
  - Increasing tachycardia and fever.
  - Failure to improve clinically or radiologically (i.e. colon diameter decreasing) after 24 hours.
  - Signs of perforation (these may be very minimal: steroids mask physical signs of perforation).
  - Mucosal islands seen on X-ray.

Complications

Worldwide the majority of deaths result from dehydration and acidosis. Complications of infection, especially by invasive pathogens, include:

- Haemolytic–uraemic syndrome.
- Non-septic arthritis and Reiter's syndrome.
- Guillain–Barré syndrome.
- Septic arthritis.

Acute liver failure

Definition

Development of <u>hepatic encephalopathy </u>(HE) within 12 weeks of onset of jaundice in patient with no history of liver disease. Subdivided into 'hyperacute' and 'subacute' ALF, with intervals from jaundice to HE of < 7 days and 5–12 weeks respectively. Previous definition of ALF extended only up to 8 weeks, with no subdivision.

Clinical syndrome

ALF is a systemic condition, characterized by:
- **Hepatic encephalopathy/cerebral oedema.** All patients with ALF have <u>HE</u> due mainly to poor liver function and cerebral oedema (present in > 80% of comatose patients as main causes), rather than <u>portal hypertension</u>.
- **Acute renal failure.** Occurs in > 50% of ALF cases, including toxin-related acute tubular necrosis (e.g. <u>paracetamol overdose</u>), renal vasculitic injury (e.g. <u>leptospirosis</u>) or type 1 <u>hepatorenal syndrome</u>, as a consequence of the severity of liver injury (also see <u>Approach to cirrhosis and chronic liver disease</u>).
- **Metabolic derangement.** Hypoglycaemia is common, and may be confused for encephalopathy. Metabolic acidosis common following <u>paracetamol overdose</u>, but carries poor prognosis whatever the cause (day 3 Ph < 7.3 predicts > 90% mortality without <u>liver transplantation</u> after paracetamol overdose). ↑Serum lactate may reflect tissue hypoxaemia.
- **Haemodynamic changes.** Characterized by peripheral vasodilatation and hyperdynamic circulation (i.e. ↑HR, ↓systemic vascular resistance (SVR), ↑cardiac output (CO), ↓mean arterial pressure (MAP)). May mask/mimic changes of systemic sepsis.
- **Pulmonary complications** occur in 50% due to range of causes: effects of cerebral oedema; gastric aspiration in confused/comatose patient; pneumonia; non-cardiogenic pulmonary oedema (especially with <u>paracetamol overdose</u>).
- **Infection** is very common and often clinically masked due to ALF. In patients with ALF and > grade 1 encephalopathy, >80% have bacterial infections, > 30% fungal infection (e.g. *Candida albicans, Aspergillus* spp), and infection associated with 50% of ALF deaths.
- **Haematological abnormalities.** Prothrombin time (PT) is one of best indicators of severity of liver failure (after exclusion of vitamin K deficiency); platelets < 100×10^9/l in 70%.

Causes of acute liver failure

Cause	Diagnosis in ALF	Comments
Hepatitis A	Anti-HAV IgM	Possible increased rate of ALF in hepatitis A in association with chronic hepatitis C
Hepatitis B	IgM Anti-HB core (HBsAg may be –ve in ALF)	ALF in 1% of acute infections. May occur with hepatitis D virus infection
Hepatitis C	HCV RNA (anti-HCV Ab often -ve)	Extremely rarely causes ALF
Hepatitis E	Anti-HEV	ALF in 20% of women infected in pregnancy in S Asia
Other infection (e.g. EBV, HSV, leptospirosis)	e.g. anti-Leptospira IgM, anti-HSV IgM, anti-EBV VCA IgM	
Paracetamol overdose (acetaminophen)	Blood levels	Commonest cause of ALF in UK
Drug reactions: e.g. NSAIDs, isoniazid, rifampicin, herbal remedies, 'ecstasy'	Drug history, eosinophils Blood/urine analysis	See drug-induced hepatotoxicity
Toxins (e.g. *Amanita phalloides* mushrooms)	History of ingestion	
Acute fatty liver of pregnancy	History, bloods	Mainly clinical diagnosis. See A–Z entry
HELLP syndrome	History, bloods	Mainly clinical diagnosis. See A–Z entry
Wilson's disease	Urinary copper, caeruloplasmin	Usually presents with ALF < 20 years of age
Hepatic ischaemia	↑AST/ALT (> 1000 U/L), imaging	Especially following episode of hypotension
Budd–Chiari syndrome	Imaging	May present with ascites
Autoimmune hepatitis	AutoAbs, Igs	20% of patients present with jaundice, but ALF unusual
Malignant infiltration	Imaging, histology	
'Seronegative hepatitis'	All above excluded	Approximately 20% of cases

Making the diagnosis

- ALF is a clinical diagnosis, based on demonstrating HE in a patient with acute liver disease. Presence of liver disease usually obvious from initial assessment and blood results (↑ bilirubin, ↑ PT, ↓ serum albumin are best blood markers of significant liver disease). See also Approach to recent-onset jaundice. Differentiating ALF from an acute presentation of decompensated chronic liver disease may be difficult, but important, as management and prognosis very different. Is there any history/ documentation to suggest more chronic disease (chat to GP/review hospital notes/check historical blood results)? Are there physical signs suggestive of chronic liver disease (e.g. spider naevi, Dupuytren's contracture, clubbing, leuconychia). Evidence of portal hypertension (splenomegaly, dilated superficial veins) is unusual in ALF.

Finding the cause (see table on previous page)

- May be obvious, but information from patient, relatives, medical attendants is vital, including: drugs (prescribed/recreational/herbal); risk of hepatitis (unprotected sex/IVDU/hepatitis contact/foreign travel/ tattoo/piercing); autoimmune diseases (e.g. thyroid/rheumatoid). Any evidence of hypotensive episode (e.g. recent surgery/↓ BP on obstetric chart/bleed/adverse cardiac event)? Any history of thrombosis or prothrombotic tendency (e.g. anti-phospholipid syndrome), precipitating Budd–Chiari syndrome?
- Breadth of investigation of cause dependent on clinical scenario (e.g. low yield on leptospira serology in 80 year old with ALF following prolonged cardiac arrest!).

Management

Optimal management depends on strict general supportive measures; consideration of specific treatments (e.g. N-acetylcysteine); defining prognosis and need for liver unit referral ± liver transplantation.

General approach

- Management in ITU/HDU setting.
- Pass urinary catheter and monitor hourly urine output.
- Monitor vital signs (HR/BP/temp) ½–2 hourly.
- Daily bloods for FBC, U&E, bicarb, glucose, clotting, LFTs.
- Culture blood, urine, sputum, even if afebrile. CXR.
- Investigate cause of ALF as directed by history (see above and table). Note that paracetamol levels may be apparently subtoxic by the time of development of ALF. ↑↑ALT/AST > 1000 U/l most likely due to hepatic ischaemia, acute viral hepatitis, or drugs.
- Discuss with specialist liver unit **early**. Detailed referral criteria vary according to cause and type of ALF, but broadly include any of the following: PT > 30s; hepatic encephalopathy; creatinine > 200 µmol/l; hypoglycaemia; metabolic acidosis—pH < 7.3. If in doubt, ask: every unit prefers an unnecessary call to a late call for patients with ALF.

- Avoid all potentially hepatotoxic drugs (e.g. NSAIDs), and those that worsen complications of ALF (e.g. ACE-inhibitors, opiates).
- Maintain nutrition, as ALF catabolic state. NG feeding preferable, as may prevent bacterial translocation, but ileus may preclude this.
- CVP for fluid monitoring (correction of coagulopathy not needed if internal jugular approach used and experienced technician).
- Ensure adequate intravascular filling with colloid, crystalloid, blood products. If mean arterial pressure (MAP) < 60 mmHg despite filling consider noradrenaline 0.2–1.8 mg/kg/min, but specialist inotrope management will be required.
- Monitor blood glucose, and give 10–20% dextrose infusions if hypoglycaemic.
- N-ACETYLCYSTEINE may be of benefit even in non-paracetamol-induced ALF, including hepatic ischaemia.
- Vitamin K 10 mg IV/day for 3 days (but usually has no effect on PT, unless vitamin K deficiency related to prolonged biliary obstruction). PT/INR very useful markers of clinical course/prognosis, so only give fresh frozen plasma (FFP) if actively bleeding. Maintain platelet count > 20 × 10^9/l with infusions.
- Acid suppression reduces risk of haemorrhagic gastritis. Usually give oral/NG PPI (e.g. omeprazole 20 mg od), although clear evidence relates to IV H2-receptor antagonists.
- Prophylactic broad-spectrum IV antibiotics reduce frequency of infections but not mortality, and are associated with resistant organisms, but are nevertheless often given. Prophylactic fluconazole ± liposomal amphotericin reduces risk of systemic fungal infection (see ANTIFUNGALS). Irrespective of use of antimicrobial prophylaxis, meticulous nursing and care of lines/pressure areas, etc. are essential.

Specific management

Cerebral oedema/hepatic encephalopathy
- Consider CT brain scan to exclude cerebral bleed.
- 20% Mannitol 0.5 g/kg IV bolus, repeated as necessary (but not if serum osmolality > 320 mOsm/l).
- Have a low threshold for intubation/mechanical ventilation in view of risk of aspiration and agitation in patients with cerebral oedema/ encephalopathy.
- Controlled hyperventilation may help to control surges of raised intra cranial pressure (ICP) in patients unresponsive to mannitol.
- In specialist unit, ICP monitor may be inserted in comatose patient, to accurately measure degree of cerebral oedema (but risk–benefit ratio of ICP monitoring much debated).
- Avoid sedatives (e.g. benzodiazepines, opiates).
- N-ACETYLCYSTEINE infusion in paracetamol-related ALF has been shown to reduce signs of cerebral oedema.

Renal failure
- Important to involve renal team early.
- Management includes stopping all potentially nephrotoxic drugs; correcting hypovolaemia; excluding and treating infection.
- Patient may require continuous haemofiltration. Standard indications include K^+ > 6.0 mmol/l, bicarb < 15 mmol/l, creatine > 400 µmol/l, but may be considered earlier in patient with liver and renal failure, as associated with less haemodynamic instability.

Artificial liver support
- Range of <u>liver support devices</u> and techniques have been developed over last 30 years to act as 'bridge' to <u>liver transplantation</u>, or even to allow time for native liver to spontaneously recover. None reliably effective to date, but search goes on.

Prognosis and liver transplantation

- Spontaneous recovery more likely with hyperacute than subacute presentation. In patients with ALF and grade III–IV hepatic encephalopathy treated with medical therapy alone, survival 10–40%.
- With <u>liver transplantation</u>, survival from ALF now 60–80%. This reinforces need to discuss case early, and consider liver transplantation criteria (see <u>liver transplantation</u>).

Acute lower gastrointestinal bleeding

Definition

Blood originating from below the ligament of Treitz (often quoted landmark: a fibromuscular band that originates from the right diaphragmatic crus and fixes the duodenal–jejunal flexure).

Clinical presentation

- Blood in the stool implies a lower GI cause unless there is very rapid bleeding from an upper GI source (this will produce haemodynamic instability and usually a raised blood urea).
- Blood in the bowel for over about 14 hours is converted to black melaena: up to 35% of patients with melaena have a bleeding point distal to duodenal–jejunal flexure.
- The patient may be hypotensive and shocked without overt evidence of bleeding: do a rectal exam.

Diagnosis

History

There may be a history of haemorrhoids, inflammatory bowel disease, radiation, or iatrogenic causes (bleeding from polypectomy can be delayed up to 10 days).

- Ask about prior episodes, presence of liver or renal disease, drug usage (anti-platelet drugs, NSAIDs, warfarin).
- Ask whether the blood is mixed with or separate from the stool (bright red blood suggests an anorectal cause) and about an associated change in bowel habit.
- In the West, common causes include bleeding from <u>diverticula</u> (40%), inflammatory bowel disease including infectious and ischaemic colitis as well as Crohn's and ulcerative colitis (20%), benign anorectal disease (10%), and arteriovenous malformations including <u>angiodysplasia</u>.

Rare causes include radiation, <u>Meckel's diverticulum</u>, and varices.

Management

Most (90%) lower GI bleeds stop spontaneously: 35% need transfusing; 5% need urgent surgery. Resuscitation is as for <u>acute upper GI bleeds</u>: there is usually time to transfuse if necessary and correct clotting abnormalities. Investigation of a stable patient gives a better chance of effective diagnosis and therapy.

Investigation

In patients who stop bleeding spontaneously, elective colonoscopy after routine preparation is indicated. In continued bleeding, urgent diagnosis is needed. If there is doubt about a lower GI source of the bleeding, upper GI endoscopy can be useful. Simple sigmoidoscopy may be useful if there is a perianal or rectal source, but for most colonic bleeding, colonoscopy is required (more sensitive than barium, and allows biopsy and therapy)

Colonoscopy in acute lower GI haemorrhage. Intestinal lavage using nasogastric intubation followed by giving 2–4 litres of an osmotic laxative such as Kleenprep allows adequate preparation. The traditional view that colonoscopy is impractical in severe bleeding is wrong, provided rapid cleansing is used (Jensen, DM and Machicado, GA. (1988) *Gastro-enterology* **95**: 1569). Angiography offers accurate diagnosis and therapy if the bleeding is brisk (over about 3 ml/min).

Treatment For in depth review see Zuckerman, GR and Prakash, C. 1999 *Gastrointest. Endosc.* **49**: 228.

- **Electrocoagulation or mechanical endoscopic techniques** (clipping, placing of loops around bleeding vessels) at colonoscopy can be useful for bleeding angiodysplasia and arterial lesions.
- Intra-arterial **vasopressin** stops bleeding from diverticula and angiodysplasia in 90% but has a complication rate of 5–15% (cardiovascular toxicity, indwelling catheter). Its use is not recommended.
- **Selective embolization** can be very effective in expert hands.
- **Surgery**. The success and postoperative bleeding rate depends on accurate pre-operative localization. Mortality in recent series is 5–10%.

Acute upper gastrointestinal bleeding

Definitions

Haematemesis refers to the vomiting of blood. Occurs in 40–50% of cases of upper GI bleeding, and indicative of bleeding point proximal to jejunum. Melaena stool is black, tarry, and smells sickly sweet. Occurs in 70–80% of upper GI bleeds. Usually results from bleeding proximal to caecum, but may sometimes occur in colonic bleeding, particularly from right colon. Haematochezia refers to red blood per rectum.

Causes of acute upper GI bleeding

- <u>Peptic ulceration</u> (25–50% of cases of non-variceal upper GI bleeding)
- Gastroesophageal varices (5% of cases, but 80% of deaths due to acute upper GI bleeding—also see <u>portal hypertension</u>)
- <u>Gastritis</u>/gastric erosions
- <u>Oesophagitis</u>
- Duodenitis
- <u>Mallory–Weiss</u> tear
- <u>Gastric antral vascular ectasia</u> (GAVE) ('watermelon stomach')
- <u>Dieulafoy lesions</u>
- <u>Hereditary haemorrhagic telangiectasia</u> ('Osler–Weber–Rendu syndrome')
- <u>Gastrointestinal stromal tumour</u> (<u>GIST</u>)
- <u>Angiodysplasia</u>
- Portal hypertensive gastropathy
- Upper GI tumours (e.g. <u>oesophageal</u>, <u>gastric cancer</u>)
- <u>Aorto-enteric fistula</u>
- Causes of <u>haemobilia</u>

Initial assessment and management

Estimate extent of blood loss

- Ask about the duration of bleeding; the volume, colour, and frequency of melaena or haematemesis (e.g. 'two cupfuls, bright red vomit'); was there associated dizziness, lightheadedness, shortness of breath, altered consciousness (suggesting large bleed)? 1000 ml of blood represents 20% of blood volume.

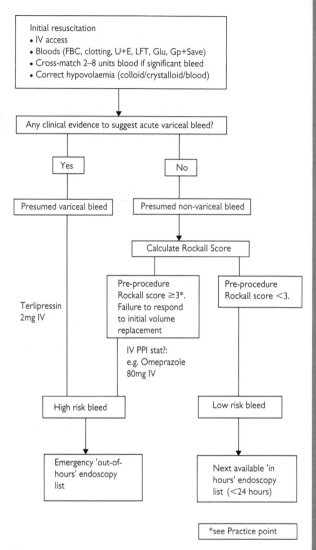

Fig. 4.1 Initial management in acute upper GI bleeding.

- Has blood loss been witnessed? 'Coffee ground vomit'—see it for yourself, as any dark vomitus tends to get this label, and dip-stick tests for blood are useless, as almost always positive. Check what's being meant by 'melaena' (examine bedpan, do rectal examination), as term often wrongly used to refer to any blood per rectum). Haematochezia in presence of haematemesis suggests large bleed and rapid luminal transit.
- Look for signs of hypovolaemia (pallor, cool peripheries, weak pulse, HR > 100 bpm, ↓BP, ↓JVP, confusion, ↑respiratory rate). Measure postural drop in BP (> 10 mmHg fall after standing for 30 s), but not in shocked patient who is hypotensive even when supine, as may precipitate cerebral hypoperfusion.

Initial resuscitation

- Establish good IV access (preferably ×2 14–16G cannulae in antecubital fossae—not a single 20G line in dorsum of the hand).
- Send bloods for: FBC, clotting, U&Es, LFTs, glucose, group and save. Note that Hb and haematocrit may not fall immediately, due to loss of whole blood, with fall only occurring after reactive plasma volume expansion and haemodilution. If significant bleed cross-match 2–8 units, according to severity, and always have 2 units available for patient with ongoing bleeding.
- If hypovolaemic give 500 ml of crystalloid (e.g. 0.9% saline) or colloid (e.g. Haemaccel®, Gelofusin®), and review haemodynamic response. Repeat if necessary whilst waiting for blood. Remember that colloid/crystalloid causes haemodilution (approximately 10% fall in Hb for each litre of fluid), and that the patient is hypovolaemic due to blood loss, which may need to be replaced. Nevertheless, only in very rare circumstances of massive exsanguinating blood loss and delayed availability of cross-matched blood, does use of un-crossmatched, blood (group O Rh neg), need to be considered.
- Do not attempt CVP line insertion prior to initial volume expansion, as wastes time and failure/complications (e.g. pneumothorax, carotid artery puncture) more likely. Initially use large-bore peripheral cannulae. However, subsequent central line insertion should be considered for those with major haemorrhage at presentation, especially in association with cardiac failure/ischaemic heart disease, renal failure, failure to respond to resuscitation, or inadequate venous access.
- Insert urinary catheter in patients with a large bleed, haemodynamic compromise, or evidence of renal impairment. Monitor hourly output.

- Monitor vital signs ¼ –2 hourly, dependent on haemodynamic stability.
- Transfuse up to a Hb of 10 g/dl. Ensure repeat clotting is checked after 4 units of blood are given and correct clotting accordingly.
- Ensure that nursing staff know to keep the patient nil by mouth.

Establish likely cause of bleed

- Important to identify patients with suspected variceal bleed. (see below)
- Ask about a history of liver disease and varices, or risk factors: alcohol excess; previous jaundice; abdominal surgery/pancreatitis. Thrombophilia may suggest portal vein thrombosis. Unexplained thrombocytopenia may point to hypersplenism due to portal hypertension.
- Consider non-variceal causes: ask about previous episodes (? angiodysplasia); preceding epigastric pain (? peptic ulceration); reflux symptoms (? oesophagitis); weight loss, fatigue (? malignancy); medication (e.g. aspirin, NSAIDs, SSRIs, warfarin, heparin); surgery (? aortic graft, with risk of aorto-enteric fistula); timing of bleeding (e.g. haematemesis after episodes of retching suggests Mallory–Weiss tear).
- On examination look for signs of liver disease (e.g. jaundice, clubbing, palmar erythema, spider naevi, tattoos, splenomegaly, ascites, hepatic encephalopathy). Hints to non-variceal causes include mucosal telangiectasia (hereditary haemorrhagic telangiectasia), left supraclavicular lymph node (Virchow's node—suggests gastric/oesophageal cancer); scars of previous abdominal surgery.

Decide on likeliest cause

- Non-variceal acute upper GI bleed.
- Variceal acute upper GI bleed.

Suspected non-variceal acute upper GI bleed

Ongoing management

- 80% of non-variceal bleeds settle spontaneously.
- Rockall score (see table) predicts risk of mortality, and so allows stratification into low- and high-risk bleeds.
- Calculate pre-endoscopy Rockall score. If score 0–2 arrange endoscopy on next available 'in hours' list (may even discharge score 0 patients). If ≥3 patient has had a high risk bleed.
- Inform on-call surgical team early about all high-risk bleeds (and encourage them to witness endoscopy—will focus minds if surgery needs to be considered).

Endoscopy

- Definitive procedure to make diagnosis and treat, and most accurately predicts prognosis (based on final Rockall score and Forrest classification—see below). Do not perform endoscopy before attempts to adequately resuscitate.

- Emergency out-of-hours endoscopy indicated in all high-risk bleeds: pre-endoscopy Rockall score ≥3 (with provisos—see practice point); suspected variceal bleed; or in any patient with large bleed and persistent hypovolaemia despite 4 units of blood/fluid.
  - Endoscopic therapy indicated in patients with active bleeding or stigmata of recent haemorrhage (see Forrest classification below).
  - Two modalities of endotherapy are most likely to be better than one (e.g. adrenaline 1:10 000 injection around ulcer + <u>heater probe</u>/haemoclip).
- In patients with bleeding <u>peptic ulcers</u>, antral CLO test biopsy for *Helicobacter pylori* taken (little evidence that 'acute' eradication effects natural history of bleeding ulcer, but will reduce recurrence).

Pharmacotherapy

- Debate continues as to what proton pump inhibitor (PPI) to use, what route, and when. Clear evidence for PPI efficacy in all suspected non-variceal bleeders prior to endoscopy is still lacking. In a patient with a significant bleed, primary goal (after resuscitation) is endoscopy, which allows diagnosis and definitive management. Nevertheless, single IV (or high-dose oral) dose of PPI in significant bleeders, prior to endoscopy, is a pragmatic approach used by many, with further PPI determined by endoscopic findings.
- High-dose proton pump inhibitor regimen reduces rebleeding rates, but minimal effect on mortality. In patients with high-risk bleeds, give omeprazole 80 mg in normal saline 100 ml IV over 30 min, then 8 mg/hour in same infusion (i.e. 10 ml/hour) for 72 hours. IV pantoprazole may be an alternative.
- Oral regime (e.g. Lansoprazole 30 mg bd) may be similarly effective, but not directly compared. Expert opinion suggests IV regimens for Forrest I, IIa, and IIb bleeds, and oral regimens for IIc and III endoscopic findings (based on risk of rebleed).
- Tranexamic acid is not used as standard treatment, although meta-analysis has suggested a survival advantage over placebo. Usual regimen is 3–6 g × 1/day IV for 2–3 days, then orally 3–5 days.

Rockall score

Variable	Score			
	0	1	2	3
Age (years)	< 60	60–79	≥ 80	
Shock	No shock Syst BP > 100 HR < 100	Tachycardia Syst BP > 100 HR > 100	Hypotension. Syst BP < 100	
Comorbidity	Nil major		Cardiac failure, IHD	Renal failure, disseminated malignancy

Post-endoscopy criteria

Diagnosis	Mallory–Weiss tear, no lesion, no stigmata	All other diagnoses	Upper GI malignancy	
Major stigmata	None, or dark spots		Blood in upper GI tract, clot, visible vessel	

Predicted mortality related to Rockall score

Score	Pre-endoscopy (%)	Post-endoscopy (%)
0	0.2	0.0
1	2.4	0.0
2	5.6	0.2
3	11.0	2.9
4	24.6	5.3
5	39.6	10.8
6	48.9	17.3
7	50.0	27.0
8+		41.1

Practice point: Rockall score and risk stratification

Don't be a slave to clinical grading systems. The Rockall score is clinically useful, but was never designed to predict who will rebleed or die. For example: an 80 year old patient with a chest infection and stable angina, who has an equivocal 'coffee ground vomit', will have a Rockall score > 3. Out-of-hours endoscopy in this situation may not only be unnecessary, but dangerous. Emergency endoscopy is indicated for those with large continuing bleeding. The Rockall score should support, not replace, good clinical assessment.

Post-endoscopy care
- Patient can eat and drink at 4–6 hours if haemodynamically stable.
- Daily bloods until stable (FBC, U&Es).
- Rebleeding indicated by new signs of hypovolaemia (compensatory tachycardia is an early sign), fall in Hb > 2 g/dl over 24 hours, or development of fresh haematemesis or melaena. Decision needed between repeating endoscopy and early surgery (see below).
- No clear role for repeating endoscopy in bleeders who have settled, prior to discharge (but all gastric ulcers need re-scoping ± biopsy in 6 weeks to check for resolution, because of risk that ulcer is malignant).
- See peptic ulceration for treatment after recovery from bleed.

Surgery
- Criteria for surgery are not absolutes, but crucial factors are **the severity of bleed, endoscopic findings, and comorbidity**.
  - High risk stigmata of rebleeding on endoscopy, and failed endoscopic control (e.g. spurting artery).
  - 1st rebleed in patient > 60 years (elderly patients tolerate further episodes of hypotension and haemorrhage poorly, and so require surgery earlier, not later, than younger patients). But consider patient's 'biological age', remembering how many > 60 year olds run the marathon!
  - 2nd rebleed in patient < 60 years (there is rarely a role for a 3rd attempt at endoscopic treatment, unless endoscopist missed the true lesion first time, or treated inadequately, or if surgeon feels that the patient is truly unfit for surgery).
  - Continued bleeding after 6 units of blood in patient > 60 years, 8 units in <60-year-old.
  - Surgery usually involves oversewing the bleeding vessel in the stomach or duodenum, vagotomy with pyloroplasty, or partial gastrectomy.
  - Alternative to surgery, particularly in patients with very poor surgical prognosis, is angiography, with embolization of feeding vessel.

Non-ulcer bleeding
- Endoscopic therapy may be effective in controlling bleeding due to Mallory–Weiss tear (although stops spontaneously in 50–80% of cases), and Dieulafoy lesions (96% controlled with primary haemostasis). Bleeding from gastric antral vascular ectasia (GAVE)) may be controlled with argon plasma coagulation (APC).
- In patient with previous aortic graft, sentinel bleed may precede catastrophic bleed due to aorto-enteric fistula. Emergency endoscopy, with views round to duodeno-jejunal flexure ± CT scan, may make diagnosis. Emergency surgery (peri-operative mortality 25–90%) or endovascular stenting may be necessary.

Endoscopy 'negative' upper GI bleeding
Further management depends on findings at first endoscopy:
- No blood and no lesion seen: may be explained by:
  - Trivial lesion that has stopped bleeding by the time of endoscopy (e.g. Mallory–Weiss tear). Suggested by no evidence of ongoing blood loss.

- Bleeding distal to scope view (e.g. small bowel <u>angiodysplasia</u>; <u>gastrointestinal stromal tumour (GIST)</u>; <u>Meckel's diverticulum</u>, <u>aorto-enteric fistula</u>). Further investigations include small bowel ('push') <u>enteroscopy</u>, mesenteric angiography (requires blood loss of 1 ml/min to demonstrate active bleeding) ± embolization of bleeding point, technetium labelled red cell scan, or capsular endoscopy. If bleed is continuous, exploratory laparotomy may be necessary.
- Blood seen, but no lesion: may be explained by:
  - Bleeding arising from 'unusual site' (e.g. <u>haemobilia</u> due to bleeding from biliary tree; gastric fundal Dieulafoy lesion).
  - Blood obscuring adequate view on initial endoscopy.
  - Repeat procedure by senior endoscopist within 24 hours. Consider stimulating gastric emptying (e.g. erythromycin 250 mg IV, metoclopramide 10 mg IV 20 min prior to procedure). If possible haemobilia, have duodenoscope available for optimal views of papilla.

Prognosis
- Overall mortality from non-variceal upper GI bleed approximately 10%. Lack of significant reduction in mortality over last 30 years likely to relate to increasing age of patients, and so worse comorbidity.
- Mortality 3% in patients aged 21–31; 10% age 41–50; 14% age 71–80 years.

Forrest classification of rebleeding risk

Class	Endoscopic finding	% Rebleeding rate
Ia	Spurting artery	80–90
Ib	Oozing	55–80
IIa	Non-bleeding visible vessel	50–60
IIb	Adherent clot	25–35
IIc	Black spot in ulcer base	0–8
III	Clean ulcer base	0–12

Suspected acute variceal bleed

Varices due to <u>portal hypertension</u> develop in 60% of patients with advanced cirrhosis (see <u>Approach to cirrhosis and chronic liver disease</u>). First bleed carries 25–50% mortality. Varices in distal oesophagus, gastro-esophageal junction, or gastric fundus most usually bleed, but ectopic variceal bleeding (e.g. rectum, stomas, surgical anastomoses) may occur.
- Risk factors for bleeding include:
  - Poor liver function (indicated by <u>Child–Pugh score</u>).
  - Large varices.
  - Endoscopic stigmata (e.g. 'red signs' on varices).
  - Bacterial infection.
  - Hepatic venous pressure gradient (HVPG) > 16 mmHg (see <u>portal hypertension</u>).

- Death from variceal bleed related to severity of initial bleed; rebleeding (30–50% within 1 week); infection; comorbid cardiorespiratory/renal disease.

Ongoing management

- If you suspect a variceal bleed, call gastroenterologist on-call immediately, as experienced staff are essential. Involve anaesthetist, as risk of aspiration if patient encephalopathic and large bleed, and may need intubation prior to endoscopy.
- Manage in ITU/HDU setting, by staff experienced in care of these patients.
- If still hypovolaemic after initial fluid resuscitation, give blood if ready, otherwise further colloid (e.g. Haemaccel®, Gelofusin®). Avoid overfilling, as may increase risk of rebleeding (↑ portal venous pressure), but vital to ensure adequate renal perfusion and urine output. Aim for CVP 4–8 cm H_2O, and Hb 9–10 g/dl.
- Give platelets if < 50 × 10^9/l, fresh frozen plasma (FFP) if PT > 20 s (and for every 4 units blood). Discuss with haematologists re dose.
- Vitamin K 10 mg IV od for 3 days.
- Give cryoprecipitate 10 units if fibrinogen <75 mg/dL.
- Insert central line after initial fluid resuscitation, and preferably (but not essential) after clotting factors given. However, withhold insertion in: agitated patient (e.g. with hepatic encephalopathy); if it will delay essential emergency endoscopy; and in patient with large ongoing haematemesis who risks aspiration on lying supine.
- Give broad spectrum IV cover (e.g. Cefotaxime 1 g bd IV + metronidazole 500 mg tds for 5 days). Bacterial sepsis is common, risk of aspiration is high, and sepsis is associated with initial bleeding/rebleeding.
- Give TERLIPRESSIN 2 mg stat (bolus over 3–5 min), then 1–2 mg every 4–6 hours for 72 hours, or until bleeding stops. May cause ischaemia, so contraindicated in patients with ischaemia on ECG, or history of vascular disease. Vasoactive drugs may help to control bleeding (79% of cases in pooled data of patients treated with terlipressin), and may reduce mortality, but their use does not replace necessity of endoscopy.

Endoscopy

- Essential for definitive treatment and investigation. Perform within 6 hours, ideally after haemodynamically stable.
- Ensure anaesthetist present. Have **low** threshold for intubation prior to endoscopy.
- Protect youself with face mask ± double gloves if any risk of parenteral virus transmission.
- At endoscopy, full examination of upper GI tract performed, as 26–56% of patients with portal hypertension and GI bleed have non-variceal cause (e.g. peptic ulceration).

Gastro-oesophageal varices. Variceal band ligation (VBL) should be performed. This involves placement of rubber bands around the base of the varix (see portal hypertension). Control of bleeding may occur through subsequent tamponade at the gastro-oesophageal junction or development of variceal thrombosis. Sclerotherapy, involving a needle puncture in or adjacent to the varix, with the injection of sclerosant (e.g. 5 ml 5% ethanolamine oleate) may be used if VBL fails (or if limited endoscopist experience of VBL). However, VBL associated with a 50% lower rebleeding rate compared to sclerotherapy.

Gastric varices account for approximately 10% of variceal bleeds, with higher rate of uncontrolled and rebleeding, and decreased survival, compared with gastro-oesophageal varices. VBL and sclerotherapy with standard sclerosants not effective. Variceal injection of cyanoacrylate ('super-glue') may be effective (90% initial haemostasis, compared with 67% for ethanolamine), but has been associated with cerebral embolism due to glue migration. Thrombin may be effective and safer, but still high rebleeding rates. In view of suboptimal haemostatic control with endoscopy or <u>Sengstaken–Blakemore tube</u> (SBT) inflation (especially if gastric varices not bleeding from high in gastric fundus), contact should be made early with specialist liver unit, for consideration of further management (see below).

Uncontrolled bleeding/early rebleeding

- 10–15% of patients have continuing variceal bleed despite initial medical and endoscopic therapy. Early rebleeding (recurrence of bleeding within 5 days of endoscopy) occurs in 30–50%, and is a strong predictor of death. Little benefit in performing > 2 endoscopies in patients with ongoing bleeding.
- In patient with an exsanguinating bleed that cannot be controlled endoscopically, SBT should be inserted. This controls acute bleeding from gastro-oesophageal varices in 90% of cases, but recurrent bleeding occurs in 50% on deflation of balloon. Endotracheal intubation should be performed prior to tube insertion. Tube should be deflated and removed within 24 hours, and repeat endoscopy performed.
- If bleeding continues despite repeat endoscopy, or failure to achieve control with SBT, contact liver unit to discuss insertion of <u>TIPSS</u> (transjugular intrahepatic portosystemic shunt).

Further management

- Keep NBM for 4 hours following VBL.
- NG tube insertion should probably be avoided for 48 hours after VBL (but little evidence of absolute risk of dislodging bands).
- Retrosternal discomfort common after endoscopic therapy, and usually responds to simple analgesia.
- Post-VBL/sclerotherapy ulceration may occur and is treated with <u>SUCRALFATE</u> 1 g qds and PPI (e.g. Lansoprazole 30 mg od). It is also a cause of re-bleeding, and then may be difficult to control.
- Prior to discharge, address the following:
  - The cause of varices and severity and aetiology of any underlying liver disease. Rebleeding is less common, and less severe, in patients with non-cirrhotic portal hypertension (e.g. <u>portal vein thrombosis</u>), and recurrence in those with liver disease is strongly linked to <u>Child–Pugh score</u>.
  - The precipitant to bleed (e.g. recent infection, alcohol binge, NSAID use).
  - Treatment of underlying liver disease, and other manifestations of decompensation (e.g. <u>hepatic encephalopathy</u>).
  - The need for secondary prophylaxis against further bleeds. Don't forget this. See <u>portal hypertension</u>.

Gastrointestinal foreign bodies

Management in this area is based on experience and not controlled trials. Before intervention, consider the type of object ingested, the organ involved, the patient's condition, and the type of symptoms. Co-operation and sedation are essential for safe removal: general anaesthesia is needed for children or the uncooperative. The young, the old, and the mentally impaired are most at risk.

Sharp objects can perforate and are most likely to do so at the sites shown in figure opposite. The ileocaecal region is the most frequent site beyond the oesophagus.

Swallowed foreign bodies

Clinical features. The location of any discomfort correlates poorly with anatomical impaction. If the object is impacted in the fauces, get ENT advice. Excess salivation or regurgitation may accompany total oesophageal obstruction.

Diagnosis. Plain X-rays (frontal and lateral) can help (look for surgical emphysema) but some objects (aluminium, wood, fish bones) are radio-lucent. Remember that foreign bodies may impact in the airway not the oesophagus. Gastrograffin studies may help. If pain or symptoms persist, endoscopy (with careful intubation under direct vision) is indicated.

Management. If ingestion is recent and the object needs to be removed (see below) laying the patient in the left lateral position may reduce the chances of passage through the pylorus. Glucagon has been suggested to relax the lower oesophageal sphincter: it is rarely effective but relatively safe. Endoscopic techniques are well described (see, for example, Cotton, PB and Williams, CB (2003). *Practical gastrointestinal endoscopy*, 5th edn. Blackwell Publishing, Oxford). Small coins, frequently swallowed by children, can generally be left to pass provided they are not lodged in the oesophagus (but if still in the stomach after 7–14 days may need endoscopic removal). Sharp objects require an experienced endoscopist and use of an overtube is advised.

Colonic and rectal foreign bodies

The range of objects retrieved is a tribute to the richness of human sexual imagination. Retrieval is usually possible: if an inserted object is beyond reach of sigmoidoscope and there is no evidence of perforation or obstruction, observation for 12–24 hours may allow descent to a reachable level. Do not use enemas or cathartics. Sigmoidoscopy after removal is necessary to exclude mucosal injury.

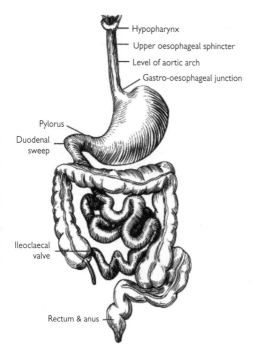

Hypopharynx
Upper oesophageal sphincter
Level of aortic arch
Gastro-oesophageal junction

Pylorus
Duodenal sweep

Ileoclaecal valve

Rectum & anus

Fig. 4.2 Common areas of luminal narrowing and angulation in the GI tract leading to foreign body impaction. (Used with permission from Feldman, M, Friedman, LS, Sleisenger, MH, and Scharschmidt, BF (ed.) (1998). *Sleisenger and Fordtran's gastrointestinal and liver disease*, 7th edn, p. 387. Saunders, Philadelphia.)

Special considerations

Alkaline batteries. These can disintegrate with local release of toxic contents. Oesophageal impaction should be managed by urgent endoscopic removal. There is less agreement if the button is in the stomach: if a plain X-ray shows separation of button components or if the button remains for more than 24 hours, endoscopic search and rescue is reasonable. Once in the small intestine, it is usually safe to wait for passage of the battery.

Body packers. Illegal drugs can be packaged and swallowed or inserted PV or PR. Intact packets can cause obstruction; burst packets can cause lethal overdose (look for symptoms of opiate or cocaine overdose). It is probably best not to give cathartics and do not attempt endoscopic removal which can rupture packets. Symptoms are an indication for surgical removal.

Ethical considerations. Treat the patient first. Inform the police and hospital administrator. Questioning of the patient must be sanctioned by a senior doctor. The patient must be aware of their right to legal advice, through an interpreter if necessary.

Oesophageal obstruction

Causes

- Swallowed foreign bodies (see gastrointestinal foreign bodies).
- Sudden occlusion by tumour, e.g. cancer of the oesophagus.
- Intramural rupture of the oesophagus (see intramural haematoma).
- Acute bolus obstruction. This may occur in a normal oesophagus after inadequate chewing, but is more common in patients with pre-existing:
  - Oesophago-gastric cancer.
  - Oesophageal ring stricture.
  - Motility disorder.
  - Patients with oesophageal stents or endoprostheses.

Difficulty in swallowing (dysphagia) is discussed in Approach to the mouth and swallowing.

Clinical features

Ask about and look for:
- **Pain**. Oesophageal pain can mimic that of acute myocardial infarction, but the close temporal relation to eating, combined with dysphagia, usually helps to distinguish the two.
- The patient's ability to swallow his/her own saliva.
- **Duration of symptoms** before obstruction.
- **Predisposing disease** (stricture, carcinoma, oesophageal ring).
- **Triggering factors** (classically steak and bread; also tablets).
- **Dehydration.**
- **Weight loss** (suggests malignancy).
- **Supraclavicular nodes** (e.g. gastric cancer).
- **Complications** (aspiration, perforation).

Management

- Contact the on-call endoscopist.
- Bloods: FBC (anaemia may suggest chronic bleeding lesion), U & E to look for dehydration.
- Chest X-ray to look for mediastinal fluid level, or evidence of signs of aspiration pneumonia oesophageal rupture.
- Intravenous fluids.

Defining the cause

- Endoscopy is better than barium swallow (which risks aspiration) but must be done by an experienced endoscopist.
- Carbonated drinks can occasionally disimpact a food bolus.

- Endoscopic removal of the bolus can be followed immediately by dilatation of any strictures or biopsy of a suspicious mucosal lesion.
- If there is an oesophageal stent or prosthesis in place, assessment of tumour ingrowth, overgrowth, or stent migration is essential.
- Endoscopic placement of a fine-bore feeding tube may be necessary after disimpaction if dilatation is delayed.
- Intravenous antibiotics for aspiration (cefuroxime 750 mg tds, METRONIDAZOLE 500 mg tds).

Oesophageal rupture

Causes

- **Spontaneous** (usually caused by vomiting; first described by Herman Boerhaave in 1724: see <u>Boerhaave's syndrome</u>), but also reported with foreign bodies such as bones, batteries, and bottle tops; caustic ingestion; and trauma.
- More than 50% cases are caused by medical procedures (see <u>endoscopic complications</u>. The oesophagus is said to be at increased risk because it lacks a serosal layer.
- <u>Intramural haematoma</u> can result from sudden increases in intra-oesophageal pressure.

Procedure	Risk of perforation	Site and comments
Rigid oesophagoscopy	1/10	Proximal oesophagus (associated with arthritic cervical spine or a pharyngeal pouch)
Flexible endoscopy	<1/1000	Usually at intubation or in attempted passage through narrowings
Balloon dilatation of achalasia	Less that 2% with balloons <35 mm: up to 5% with 40 mm balloon	
Dilatation of malignant strictures	Up to 10% in old series using rigid prostheses: much less with softer expanding stents	

Diagnosis

Early diagnosis is crucial: clinical signs may be minimal as the perforation is usually small, the patient is often fasted (and sedated), and the instruments should be clean if not sterile. Perforation may be apparent at the time of procedure, but surgical emphysema, tachycardia, cyanosis, and pain (especially after swallowing) should arouse suspicion.

Radiology

Plain films may show pneumomediastinum, pneumoperitoneum, or left pleural effusion, but can be normal. Late changes of air–fluid collections are better assessed by CT, but contrast studies using water-soluble media are conventionally used to define the site and length of perforation.

Management

- **Get a surgical opinion**: mortality is high and non-operative approaches apply only to specific situations and require experience.
- If the perforation is small (<1 cm), recognized early, and not associated with gross contamination, conservative management can be successful and includes nil by mouth, IV broad-spectrum antibiotics (e.g. cefuroxime 750 mg tds, <u>METRONIDAZOLE</u> 500 mg tds), and parenteral feeding. Exceptions are perforations into the abdominal or pleural cavities, which need surgical repair.
- Spontaneous ruptures are usually associated with gross contamination and surgery is usually advised.
- Perforations associated with balloon dilatation are often contained within the oesophageal wall and may be managed without surgery.
- **Perforation of oesophageal cancer** at endoscopy is a difficult problem, with a higher mortality of up to 50%. The perforation site can sometimes be protected by an endoscopically placed covered metal stent. Give antibiotics and start nutritional support.

Clinical factors determining outcome

- The delay in diagnosis.
- The size of hole.
- The degree of soiling of mediastinum or pleural cavity with stomach contents.

Appendices

CT images of the abdomen

Normal abdominal CT

There's never a substitute for sitting down and reviewing imaging with your friendly radiology colleagues, but it's often worth knowing where normal anatomy resides on an abdominal CT scan.

Few tips:
- Film usually taken with patient supine, and viewed from caudal position (ie below, with right side of abdomen appearing on left)
- Air, water, and fat appear dark/black on CT.
- Oral contrast (positive: eg dilute barium; negative: ie water) may be given to delineate stomach and upper GI tract from surrounding structures.
- Structures with high density (eg bones, calcified vesseles) appear white.
- After intravenous contrast, images can be taken during arterial phase (bright aorta and branches) and venous phase (bright hepatic and portal veins)

The following sequence of CT scans show sequential cuts through the abdomen from diaphragm to pelvis.

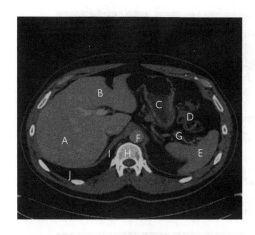

A: Right lobe of liver

B: Left lobe of liver

C: Stomach

D: Colon (splenic flexure)

E: Spleen

F: Aorta

G: Splenic artery

H: Vertebra

I: Diaphragmatic crura

J: Right lung base

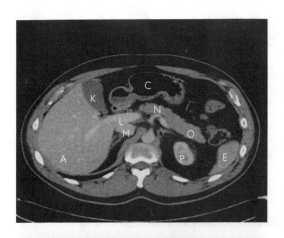

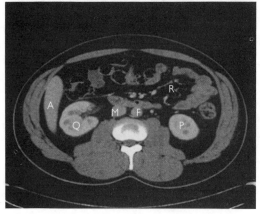

K: Gall bladder

L: Portal vein

M: Inferior vena cava

N: Body of pancreas

O: Tail of pancreas

P: Left kidney

Q: Right kidney

R: Small bowel mesentery

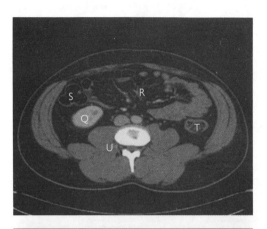

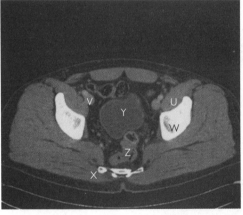

S: Ascending colon

T: Descending colon

U: Psoas muscle

V: External iliac vessels

W: Acetabulum

X: Sacrum

Y: Bladder

Z: Rectum

BMI calculator and height converter

Height in metres

Weight (kg)	1.36	1.40	1.44	1.48	1.52	1.56	1.60	1.64	1.68	1.72	1.76	1.80	1.84	1.88	1.92	1.96	2.00
125	68	64	60	57	54	51	49	46	44	42	40	39	37	35	34	33	31
123	67	63	59	56	53	51	48	46	44	42	40	38	36	35	33	32	31
121	65	62	58	55	52	50	47	45	43	41	39	37	36	34	33	31	30
119	64	61	57	54	52	49	46	44	42	40	38	37	35	34	32	31	30
117	63	60	56	53	51	48	46	44	41	40	38	36	35	33	32	30	29
115	62	59	55	53	50	47	45	43	41	39	37	35	34	33	31	30	29
113	61	58	54	52	49	46	44	42	40	38	36	35	33	32	31	29	28
111	60	57	54	51	48	46	43	41	39	38	36	34	33	31	30	29	28
109	59	56	53	50	47	45	43	41	39	37	35	34	32	31	30	28	27
107	58	55	52	49	46	44	42	40	38	36	35	33	32	30	29	28	27
105	57	54	51	48	45	43	41	39	37	35	34	32	31	30	28	27	26
103	56	53	50	47	45	42	40	38	36	35	33	32	30	29	28	27	26
101	55	52	49	46	44	42	39	38	36	34	33	31	30	29	27	26	25
99	54	51	48	45	43	41	39	37	35	33	32	31	29	28	27	26	25
97	52	49	47	44	42	40	38	36	34	33	31	30	28	27	26	25	24
95	51	48	46	43	41	39	37	35	34	32	31	29	28	27	26	25	24
93	50	47	45	42	40	38	36	35	33	31	30	29	27	26	25	24	23
91	49	46	44	42	39	37	36	34	32	31	29	28	27	26	25	24	23
89	48	45	43	41	39	37	35	33	32	30	29	27	26	25	24	23	22
87	47	44	42	40	38	36	34	32	31	29	28	27	26	25	24	23	22
85	46	43	41	39	37	35	33	32	30	29	27	26	25	24	23	22	21
83	45	42	40	38	36	34	32	31	29	28	27	26	25	23	23	22	21
81	44	41	39	37	35	33	32	30	29	27	26	25	24	23	22	21	20
79	43	40	38	36	34	32	31	29	28	27	25	24	23	22	21	21	20
77	42	39	37	35	33	32	30	29	27	26	25	24	23	22	21	20	19
75	41	38	36	34	32	31	29	28	27	25	24	23	22	21	20	20	19
73	39	37	35	33	32	30	29	27	26	25	24	23	22	21	20	19	18
71	38	36	34	32	31	29	28	26	25	24	23	22	21	20	19	18	18
69	37	35	33	31	30	28	27	26	24	23	22	21	20	19	19	18	17
67	36	34	32	31	29	28	26	25	24	23	22	21	20	19	18	17	17
65	35	33	31	30	28	27	25	24	23	22	21	20	19	18	18	17	16
63	34	32	30	29	27	26	25	23	22	21	20	19	18	17	16	16	16
61	33	31	29	28	26	25	24	23	22	21	20	19	18	17	17	16	15
59	32	30	28	27	26	24	23	22	21	20	19	18	17	16	15	15	15
57	31	29	27	26	25	23	22	21	20	19	18	17	16	15	15	15	14
55	30	28	27	25	24	23	21	20	19	19	18	17	16	16	15	14	14
53	29	27	26	24	23	22	21	20	19	18	17	16	16	15	14	14	13
51	28	26	25	23	22	21	20	19	18	17	16	16	15	14	14	13	13
49	26	25	24	22	21	20	19	18	17	17	16	15	14	14	13	13	12
47	25	24	23	21	20	19	18	17	17	16	15	14	14	13	13	12	12
45	24	23	22	21	19	18	18	17	16	15	15	14	13	13	12	12	11
43	23	22	21	20	19	18	17	16	15	15	14	13	13	12	12	11	11

Weight in kilograms

- BMI <18.5 – underweight
- BMI 18.5–24.9 – acceptable weight
- BMI 25–29.9 – overweight
- BMI 30–39.9 – obese
- BMI >= 40 – morbid obesity

Height converter	
Height (ft and in)	Height (m)
5'0"	1.52
5'1"	1.55
5'2"	1.58
5'3"	1.60
5'4"	1.63
5'5"	1.65
5'6"	1.68
5'7"	1.70
5'8"	1.73
5'9"	1.75
5'10"	1.78
5'11"	1.80
6'0"	1.83
6'1"	1.85
6'2"	1.88
6'3"	1.90
6'4"	1.93
6'5"	1.96
6'6"	1.98

BMI = weight (kg)/height (m^2)

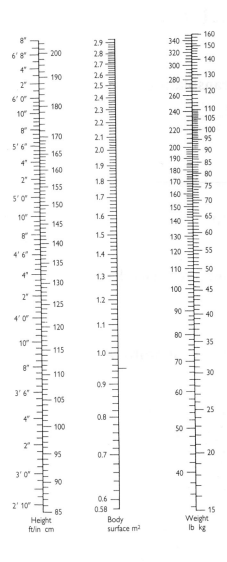

Height ft/in cm	Body surface m²	Weight lb kg

Useful links

UK liver transplant units

Royal Free Hospital, London	0207 794 0500
Adenbrookes, Cambridge	01223 245 151
Freemans Hospital, Newcastle	0191 284 3111
Queen Elizabeth Hospital Birmingham	0121 472 1311
St James Leeds	0113 243 3144
Edinburgh Royal Informary	0131 536 1000
Kings College Hospital London	0207 737 4000

Poisons unit

National Helpline	0870 600 6266

Tropical and infectious diseases

London	0207 387 4411
Liverpool	0151 708 9393
Glasgow	0141 21 1000

Virus reference laboratory

Colindale, London	0208 200 4400

General journals

British Medical Journal *www.bmj.com*
The Lancet *www.thelancet.com*
New England Journal of Medicine *www.nejm.com*
National Library of Medicine (PubMed)
www.ncbi.nlm.nih.gov/entrez/query.fcgi
Free medical journals site *www.freemedicaljournals.com*

GI and hepatology journals

Gastroenterology *www.gastrojournal.org*
Gut *http://gut.bmjjournals.com*
Hepatology *www3.interscience.wiley.com*
Alimentary Pharmacology and Therapeutics *www.blackwellpublishing.com/ journal.asp?ref−0269-2813*
Current Opinion in Gastroenterology *www.co-gastroenterology.com*

GI and hepatology societies

British Society of Gastroenterology (BSG) *www.bsg.org.uk*
British Association for the Study of the Liver (BASL) *www.basl.org.uk*
American Association for the Study of Liver Disease (AASLD) *www.aasld.org*
American Gastroenterology Association (AGA) *www.gastro.org*
European Association for the Study of the Liver (EASL) *www.easl.ch*
Pancreatic Society of Great Britain and Ireland *www.pancsoc.org.uk*

Patient support and charitable organizations

Barrett's Oesophagus Foundation *www.barrettsfoundation.org.uk*
British Liver Trust (BLT) *www.britishlivertrust.org.uk*
Cancer Research UK *www.cancerresearchuk.org*
Coeliac UK *www.coeliac.co.uk*
National Association for Colitis and Crohn's Disease (NACC) *www.nacc.org.uk*
CORE (formerly Digestive Disease Foundation) *www.digestivedisorders. org.uk*
Patient UK *www.patient.co.uk*
PBC Foundation *www.pbcfoundation.org.uk*
UK Transplant *www.uktransplant.org.uk*

Clinical information and teaching

National Institute for Health and Clinical Excellence (NICE) *www.nice.org.uk*
National Digestive Diseases Information Clearinghouse *digestive.niddk.nih.gov*
Simple anatomy site *anatomy.uams.edu*
Evidence based medicine *www.jr2.ox.ac.uk/bandolier*
Medical acronyms *www.whonamedit.com*

Normal laboratory ranges

Haematology

Haemoglobin	Male: 13–18 g/dl
	Female: 11.5–16 g/dl
Mean cell volume (MCV)	78–98 fl
Haematocrit	0.36–0.46
White blood cells	$4–11 \times 10^9/l$
Neutrophils	$2–7.5 \times 10^9/l$
Lymphocytes	$1.5–4 \times 10^9/l$
Eosinophils	$0.04–0.4 \times 10^9/l$
Platelets	$150–400 \times 10^9/l$
Erythrocyte sedimentation rate (ESR)	1–12 mm/hour

Biochemistry

Sodium	135–145 mmol/l
Potassium	3.6–5 mmol/l
Urea	2–7.5 mmol/l
Creatinine	50–120 µmol/l
Uric acid	0.1–0.4 mmol/l
Calcium	2.15–2.6 mmol/l
Phosphate	0.8–1.48 mmol/l
Glucose	3.6–7 mmol/l
Bicarbonate	22–28 mmol/l
C-reactive protein (CRP)	0–10 mg/l
Amylase	20–80 U/l
Total immunoglobulin (Ig)	15–35 g/l (IgG 5.3–16.5; IgA 0.8–4; IgM 0.5–2)
Cholesterol	3.3–7.3 mmol/l
Triglycerides	0.8–2.0 mmol/l

Liver function tests

Bilirubin	3–17 µmol/l
Alanine transaminase (ALT)	5–50 IU/l
Aspartate transaminase (AST)	5–45 IU/l
γ-glutamyl transferase (GGT)	10–60 IU/l
Alkaline phosphatase (ALP)	40–165 IU/l
Total protein	60–80g/l
Albumin	35–50 g/l

Haematinics

Serum iron	10–32 µmol/l
Ferritin	11–307 ng/ml
Total iron binding capacity (TIBC)	45–72 µmol/l
Red cell folate	100–600 µg/l
Vitamin B12	150–700 ng/l